Advances in
Modern Environmental Toxicology

VOLUME IX

Inorganics in
Drinking Water and
Cardiovascular Disease

Editors:

EDWARD J. CALABRESE
ROBERT W. TUTHILL
LYMAN CONDIE

Published by:

PRINCETON SCIENTIFIC PUBLISING CO., INC.
Princeton, New Jersey

ACKNOWLEDGEMENT

This conference was supported by an Environmental Protection Agency Grant to Dr. Edward J. Calabrese, EPA grant # 810838-01-0.

Printed and bound in the United States of America.

PRINCETON SCIENTIFIC PUBLISHING CO., INC.
P.O. Box 2155
Princeton, New Jersey 08540
Tel.: 609/683-4750

LIBRARY OF CONGRESS CATALOG NUMBER: 85-062107
ISBN 0-911131-10-8
Cover Art: From Chapter 18, Kopp et al., Fig. 5.

TABLE OF CONTENTS

INTRODUCTION

In October of 1979, the United States Environmental Protection Agency sponsored a symposium which addressed the relationship between inorganics in drinking water and cardiovascular disease (CVD). At that conference, papers were presented in a number of areas, including the hard water-soft water controversy; the relationship of sodium in drinking water to blood pressure in children; and the influence of heavy metals, including cadmium, copper, and lead, on cardiovascular function in animal models.

The proceedings of the present conference, which was held May 1-3, 1984 at the University of Massachusetts, represent an effort to assess scientific progress in the area of inorganics in drinking water and CVD and to identify areas of continuing and potential research concern over the four years since the original conference. From 1979 to 1984, considerable efforts were made in addressing, from an epidemiological aspect, the relationship of sodium in drinking water and its effects on blood pressure. The conference brought together the principal researchers in the sodium area from Europe, Australia and the United States to present, debate and assess their findings in relation to each other's results. In addition, the conference addressed the issue of the public health significance of modest (5mmHg) increases in blood pressure on cardiovascular morbidity/ mortality. The regulatory impacts of these findings were discussed with respect to both the United States and Canada.

The conference also devoted considerable time to understanding the public health impacts on cardiovascular disease of a number of toxic heavy metals, including barium and cadmium, with particular emphasis on using toxicologic and epidemiologic methodologies. Animal model studies provided a major new observation, showing that consumption of water with chlorine may contribute to increased cholesterol absorption by the intestine and increased cholesterol deposition in blood vessels. Finally, it is hoped that the findings presented in these Conference Proceedings will be of considerable assistance to EPA in assessing the impact of drinking water factors on CVD and in addressing future research needs in this area.

Edward J. Calabrese
Robert W. Tuthill
Lyman Condie

THE MASSACHUSETTS BLOOD PRESSURE STUDY, PART 1. ELEVATED LEVELS OF SODIUM IN DRINKING WATER AND BLOOD PRESSURE LEVELS IN CHILDREN

Edward J. Calabrese and Robert W. Tuthill

Division of Public Health
University of Massachusetts
Amherst, Massachusetts

ABSTRACT

Continuing epidemiologic studies at the University of Massachusetts have examined the hypothesis that elevated levels of sodium (Na) in drinking water contribute to elevations of blood pressure (BP). Comparing tenth graders from a town with 107 mg Na/L in the drinking water to those from a town with 8 mg Na/L revealed statistically significant and medically important higher BP distributions among the high Na town students relative to their low Na town peers for both systolic and diastolic BP in both boys and girls. The differences were upheld when potentially confounding factors, including dietary Na intake and other water factors occurring differentially in the two water supplies, were controlled in the analysis. A replication study among third graders in the same communities showed similar results.

INTRODUCTION

Attempts to derive a sodium standard as a result of the National Safe Drinking Water Act of 1974 have been hampered by a dearth of definitive human population studies demonstrating the effects on health of sodium in the drinking water. For this reason, the U.S. Environmental Protection Agency did not propose a maximum concentration limit for sodium in drinking water (Federal Register, 1975). The American Heart Association (1957) implied that a limit of 20 mg Na/L be adopted as a standard in order to afford protection to those individuals with heart or kidney ailments who require a low sodium diet.

1

Similarly the EPA has recently recommended that a level of 20 mg Na/L be a goal for public water systems, while proposing a requirement for monitoring sodium levels in water supplies (Federal Register, 1979).

Nearly all of the previous studies of the relationship between hypertension and sodium intake have considered the contribution of sodium from food rather than from water. This is understandable in light of the fact that water contributes from less than 0.15 percent to 9.0 percent of the total sodium an individual consumes with the important exception of persons on a restricted salt diet (Schroeder, 1974; American Heart Association, 1957).

The present paper represents a summary of the past three years of research which has been designed to assess whether elevated levels of sodium in the community drinking water could bring about an increase in the blood pressure (BP) levels of elementary (third grade) and high school (tenth grade) students.

TENTH GRADE STUDY

The authors compared BP distributions among students in two geographically contiguous Massachusetts communities markedly similar with regard to size, income, education, and recent rate of growth (Calabrese and Tuthill, 1977; Tuthill and Calabrese, 1979). One community had low levels of sodium in the public drinking water while the other had considerably higher levels at 8 mg/L and 107 mg/L, respectively (Table 1). These differences in sodium levels have existed since 1962.

Methods. The tenth grade class of the public high schools in the two communities was chosen as the population to be surveyed. Of approximately 850 tenth grade students in the schools, 606 obtained permission to be screened, for an overall response rate of approximately 67 percent and 76 percent of the high and low Na groups, respectively. In the high sodium community 300 students participated and 306 participated in the low sodium community.

The screenings were scheduled such that 150 students were screened on each of the four days, two successive days in one community and on the same two

TABLE 1
Socioeconomic Comparisons of the High and Low Sodium Communities*

	High Sodium Community	Low Sodium Community
1970 Population	low 20,000's	low 20,000's
Percent Population Change 1960–1970	17.0	16.3
Median Family Income	$13,434	$12,281
Median School Years	12.7	12.5
Percent Black	0.4	0.7
Percent Foreign Born	6.0	5.7
Water Sodium Level (1976)	107 mg/L	8 mg/L

*1970 U.S. Census Data

days of the week the following week in the second community. Thus, the screenings were conducted equally on mornings and afternoons in each town.

Four highly skilled and carefully standardized nurses took the BP of the students, with three working at a time on a 45 minute rotation. The same nurses took the BP readings at both schools on all four days. The aneroid manometers used were standardized twice each day. In order to minimize the effects of recent food intake and exercise on BP, the students were screened at least 45 minutes after a meal and they did not attend gym class at least one hour before being screened. The students were brought quietly to the screening area and spent at least six minutes seated, completing a questionnaire, before proceeding to the BP stations where they progressed to each of the nurses for a casual, seated BP reading on the left arm. Each successive nurse was blind to the previous reading for each person. Thus, three readings were obtained for each student, and these measurements were averaged to provide an estimate of the BP for each individual. The pulse rate for each child was recorded by the nurse at the first station.

The questionnaire completed by each student was designed to provide information in regard to variables known to affect BP. If any of these factors differed significantly between the two communities they could then be controlled in the analysis. Thus, information was obtained on age, height, weight, length of residence in town, smoking history, length of time since last cigarette and last meal, recent excessive weight gain or loss, whether on a low sodium diet, eating habits in relation to salty items, amount of community water drunk either plain or as mixed in something such as orange juice, health status, occupation and education of the family's main wage earner, and whether they were currently taking BP medication.

Results. The students of the high sodium community showed the hypothesized upshift along their entire BP distribution when compared to the low sodium community students. Figure 1 illustrates this upshifted distribution, which occurred for both systolic and diastolic BP and was consistent for both sexes, although more pronounced for females. The mean systolic and diastolic BP for females in the high sodium community was 113.5/67.8 mmHg compared to 108.4/62.7 mmHg in the low sodium community. The difference between the two groups of females for both mean systolic and diastolic BP was 5.1 mmHg, a difference statistically significant at the $p < 0.001$ level. The same upshift in the population distribution for BP occurred with the high sodium males as with the females, but not to the same degree. Among males the mean systolic and diastolic BP in the two communities was 123.1/65.2 mmHg in the high sodium community and 119.5/62.5 mmHg in the low sodium community. The difference in mean systolic and diastolic BP between the two male groups was 3.6 mmHg and 2.7 mmHg, respectively. Both of these differences were statistically significant at $p < 0.001$.

Statistical analyses designed to evaluate the possibility of confounding revealed no variables which were statistically significantly different between the tenth grade groups from the two communities which were also statistically significantly related to BP within the population.

Other statistical analyses which were designed to adjust mean BP simultane-

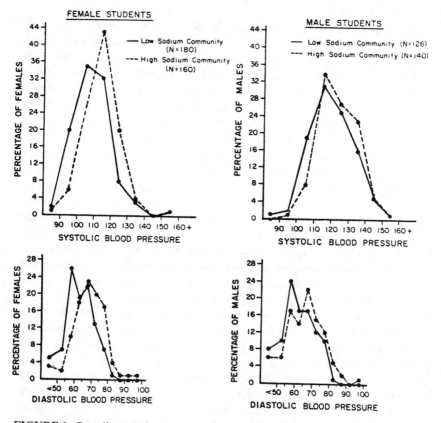

FIGURE 1. Systolic and diastolic blood pressure distributions by sex for tenth grade students from high (107 mg/l) and low (8 mg/l) sodium communities.

ously for any differences between communities' student groups in regard to eighteen variables on the pupil questionnaire were carried out. Although minor changes in the mean values occurred as a result of these statistical analyses, the fundamental findings of the study were supported.

Blood pressure is known to rise with age in Western societies (Smith, 1977; Fries, 1976). Several studies among adolescents in the U.S. report a 0.5 mmHg/year increase in BP for males from 15 to 17 years; however, systolic BP shows a yearly increase of approximately 2 mmHg/year and diastolic, an increase of about 1.5 mmHg/year for females of the same age group (NCHS, 1977; NCHLBI, 1977; Silverberg et al., 1975; Swartz and Lietch, 1975). Therefore, the upward shift in the high sodium males' systolic and diastolic BP is characteristic of an age group about two years older when compared to the low sodium control group. However, the 4 to 5 mmHg upshift in systolic and diastolic BP among the high sodium girls is suggestive of a group 10 years older when compared to their low sodium peer group based upon the 1970–74 National Center for Health Statistics BP data. Since an individual tends to maintain his or her position on the blood pressure curve over time (Oberman et al., 1967; Smith, 1977) these data suggest that those individuals on the high end of the blood pressure distribution in the high sodium community may become hypertensive years earlier than their counterparts in the low sodium community.

A follow-up study (Calabrese and Tuthill, 1978) among approximately 80 students from each of the communities examined distribution system and household water samples for 9 heavy metals known to or suspected of affecting cardiovascular function. This study was designed to determine if the presence of confounding variables with respect to drinking water could have affected the interpretation of the original study. However, the results indicated elevated drinking water sodium levels to be the prime explanatory factor in the differences in BP distribution between the two towns.

THIRD GRADE REPLICATION STUDY

A third grade study in the same two communities was carried out to confirm the earlier findings by possibly replicating the tenth grade differences and to rule out potentially confounding variables in the first study, such as possible differential illicit drug use in the two high school populations.

Methods. There were seven elementary schools in each community with 384 third graders in the high sodium community and 301 third graders in the low sodium community. In the high sodium community 346 out of 384 children were screened, and in the low sodium community 262 out of 301 children were screened, for a net participation rate of 90.1 percent and 87.0 percent, respectively.

The screenings were conducted in fourteen sessions over eight school days within a two week period. Careful attention was paid to ensure that the towns were screened equally on mornings and afternoons to eliminate diurnal variation in BP as a possible confounding variable. In each town, four schools were screened in the morning and three in the afternoon. This resulted in 65.2 percent of the high sodium community children being screened in the morning, compared to 69.7 percent in the low sodium community.

Five nurses who had been carefully standardized were available to do the screening. The same four nurses did the screening at eleven of the sessions with the fifth nurse substituting during three of the sessions. Three children at a time were screened at three different stations, each child moving from station to station, so that three casual BP readings on the left arm using a mercury sphygmomanometer at eye level were recorded for each child. Each reading was taken by a different nurse who was blind to the readings of her colleagues. The nurses rotated through the stations on a time schedule, with only three of the four working at a time, one at each station, with pulse rate recorded by the nurse working at the first station, procedures similar to those previously described.

The children were brought to the screening area (usually a gym, auditorium, extra room, or school nurse's office) slowly and quietly, and were seated quietly for several minutes before being screened. No gym classes were scheduled in the hour prior to the screening, and meals were consumed at least 45 minutes before the screening. Age, height, and weight were recorded from current school

5

records. In both towns, height and weight had been measured in the immediately preceding months by the school nurses. The school scales were checked for accuracy at the time of screening, and all weighed to within 1 lb. of a 40 lb weight (which approximated the weight of these children).

Additional information on factors related to BP was obtained for each child from a short questionnaire completed by the parents in conjunction with the permission slip. The questionnaire provided information on family history of high BP, source of drinking water, length of residence in town, medications being taken by the child which may affect BP, infant feeding habits, and the education level and occupation of the main wage earner in the family. In addition, each child was asked to complete a 24-hour dietary diary to be used to assess sodium, potassium and calcium intake. Again, the three BP readings for each child were combined to form an average reading on which the following analyses were based.

As in the tenth grade study, a subset of 100 of the individuals from each community were asked to provide household water supplies.

Dietary diary. In addition, each child was asked to fill out a twenty-four hour dietary diary which was begun in school after lunch with the teacher's help and completed at home with the parents' aid. The records indicated the portion size, whether the food was fresh, frozen, or canned; the quantity of salt added in cooking; and the amount and type of liquid consumed. The diaries were obtained several weeks after the blood pressures were recorded.

Results. The results for the third graders have supported the original high school findings; there was a statistically significant difference in mean BP between the two communities, for both boys and girls, for systolic and diastolic BP. The mean systolic and diastolic BP for boys from the high and low sodium communities was 101.3/56.3 mmHg and 98.0/53.7 mmHg, respectively. This represented a difference in systolic BP of 3.3 mmHg ($p = 0.001$) and a 2.6 mmHg difference in mean diastolic BP ($p = 0.032$). The differences in mean systolic and diastolic BP were also significant between the girls. The high sodium community girls' mean BP was 97.9/58.1 mmHg, and it was 95.3/54.5 mmHg among the low sodium community girls. The resulting systolic and diastolic BP differences were 2.6 mmHg and 3.6 mmHg, which were statistically significant at $p = 0.023$ and $p = 0.002$, respectively.

As with the tenth graders, the upshifts occurred along the entire distribution of systolic and diastolic BP for the third graders from the high sodium community relative to the low sodium community third graders for both boys and girls (Figure 2). The upshift was least marked for systolic BP for girls and more distinct for boys. However, the pattern was completely consistent for all four comparisons. When testing the statistical significance of the difference in the two distributions for each of the four comparisons, the female systolic distributions did not differ significantly between the two towns at $p = 0.14$. The female diastolic comparison and the male systolic and diastolic comparisons revealed statistically significant differences by community of at least $p = 0.008$.

These results are very similar in pattern to the differences found in the screening of the tenth grade populations of these two sexes for both systolic and diastolic BP among the third graders, and their consistency with the earlier tenth grade findings lends importance to these results in conjunction with their statistical significance.

The statistical assessment of these data upheld the initial findings. In fact, the statistical adjustment for differences in the confounding characteristics resulted in an adjusted difference in mean BP between the two towns which was even greater than when these factors were uncontrolled. That is, the net impact of adjusting for differences in height, weight, and socioeconomic status resulted in a larger difference in systolic and diastolic BP between the two towns, for both boys and girls.

The resultant adjusted differences were all statistically significant. The difference in diastolic BP between high and low sodium community boys had an associated significance level of $p = 0.014$. For the difference in systolic BP between both high and low sodium community boys and girls and for the difference in diastolic BP between high and low sodium community girls, the associated significance level was $p \leq 0.001$.

Dietary diaries. Codable twenty-four hour diaries were collected from 312 or 90.2 percent of the children in the high sodium community and 240 or 91.6 percent of those in the low sodium community. Table 2 indicates the mean dietary intake of sodium, potassium and calcium and shows the sodium/potassium ratio for the four sex/community groups. The dietary sodium intake is about thirteen percent higher and the potassium intake about eight percent higher in the high sodium community compared to the low sodium community for both sexes. Calcium intake is about twenty percent higher for males and sixteen percent higher for females whereas the sodium/potassium ratio is five percent higher for the males and about 2–3 percent higher for the females in the high sodium community.

TABLE 2
The Mean Dietary Intake of Sodium, Potassium and Calcium

	High Sodium Community (n = 160)	Low Sodium Community (n = 130)	Difference Amount	%	p-Value (2-Tail)
	MALES				
Sodium (mg)	2904	2557	347	13.6	0.004
Potassium (mg)	3239	2995	244	8.1	0.056
Calcium (mg)	1225	1023	202	19.7	0.001
Na/K Ratio	.958	.914	.044	4.8	0.366

	High Sodium Community (n = 152)	Low Sodium Community (n = 110)	Difference Amount	%	p-Value (2-Tail)
	FEMALES				
Sodium (mg)	2851	2523	328	13.0	0.015
Potassium (mg)	3036	2804	232	8.3	0.054
Calcium (mg)	1152	991	161	16.2	0.002
Na/K Ratio	1.000	.976	.024	2.5	0.610

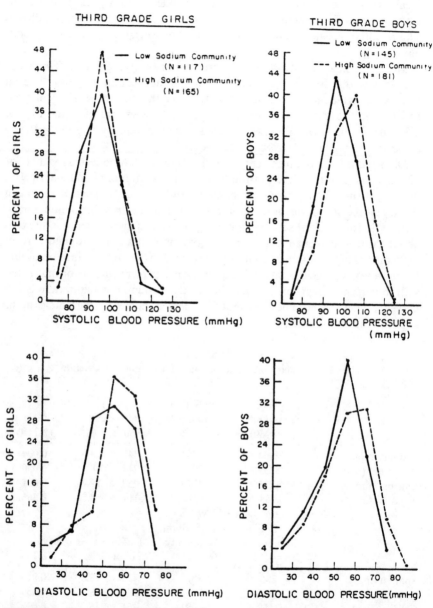

FIGURE 2. Systolic and diastolic blood pressure distributions by sex for third grade students from high (107 mg/l) and low (8 mg/l) sodium communities.

In absolute terms, the high sodium community pupils' intake is about one-third of a gram more sodium per day, one-quarter of a gram more potassium, and one-fifth of a gram more calcium. These figures do not include the sodium in the drinking water consumed either directly or when mixed with orange juice concentrate, Kool-Aid, etc. Data on liquid consumption collected at a later time indicated that the third grade high sodium pupils consumed about one liter of tap water per day, obtaining 120 mg of sodium per day from this source. Assuming a similar amount of water consumption in the low sodium community, the children there would receive eight mg of sodium per day from their drinking water daily. If the sodium obtained from water is added to both communities' total dietary intake, then about one quarter of the excess sodium intake in the high sodium community is derived from this source: 24.4 percent for males (112/459) and 25.5 percent for females (112/440 mg).

Evaluation of the drinking water for heavy metal constituents known to affect BP did not reveal any consistent difference of biological significance other than the originally defined differences in sodium values.

CONCLUSION

Epidemiologic investigations in Massachusetts have revealed that the BP of third and tenth grade students from a community with 107 mg Na/L in the drinking water was significantly upshifted as compared to similarly aged students from a closely matched, geographically contiguous community with only 8 mg Na/L.

ACKNOWLEDGEMENTS

The preliminary findings of the original Tenth Grade Study were published in the *Archives of Environmental Health* 32:200–202, 1977, followed by a more comprehensive report, *Archives of Environmental Health* 34:197–203, 1979. A brief summary of the Tenth and Third Grade reports were published in the proceedings of the Annual Conference of the American Water Works Association held in June 1979. A comprehensive report of the Third Grade Study was published in the *American Journal of Public Health* 71:722–729, 1981.

We would like to acknowledge the overall efforts of our research associates Janelle Klar and Thomas Sieger, who have been crucial to the success of this project. This research was supported by the Health Effects Research Laboratory of United States Environmental Protection Agency, Cincinnati, Ohio *Grant #R-805612-02.

REFERENCES

AMERICAN HEART ASSOCIATION. (1957). Your 500 Milligram Diet. New York.

CALABRESE, E.J. and TUTHILL, R.W. (1977). Elevated blood pressure and high sodium levels in the public drinking water. Arch. Environ. Health **32**: 200–202.

CALABRESE, E.J. and TUTHILL, R.W. (1978). Elevated blood pressure and community drinking water characteristics. J. Environ. Sci. Health **A13(10)**: 781–802.

CODE OF FEDERAL REGULATIONS. (1979). Standards of quality bottled water. Title 21, Part 103, **35**: 50–54.

FEDERAL REGISTER. (1975). National interim primary drinking water regulations. **49**: 59576–77.

FEDERAL REGISTER. (1979). Proposed regulations. **44**: 140.

FRIES, E.D. (1976). Salt volume and the prevention of hypertension. Circulation **53**: 589–595.

NATIONAL CENTER FOR HEALTH STATISTICS. (1977). Blood pressure levels of persons 6–74 years. In *Vital and Health Statistics*, Series II, Number 203. DHEW Publication No. (HRA) Washington, D.C. 78–1648.

NATIONAL HEART, LUNG, AND BLOOD INSTITUTE'S TASK FORCE ON BLOOD PRESSURE CONTROL IN CHILDREN. (1977). Pediatrics (Suppl.) **59**: 5 Part II.

OBERMAN, A., LANE, N.E., and HARLAN, W.R. (1967). Trends in systolic blood pressure in the thousand aviator cohort over a twenty-year period. Circulation **26**: 812–828.

SCHROEDER, H.A. (1974). The role of trace elements in cardiovascular diseases. Med. Clin. North Am. **58**: 381–396.

SILVERBERG, D.S., VAN NOSTRAND, C., JUSHLI, B., SMITH, E.S.O. and DORSSER, E.V. (1975). Screening for hypertension in a high school population. CMA Journal **113**: 103–108.

SMITH, W.M. (1977). Epidemiology of hypertension. Med. Clin. North Am. **61**: 467–486.

SWARTZ, H. and LEITCH, C.J. (1975). Differences in mean adolescent blood pressure by age, sex, ethnic origin, obesity and familial tendency. J. Sci. Health **45(2)**: 76–82.

TUTHILL, R.W. and CALABRESE, E.J. (1979). Elevated sodium levels in public drinking water as a contributor to elevated blood pressure levels in the community. Arch. Environ. Health **34(4)**: 197–203.

TUTHILL, R.W. and CALABRESE, E.J. (1981). Drinking water sodium and blood pressure in children: A second look. Am. J. Public Health **71**: 722–729.

CHAPTER II

THE MASSACHUSETTS BLOOD PRESSURE STUDY, PART 2. MODESTLY ELEVATED LEVELS OF SODIUM IN DRINKING WATER AND BLOOD PRESSURE LEVELS IN HIGH SCHOOL STUDENTS

Robert W. Tuthill and Edward J. Calabrese
Division of Public Health
University of Massachusetts
Amherst, Massachusetts

ABSTRACT

The blood pressure (BP) of tenth grade students from a town with 42 mg Na/L in drinking water was compared to that of comparable tenth grade students in a geographically contiguous community with 6 mg Na/L. No statistically significant difference occurred in mean BP between the two communities for males and females for diastolic BP and male systolic BP. However, the low sodium community females displayed a significantly higher BP (p < 0.05) of 1.6 mmHg. Analysis of covariance for potentially confounding variables did not significantly alter the initial findings. In summary, an average of 36 mg Na/L higher Na levels in the drinking water was not associated with an increase in BP levels in tenth grade students.

INTRODUCTION

After observing the BP differences among tenth grade and third grade students with a differential of approximately 100 mg/L Na in the drinking water (see previous paper by Calabrese and Tuthill), a study was designed to test the drinking water Na hypothesis in communities with a narrower Na differential. The hypothesis of a dose-response relationship between drinking water Na and BP was tested.

In this replication of the original school study, two newly matched communities were chosen which had a difference in Na levels in drinking water of about

TABLE 1
Socioeconomic and Demographic Comparisons of the
Medium and Low Sodium Communities*

Characteristics	Medium Sodium Community	Low Sodium Community
Population, 1970	37,406	33,180
Population Change, 1960–70 (%)	19.8	12.0
Median Family Income ($)	11,748	12,424
Median School Years	12.4	12.5
Black Population (%)	0.6	0.2
Foreign Born Population (%)	5.5	6.7
Water Sodium Level, 1976 (mg/L)	42.1	6.3

*1970 U.S. Census Data

one-third that found in the original high school study. The low Na community (LoNaC) had one water source which served the entire community and had a Na level of 6 mg/L. The medium sodium community (MdNaC) received their water from 47 different wells with Na content ranging from 33–51 mg/L. A Na determination from the water of 16 different household taps sampled throughout the town yielded an average Na level of 42 mg/L. The average difference in Na level between these communities was approximately 36 mg/L versus the 100 mg/L in the earlier study.

It was proposed that individual water samples and urine specimens be collected from participating students, but the school system in the McNaC community withheld permission to carry out this phase of the study subsequent to the measurement of BP in both communities. A 24-hour dietary diary which was to have been complete at the time of the water and urine collection was administered. The BP data were recorded in May, 1978, and the dietary diaries were collected in June, 1978.

METHODS

Selection of Communities. The test and control communities were chosen to be well-matched on social and demographic characteristics, geographically similar and close, and to have a drinking water Na differential of 50 mg/L or less. Table 1 presents the pertinent data. Both communities are suburbs north of Boston, as in the original tenth and third grade studies.

Blood Pressure. The BP of tenth graders was recorded on the same three days of the week in each community, on two consecutive weeks. As previously, five registered nurses from the regional Visiting Nurse Association served as the BP technicians in both communities. They were selected on the basis of both inter and intraobserver reliability, and were standardized and validated using the methods described for the Third Grade Study that are given immediately prior to this paper in this volume.

The BP screenings were conducted during three full days at each high school, during mornings and afternoons. The screening area in the MdNaC was a divided gym, with the waiting area for completing questionnaires on one side of a partition, and the screening area on the other side. In the LoNaC, the staging and screening areas were adjacent science rooms. Four nurses working on the rotating schedule previously described took the BP's in both towns. Procedures were again standardized as closely as possible.

As before, three BP readings were recorded independently by three nurses, blind as to each other's readings. Systolic BP was recorded as the first phase Korotkoff sounds, and diastolic was recorded as the fifth phase. The three readings were averaged for the data analysis. Pulse was recorded as the number of beats in 30 seconds multiplied by two. Height and weight were recorded by project staff on school scales at the time of BP measurement.

Questionnaire. Students completed a questionnaire at the time of the screening which provided information on a variety of factors potentially related to BP which could be confounders of an association between Na and BP. In addition, the Health Opinion Survey (HOS) was incorporated into the questionnaire in an attempt to measure differential stress as a possible confounding factor.

Dietary Diary. Dietary intake of Na was estimated from self-reports of food consumed during one 24-hour period. Information was requested which would permit classification of food items on Na content as accurately as possible using the previously described sources for nutrient content information.

RESULTS

Blood Pressure. Participation rates in the two schools were lower than in previous studies and were unequal in the two communities, and no data were available to characterize the representativeness of the participants versus non-participants. In the LoNaC, 360 of 505 (71.3%) tenth graders participated, and 362 of 703 (51.5%) participated in the MdNaC. Differential participation was partially attributed to the greater difficulty in communicating enthusiasm for the study to a larger, more dispersed group of students. It was also partially attributed to being able to communicate personally with the science teachers through whom all study communications were conveyed in the LoNaC, but only indirectly through school administrative personnel with the homeroom teachers, through whom all study communications were forwarded, in the MdNaC.

The initial results for the tenth graders revealed no statistically significant differences in mean BP between the two communities for males and females for diastolic BP and for male systolic BP. It can be seen from Table 2 that systolic BP for females was significantly different between the two communities, but the direction was opposite to that predicted in the original hypothesis. The females in the MdNaC had a significantly lower mean systolic BP than the females in the LoNaC (-1.66 mm Hg, $p = 0.043$). However, for males the difference in mean systolic BP was 0.5 mm Hg ($p = 0.349$) and for diastolic BP the difference was

TABLE 2
Mean Systolic and Diastolic Blood Pressure in the Medium and Low Sodium
Communities, for Tenth Grade Males and Females

	n	Systolic BP (mm Hg)		1-tailed p ≤	Diastolic BP (mm Hg)		1-tailed p ≤
		Mean	SD		Mean	SD	
Males							
Medium Sodium							
Community	183	116.8	11.8		60.5	10.2	
Low Sodium							
Community	163	116.3	12.1		60.0	9.2	
Difference							
In Means		0.5		.349	0.5		.324
Females							
Medium Sodium							
Community	179	106.0	8.6		61.6	7.9	
Low Sodium							
Community	197	107.6	9.9		62.0	8.5	
Difference							
In Means		−1.6		.043	−0.4		.322

0.648 mm Hg (p = .324). The difference in diastolic BP for the two female groups was not significant with a difference of −0.40 mm Hg (p = 0.322).

Figure 1 presents these findings in graphic form. No upshift of the BP curve for male systolic and diastolic BP or female diastolic BP can be seen. An upshift in the female systolic BP curve for the LoNaC can be observed. The Kolmogorov-Smirnov 2-sample test was used as well to test the significance of the differences in the distributions of BP in the two communities. No significant differences were found. For males for systolic and diastolic BP, the associated p-values were 0.924 and 0.736, respectively.

These results were not consistent with the previous tenth grade and third grade studies. This could have been due to there being no effect of Na in drinking water at this lower differential or a real difference could have been masked by confounding. For both sexes it was determined whether any other variables differed significantly between the two towns and were also significantly associated with BP. Chi-square analysis was used to test the differences in response to categorical variables between the two towns and t-tests were employed to test these differences in continuous variables. A one-way analysis of variance was used to examine the association of categorical variables with blood pressure and the Pearson Correlation Coefficient was used to determine the association of continuous variables with blood presssure. All tests were evaluated at the p = 0.05 level of significance.

For males, time elapsed since their last cigarette prior to having their BP recorded was shorter for LoNaC males than MdNaC males (p = 0.028), and it was associated with both systolic and diastolic BP such that BP's were higher

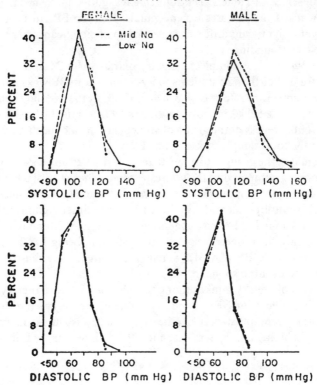

FIGURE 1. Systolic and diastolic BP distributions of tenth grade males and females from the Medium and Low Na Communities.

among those for whom less time had elapsed (p = 0.049 and 0.045, respectively). This difference would have the effect of working against the hypothesis. The HOS score for the LoNaC males was significantly higher (p ≤ 0.01), which would enhance the hypothesized relationship when controlled for.

Among females, reported level of usual physical activity and whether they recalled previously having their BP recorded were significantly different between the two communities and were related to BP. The females in the MdNaC tended to be less active than those from the LoNaC (p = 0.047), and higher diastolic BP was associated with less physical activity (p = 0.022), working in favor of the hypothesis. Fewer females in the MdNaC recalled having had their BP previously recorded (p = 0.001) and this was related to systolic BP such that females who did not recall a prior BP had lower BP (p = 0.047), working against the hypothesized relationship.

Analysis of covariance was used to control simultaneously for the net impact of the potentially confounding variables on the originally observed BP distributions. For males, time elapsed since last cigarette before BP and HOS score were included as covariates. For females, level of physical activity and recall of a prior BP being taken were the covariates. The results of the adjustment proce-

15

dure are presented in Table 3. The adjustment slightly diminished the observed differences in BP in all cases except female diastolic BP. In no case was a previously nonsignificant difference revealed to be significant after controlling for possible confounding.

Dietary Na Intake. Completed dietary diaries for a 24-hour period were available for 324 of the 722 students (44.9%) for whom BP was recorded. For males, the completion rate was 38.3% and 35.0% in the MdNaC and LoNaC, respectively. It was 52.0% in the MdNaC and 52.8% in the LoNaC for females. The representativeness of the group of students returning the dietary diaries in relation to the total sample was examined.

Among males, the group returning dietary diaries had an average systolic BP of 119.4 mm Hg compared to the nonresponders, whose systolic BP was 114.9 mm Hg, making the responders a group with 5.5 mm Hg higher mean systolic BP than the nonresponders. Diastolic BP did not differ significantly for the males, at 61.4 mm Hg for responders and 59.6 mm Hg for nonresponders. Among females, the differences were not significant, being 107.2 versus 106.4 mm Hg for systolic BP and 61.2 versus 62.6 mm Hg for diastolic BP, for responders versus nonresponders, respectively.

The pattern of dietary intake among the 324 students with dietary diaries is presented in Table 4 for Na, K, and Ca. None of the observed differences in nutrient intake were statistically significant ($p > 0.05$). Na intake in the MdNaC was 56 mg Hg higher among females, but 412 mg higher for the LoNaC among males.

CONCLUSION

No differences were observed in the BP distributions of the tenth graders from two communities with drinking water Na differential of 36 mg/L which

TABLE 3

Differences in Unadjusted and Adjusted Mean Systolic and Diastolic Blood Pressure Between the Medium and Low Sodium Communities, for Males and Females, When Controlling for Confounding Variables

	n	Systolic BP (mm Hg) Unadjusted	Adjusted	Diastolic BP (mm Hg) Unadjusted	Adjusted
Males					
Medium Sodium Community	183	116.8	116.4	60.5	60.4
Low Sodium Community	163	116.3	116.7	60.0	60.1
Difference		0.5	−0.3	0.5	0.3
p values		$p \le .35$	$p \le .41$	$p \le .32$	$p \le .39$
Females					
Medium Sodium Community	179	106.0	106.3	61.6	61.5
Low Sodium Community	197	107.6	107.4	62.0	62.1
Difference		−1.6	−1.1	−0.4	−0.6
p values		$p \le .04$	$p \le .15$	$p \le .32$	$p \le .24$

TABLE 4

Dietary Na, K, and Ca Intake Among Tenth Grade Males and Females from Medium and Low Sodium Communities

	Medium Sodium		Low Sodium		Difference in Means	2-tailed p ≤
	Mean	SD	Mean	SD		
Males	(n = 70)		(n = 57)			
Sodium (mg)	3788	1413	4200	1629	−412	0.130
Potassium (mg)	3845	1466	4230	1542	−385	0.153
Calcium (mg)	1644	780	1797	790	−153	0.275
Females	(n = 93)		(n = 104)			
Sodium (mg)	2495	1120	2439	1100	56	0.723
Potassium (mg)	2288	980	2455	917	−167	0.220
Calcium (mg)	967	471	953	467	14	0.836

could be attributed to that differential, and no variables for which data were available were revealed to be confounding a possible association. The lack of support for a dose-response effect of drinking water Na on BP was inconsistent with the previous findings among tenth graders and third graders, and it may indicate that BP sensitivity to a Na differential of 100 mg/L does not apply at a differential as small as 36 mg/L.

ACKNOWLEDGEMENTS

We would like to acknowledge the overall efforts of our research associates Janelle Klar and Thomas Sieger who have been crucial to the success of this project. This research was supported by the Health Effects Research Laboratory of United States Environmental Protection Agency, Cincinnati, Ohio *Grant #R-805612-02.

CHAPTER III

THE MASSACHUSETTS BLOOD PRESSURE STUDY, PART 3. EXPERIMENTAL REDUCTION OF SODIUM IN DRINKING WATER: EFFECTS ON BLOOD PRESSURE

Edward J. Calabrese and Robert W. Tuthill
Division of Public Health
University of Massachusetts
Amherst, Massachusetts

ABSTRACT

An experimental bottled water study assessed the effect on blood pressure of lowering Na concentration in the water of some of the high sodium community fourth graders. For three months, trios of children matched by sex, school, and baseline BP each used different water for all cooking and drinking purposes, with BP monitored bi-weekly. Pupils were randomly allocated to the three water conditions: (1) high sodium water bottled from their own community distribution system, (2) low sodium water bottled from the distribution system of the comparison community with sodium added to the level of the high sodium community water and (3) low sodium water bottled from the distribution system of the low sodium community but with no sodium added. The results indicate that BP levels among the girls but not boys on the low sodium water exhibited marked decreases in BP over the test period when compared to the other two groups.

INTRODUCTION

Subsequent to the tenth grade, third grade, and dose-response studies, a study was designed to experimentally assess the effect of drinking water Na concentration on BP. The study was structured to provide a more definitive test of the hypothesized relationship than that possible from the cross-sectional, observational studies previously undertaken. The study investigated whether the differential distribution of BP observed between students from a community with a high drinking water Na concentration (HiNaC) in comparison to students from a community with a low drinking water Na concentration (LoNaC) was attributable to the Na differential, to other unidentified differences in the two water supplies, or to factors unrelated to drinking water. Specifically, the study was designed to test whether a reduction in drinking water Na concentration in a fourth grade population resulted in a corresponding decrease in BP over a three-month period. The study was conducted only in the HiNaC which had been the focus of the original tenth and third grade studies. The fourth grade participants were from the same group of students who had participated as third graders in the cross-sectional comparison. The data were collected between March and June, 1979.

METHODS

Recruitment of Participants. Participation was solicited from the families of the fourth grade children in the HiNaC whose parents had consented to their participation in the previous year's study among the third graders. The contact initially was by letter, with a follow-up telephone call, inviting parents to attend a series of informational meetings. Subsequently, a mailing detailing what participation in the project would involve went out to all parents in conjunction with a statement of informed consent to be signed by parents indicating their willingness to have their child participate.

Water Usage Groups. The study requirements specified that for a three-month period, from early March through early June of 1979, participating families would regularly receive bottled water to be used for all of the children's drinking water and for all water used in the preparation of foods and beverages to be consumed by the children. Additionally, water of each type was provided in the classroom to serve the drinking needs of the children while at school. No control was exerted over the preparation of school lunches.

Three different types of water, distinguished for participants by cap color, were distributed and the children divided into three groups according to the type of water used. Children were matched in triads of three students each on the basis of sex, school, and baseline BP. The members of each triad were then randomly allocated to one of three bottled water conditions:

1) HI: received water bottled directly from their own HiNaC water distribution system at approximately 110 mg/L Na;

2) LO: received water bottled directly from the LoNaC water distribution system at approximately 10 mg/L Na;

3) LO+: received water from the LoNaC water distribution system, with Na added up to the 110 mg/L of the HiNaC.

It was hypothesized that the reduced Na intake from drinking water would result in a decrease in BP in the LO group. The LO+ comparison group made it possible to determine whether any difference in change in BP between the HI and LO groups over the three months was due to the reduction in Na or due to differences in other characteristics between the HiNaC and LoNaC water supplies. Participating children, their families, all school personnel, and the nurses recording BP were blind to the group assignment of the children.

Water Preparation and Delivery. Water was taken from the distribution system of each of the two towns and loaded into a 5,000 gallon stainless steel tanker truck for transport to the bottling facility. The water was bottled in one gallon polypropylene containers at an FDA approved commercial bottled water facility. The three types of water were distinguished by color coded caps and labels. Na concentrations in LO+ water were raised from 9 mg/L to approximately 110 mg/L with the addition of measured amounts of NaCl (Reagent grade Mallinkrodt Chemicals) to the appropriate tankers of LoNaC water prior to bottling. Water in the tanker was thoroughly mixed with a circulating pump to insure all the NaCl went into solution.

The water was bottled and delivered to the individual homes and schools every two weeks during the study. Computerized delivery records were maintained on the amount and type of water delivered to households and schools for the duration of the study. In the schools the water was placed in refrigerated 5-gallon capacity coolers, appropriately color coded, and placed in a location easily accessible to each student. All personnel involved in the bottling and delivery process were blind as to the type of water denoted by the color coded caps and labels.

Insuring a high standard of water quality was an important consideration throughout the study. The tanker trucks routinely used only for the transport of liquid food products designated for human consumption were thoroughly steam cleaned and inspected prior to each use. The bacteriological water quality of each bottling was monitored by fecal coliform determinations and standard plate counts using the membrane filter method. In addition, daily fecal coliform and standard plate count determinations were conducted for two weeks during the study to monitor water quality over a period corresponding to the shelf time of the water stored in the homes. The results of all fecal coliform tests were zero, and with only six of 38 standard plate determinations indicating counts greater than zero. Sodium concentrations of samples representing all the water bottled during the study were analyzed using a Perkin Elmer model 103 atomic absorption spectrophotometer. Samples were directly atomized in an air-acetylene flame at 330.2/330.3 nm. The concentration was determined by comparison of sample absorbence to a calibration curve constructed with aqueous standards. The range of Na concentrations in the three groups during the study was as follows: HI, 108–116 mg Na/L; LO+, 106–113 mg Na/L; LO, 9–10 mg Na/L.

Blood Pressure. Monitoring of BP occurred on a bi-weekly basis with the first screening in the week before beginning the twelve weeks of bottled water usage serving as the baseline pressure on which the matching of triads was achieved. Six subsequent screenings followed, at two-week intervals, for the twelve-week duration of the project. The screenings were conducted at each of the seven schools in the community, and were scheduled for four mornings and three afternoons during each screening week. All participating children in any one school were screened in a single morning or afternoon session; and, since the triads were matched by school, diurnal variation in BP was thereby controlled.

During each screening week there were a few absentees. In order to provide as complete a set of BP data as possible at the midpoint (fourth screening, after six weeks of participation) and the endpoint (seventh screening after twelve weeks of participation), extra effort was made at these times to screen absent children at home or later in the week at school if possible. Screening procedures were closely standardized among the seven schools and from screening to screening. Children were brought to a suitable, quiet location in each school for the screenings, either the nurse's office (two schools), a reading room (two schools), the principal's office (one school), the gym (one school), or auditorium (one school). They were brought to the screening area slowly and quietly, but three of the 21 classrooms of children were required to go up or down one flight of stairs. In these cases they were brought to the area early and seated quietly for at least ten minutes prior to being screened. No gym classes or active recesses were scheduled in the hour prior to screening, and meals were not consumed for 45 minutes prior to screening.

At each screening the children proceeded through three stations, with their pulse being recorded by the nurse at the first station, and a casual seated BP on the left arm being taken at each station by a nurse using a mercury sphygmomanometer. The pressure was raised approximately 30 mm Hg above the point at which the pulse disappeared and then released at a rate of 2 to 3 mm Hg/sec. Systolic pressure was recorded at the point where two consecutive Korotkoff sounds were audible and diastolic pressure at the disappearance of sound. The same nurse worked at the same station each time, and the nurse at each succeeding station was blind to the preceding readings of her colleagues. The three nurses regularly conducting the screenings, and the two back-up nurses, had been selected from a pool of nurses on the basis of their inter- and intraobserver reliability, using the standard procedures previously described.

The services of the back-up nurses were required on only two occasions out of the 49 total screening sessions (seven schools, seven bi-weekly screenings each). On one occasion one nurse substituted at an afternoon screening, and on another two nurses substituted at a morning screening.

Urinary and Dietary Data. First-morning urine specimens and two-day diet records were collected at monthly intervals: first at baseline before commencing bottled water usage, and monthly thereafter for the three-month study period, for a total of four times. Sterile sample containers and instructions for a clean-catch urine specimen were distributed each month on a Tuesday to the children at school to be taken home for Wednesday morning's use. All families were telephoned that night and arrangments made to deliver a specimen bottle to the home if it had been left at school. The specimens were returned to the schools in the morning, and were immediately collected, placed on ice, and taken to the University. The specimens were analyzed for Na and K levels using an IL flame photometer.

The diet records, designed to promote accuracy and ease in recording diet information, were distributed in school each Monday morning at monthly intervals. The children, with the aid of their teachers and parents, kept an on-going record of all food and liquids consumed for the 48-hour period from

Monday lunch through Wednesday breakfast. Teachers and parents were given special instructions at the outset on how the records should be kept. Additionally, it was emphasized to parents that the meals served to their children should not differ in any way from usual practice.

Questionnaire. Information was solicited via questionnaire to assess whether there were any changes in dietary habits, particularly salt use, over the study period, how frequently the child ate the school lunch, at which time they were exposed to the regular town water, and the socioeconomic status (SES) of the family, as defined by education and occupation of the principal wage earner. In addition, the questionnaire information gathered during the previous year provided data on the length of residence of the children in the town, family history of high BP, and the infant feeding habits regarding breast milk versus a formula preparation, commercially or home prepared solid foods, and the age at which solid food intake was instituted.

A critical factor to evaluate in determining whether the study provided a credible test of the hypothesis was compliance rates among the three groups. Parents were asked to complete a questionnaire at two-week intervals, reporting the extent to which their child adhered to the bottled water regimen during that period. Information was sought on the compliance of the children in using the bottled water for all drinks of water, and the compliance of the parents in cooking all foods and making all mixed liquids served to the children with the bottled water.

Further data collected on each child were height and weight, both at baseline and at the final screening. School scales were used, all of which weighed correctly (within 1 lb.) a 40 lb. weight, a weight lower than the average weight of the children. The same scales were used for the initial and final measurements.

RESULTS

Blood Pressure. At the initiation of the study, the families of 171 of the 353 children eligible to participate agreed to take part in the study. Due to rigorous parental involvement required, a positive response of this size was excellent. These 171 children, 87 boys and 84 girls, were grouped into triads on the basis of their initial BP measurements, by sex, and by school. Because one boy was not available for baseline measurement, the effective number of complete matches among the boys was reduced to 28 triads. There were also 28 complete matched triads for girls. Due to the number of participants in any one school not always being evenly divisible by three, the extra students from all the schools were put into matched triads, resulting in one triad of boys and two triads of girls not being matched by school. The total number of children who completed the study, regardless of triad matching, was 164, or 95.9% of the initial participants. The number of complete triads at study completion was 25 among the girls and 26 among the boys, 89.5% of the initial 57 matched triads.

For the analysis, the three BP readings per student at each screening were averaged together for one representative BP value for each screening. Further, the second and fourth week readings, the sixth and eighth week readings, and

TABLE 1
Mean Systolic and Diastolic Blood Pressure at Baseline of Three Matched Groups, for Males, Females, and Sexes Combined

Water Group	n	Systolic Mean	SD	Diastolic Mean	SD
Males					
High Sodium	26	101.0	7.7	59.0	9.3
Lo+ Sodium	26	101.2	7.4	57.8	12.2
Lo Sodium	26	101.3	9.2	58.0	9.5
Females					
High Sodium	25	97.5	8.7	56.4	11.1
Lo+ Sodium	25	97.6	9.7	56.9	10.2
Lo Sodium	25	97.7	10.1	56.1	9.2
Total					
High Sodium	51	99.3	8.3	57.7	10.2
Lo+ Sodium	51	99.4	8.7	57.3	11.2
Lo Sodium	51	99.6	9.7	57.1	9.3

the tenth and twelfth week readings were averaged to form their average monthly readings. Fourteen of the 153 children remaining in the analysis were missing one BP value and had the mean substituted for their one missing screening of the seven. This represented 1.3% of the total number of readings.

The mean baseline BP values for the three groups, presented in Table 1, indicate that there were no initial significant BP differences among the three groups, the matching having been successful. Table 2 presents a comparison of the children on other characteristics measured at baseline but not considered in the matching procedure. There was a statistically significant difference in weight among the three groups of girls, the group receiving the low Na (Lo) water

TABLE 2
Comparison of Three Matched Groups on Initial Weight, Height, and Pulse, for Males and Females

Variable	High Sodium Group Mean	SD	Added Sodium Group Mean	SD	Low Sodium Group Mean	SD
Males						
Weight (kg)	34.3	5.9	36.3	6.5	34.0	6.5
Height (cm)	138.4	6.6	139.4	4.8	137.9	6.4
Pulse (beats/min)	81.7	12.7	79.2	9.7	79.2	12.5
Females						
Weight (kg)*	32.5	5.1	33.6	6.0	29.8	4.2
Height (cm)	134.9	5.8	136.4	6.1	134.9	6.4
Pulse (beats/min)	82.9	8.6	82.4	11.4	86.9	11.9

*$p \leq 0.05$

TABLE 3
Mean Systolic and Diastolic Blood Pressure for Each Water Group
at Each Screening Period for Males and Females*

| | Systolic BP | | | | | | Diastolic BP | | | | | |
| | High Sodium | | Added Sodium | | Low Sodium | | High Sodium | | Added Sodium | | Low Sodium | |
Week	Mean	SD	Mean	SD	Mean	SD	Mean	SD	Mean	SD	Mean	SD
Males												
Baseline	101.0	7.7	101.2	7.4	101.3	9.2	59.0	9.3	57.8	12.2	58.0	9.5
2	98.5	8.0	100.7	7.9	97.9	9.7	55.9	10.5	55.9	10.8	55.6	10.5
4	97.9	5.9	97.6	6.0	98.8	8.7	55.0	9.6	55.4	7.8	51.3	12.4
6	98.7	6.3	96.8	7.7	97.4	8.2	56.5	8.9	50.9	15.2	54.3	10.2
8	98.3	7.0	97.9	8.2	98.7	9.0	53.5	8.9	51.4	12.7	52.0	11.0
10	96.6	5.7	97.3	6.8	100.6	9.5	50.6	10.9	52.3	9.5	54.4	10.5
12	98.6	6.9	98.5	6.7	98.9	8.2	53.7	10.9	55.4	10.3	56.0	9.0
Females												
Baseline	97.5	8.7	97.6	9.7	97.7	10.1	56.4	11.1	56.9	10.2	56.1	9.2
2	93.6	7.3	95.8	8.8	93.9	9.0	53.0	9.8	56.4	10.8	56.1	9.2
4	93.6	8.1	92.4	8.8	90.7	9.2	54.6	9.2	52.9	12.4	51.4	8.9
6	92.4	6.6	94.1	9.0	90.6	9.5	52.9	9.2	50.7	14.9	48.1	8.4
8	93.2	6.3	94.4	8.6	92.3	8.1	48.4	11.4	52.7	9.9	44.5	12.3
10	93.1	8.0	93.3	9.2	91.3	9.9	51.3	8.7	50.5	8.5	48.1	8.8
12	94.3	7.1	93.5	10.3	92.4	8.5	53.7	9.1	52.0	10.3	47.4	11.0

*For 14 of 1071 readings (1.3%) mean of reading on either side was substituted for missing reading.

weighing 29.8 kg, compared to 32.5 kg and 33.6 kg for the high Na (Hi) and added Na (Lo+) groups, respectively.

Table 3 presents the average BP reading for each group of the seven bi-weekly screenings for boys and girls. All three experimental groups exhibited a drop in BP over the study period, characteristic of becoming more familiar with the screening situation. Among the girls a consistent pattern of a greater drop in BP among the Lo group was evident for both systolic and diastolic blood pressure. However, there was no consistent difference among the groups in the pattern of the drop in BP among the boys. An initial effect was not sustained beyond the first month.

Graphically, the differences in BP pattern over the study period are seen in Figures 1 & 2. The random pattern of change among the boys, compared to the consistent pattern of a greater reduction in BP among the girls on low Na water relative to their high Na water counterparts, are closely reflected in the graphs. Pairs of bi-weekly values were averaged as monthly values, and the girls using low Na water show a consistently greater decline in both systolic and diastolic BP compared to the other two high Na groups; Table 4 presents the baseline values and the subsequent change in BP for these monthly follow-up periods.

Table 5 compared baseline values to the final reading during the twelfth week of the study. The pattern of difference between boys and girls in systolic and diastolic BP change was similar, with girls having a greater decrease than boys in both cases, the differences being statistically significantly different at $p = 0.033$ for the difference in change in diastolic BP. Looking at the difference between boys and girls in change from baseline compared to the average of the six subsequent readings over the twelve-week screening period, again the pattern is similar, with girls having a greater average change than boys. In this analysis the change for girls was statistically significantly different than that for boys for systolic BP at $p = 0.03$. Because there was no prior hypothesis as to whether the low Na water would have a greater impact on boys than girls, two-tailed tests of significance were used for this evaluation.

The next issue was to determine whether there were significant differences in BP changes between the two groups on high Na water: the group using their own high Na community water and the group using the low Na community water with the Na addition. Testing differences in change in systolic and diastolic BP between the two high Na water groups revealed no significant differences for either boys or girls, for either systolic or diastolic BP. The range of p-values was $0.32 < p < 0.84$. The same comparison but using a paired t-test analysis to take into account the matching, likewise yielded no significant differences between the two groups of students in the degree of BP change. The range of p-values was $0.20 < p < 0.83$. A similar analysis was performed using the average changes in the six treatment readings against baseline as the index of change. With a range of p-values of $0.70 < p < 0.90$, no significant differences between the two groups using high Na water, either among boys or girls or for systolic or diastolic BP, were found.

A further analysis compared the change of BP among the students using the low Na water to the combined average change in BP among the two groups

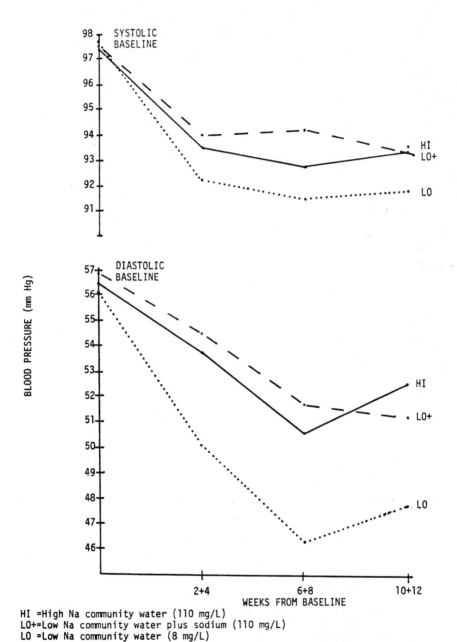

FIGURE 1. BP adjusted for baseline weight and pulse, combined readings—girls (25 trios).

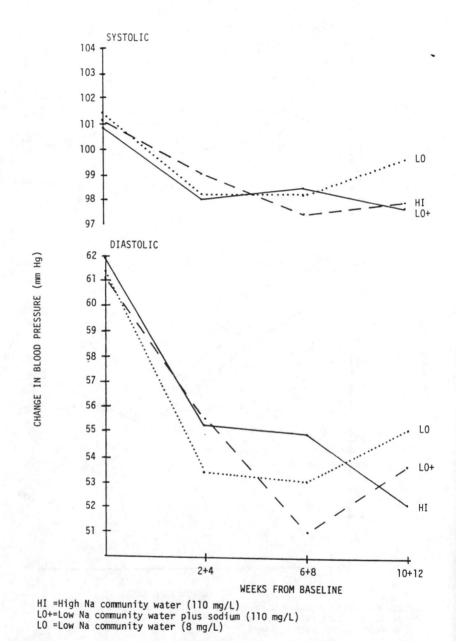

FIGURE 2. BP adjusted for baseline weight and pulse combined readings—boys (26 trios).

TABLE 4
Mean Decline in Systolic and Diastolic Blood Pressure for the Water Groups by Combined follow-up Periods

Group	Baseline	Weeks 2–4	Weeks 6–8	Weeks 10–12
Systolic		**MALES**		
High	101.0	−2.8	−2.5	−3.2
Low+	101.2	−2.0	−3.8	−3.3
Low	101.3	−3.0	−3.3	−1.5
Diastolic				
High	59.0	−3.6	−4.0	−6.8
Low+	57.8	−2.1	−6.7	−4.0
Low	58.0	−4.6	−4.9	−2.8
Systolic		**FEMALES**		
High	97.5	−3.9	−4.7	−3.8
Low+	97.6	−3.5	−3.4	−4.2
Low	97.7	−5.4	−6.3	−5.9
Diastolic				
High	56.4	−2.6	−5.8	−3.9
Low+	56.9	−2.3	−5.2	−5.7
Low	56.1	−5.3	−9.8	−8.4

using high Na water. The rationale for this combination was that the high and added Na groups did not differ statistically significantly from each other. The finding of no difference between these two groups was consistent with the hypothesis that the two groups on high Na water would not differ in BP experience unless some water factor other than Na were contributing to the differences observed previously among tenth graders and third graders. These findings are presented in Table 6. As previously, the analysis considered both

TABLE 5
Differences Between Males and Females Using Low Sodium Water in Amount of Blood Pressure Change From Baseline to the Twelfth Week Reading: And Comparing the Baseline Reading to the Average of the Six Subsequent Readings over the Treatment Period

Comparison	Males Mean Change	SD	Females Mean Change	SD	2-tailed t	$p \leq$
Baseline to 12th Week						
Systolic	−2.44	6.0	−5.33	6.6	1.64	.108
Diastolic	−2.05	6.4	−8.67	13.5	2.23	.033
Baseline to Other Weeks						
Systolic	−2.62	5.7	−5.86	4.6	2.23	.030
Diastolic	−4.09	6.2	−7.81	8.0	1.85	.071

TABLE 6
Differences Between Students Using Low Sodium Water and the Average
of Students Using High and Added Sodium Water in Amount of Blood
Pressure Change from Baseline to the Twelfth Week Reading and from Baseline to
the Average of the Six Subsequent Readings

Comparison	Low Sodium		High Added Sodium Average		1-tailed	
	Mean Change	SD	Mean Change	SD	t	p ≤
Baseline to 12th Week			**MALES**			
Systolic	−2.44	6.0	−2.54	3.9	−.10	.462
Diastolic	−2.05	6.4	−3.80	8.6	−.87	.197
Baseline to All Other Weeks						
Systolic	−2.62	5.7	−2.95	3.8	−.36	.360
Diastolic	−4.09	6.2	−4.50	5.8	−.28	.392
Baseline to 12th Week			**FEMALES**			
Systolic	−5.33	6.6	−3.60	3.9	1.39	.088
Diastolic	−8.67	13.5	−3.80	5.0	1.87	.037
Baseline to All Other Weeks						
Systolic	−5.86	4.6	−3.88	4.3	2.37	.013
Diastolic	−7.81	8.0	−4.21	4.6	2.58	.008

change from baseline to final reading and from baseline to the combined average of all subsequent readings. From the table a pattern emerges confirming the differential effect of the low Na water on the BP of boys versus girls. Among the girls, the group on the low Na water displayed a consistently greater decrease in BP than the average of their counterparts on the two high Na waters. The difference among the girls for the various comparisons ranged from a 1.73 mm Hg to a 4.87 mm Hg greater decrease in BP among the girls in the LoNa group, with associated p-values in the range of $0.008 < p < 0.088$. The effect of the low Na water on BP was more marked for diastolic BP than for systolic BP, at $p < 0.002$ and $p < 0.030$, respectively.

Further analyses of the relationship between Na and BP over the study period considered the effect of potentially confounding variables on the BP pattern. All variables were evaluated for any differences among the water groups and in relation to systolic and diastolic BP, including height, weight, pulse, sociodemographic and family history information, and compliance rates as assessed via the bi-weekly questionnaires. Among the boys, only pulse at the sixth screening and weight were both significantly different between the water groups ($p < 0.05$)

and significantly correlated with BP (p < 0.01). Only weight was significantly different between the water groups (p < 0.01) and significantly correlated with BP (p < 0.01) among the girls. However, for consistency in analysis, both weight and pulse at each screening were included as covariates for both sexes.

An analysis of repeated measures was performed with baseline BP and weight used as covariates, remaining constant over the three averaged follow-up screenings. Pulse, which varied over the study period, was controlled at each BP reading.

The results of the analysis of repeated measures for the low versus the combined high Na groups for boys showed no significant differences in systolic or diastolic BP. For girls, differences in systolic BP for the low versus the combined high Na groups had an associated significance level of p < 0.08. The same comparison for diastolic BP was significant at p < 0.01. The same analysis for the six separate follow-up periods produced results similar to the analysis for the three averaged follow-up periods for both boys and girls, with only the pattern for the girls being statistically significant.

Na Intake and Excretion. A comparison of the Na exposure of the three water groups was assessed via the two-day dietary diaries and first-morning urine specimens which were collected at baseline and at the three bi-weekly follow-up intervals. Table 7 presents the mean urinary Na and K values for the three water groups for boys and girls. None of the differences were statistically significant over the study period among the groups nor was there a significant correlation between Na excretion and BP. Na excretion levels did not differ significantly between the sexes.

TABLE 7
**Mean Urinary Na and K Excretion (MEQ) at Baseline
and Three Bi-Weekly Follow-Up Periods**

Group	Baseline	Week 4	Week 8	Week 12
		SODIUM		
Males				
High	109.5	141.2	143.3	123.2
Low+	133.5	140.3	129.8	127.6
Low	148.8	134.6	133.9	127.2
Females				
High	110.3	131.7	107.4	109.0
Low+	132.6	133.3	130.0	135.8
Low	132.7	135.3	132.6	128.6
		POTASSIUM		
Males				
High	51.3	49.4	38.6	33.6
Low+	44.2	47.9	34.0	42.4
Low	52.2	57.4	38.6	36.8
Females				
High	45.7	43.3	29.1	34.9
Low+	49.1	37.9	33.5	36.0
Low	42.0	37.6	36.3	32.2

TABLE 8

Average Daily Na Intake at Baseline and Three Follow-Up Periods and Summary
Intake, by Water Groups for Males and Females

Group	Baseline	Week 4	Week 8	Week 12	Overall
Males					
High (15)	3290	3242	2613	2711	2964
Low+ (16)	3684	3736	3209	2929	3390
Low (15)	4267	3688	3661	2908	3631
Females					
High (15)	2737	2634	2199	2479	2512
Low+ (14)	3515	3140	2291	2831	2944
Low (15)	3170	3401	2987	2970	3132

In regard to dietary Na intake, completed dietary records over the study period were available for 90 of the 153 participants. Although this group represented only 59% of the total, there were no significant average BP differences at baseline or at any of the three bi-weekly follow-up periods between those for whom dietary data was available and those for whom it was not. Since the volume of dietary information to be coded for nutrient value required that two separate coders be involved, and since the number coded by each coder varied by group, all values presented were coder adjusted. If codable nutrient intake information was missing for a participant for a bi-weekly period, the mean of all other periods was substituted for the missing value.

The average daily Na intake at baseline and the three follow-up periods is presented in Table 8. Also shown is the overall average daily Na intake during the study, which was represented by the average of the four two-day values. Thus, the overall average is a summary figure which characterized daily Na intake among this group of students, for boys and girls. It can be seen that average daily Na intake differed between the groups. Although the differences were not statistically significant due to sample size considerations, daily Na intake at each interval was used as a covariate in a repeated measures analysis of variance in order to assess the water group effect while controlling for dietary Na intake. The unadjusted differences in change in BP from baseline are presented in Table 9. It is clear that the adjustment for dietary Na intake had little effect on the pattern of BP change among the three water groups for either male or females, and the overall picture of no association among the boys in contrast to an observed association among the girls was maintained. Although not statistically significant at these smaller sample sizes, the pattern of BP change of those with diet records among the girls on the low Na water compared to the girls on the high Na water was striking.

CONCLUSION

In sum, the female data seemed to indicate a sensitivity of BP to reduction of small amounts of Na in the drinking water. However, the male data did not provide support for this effect. Whether these differences in effect by sex may

TABLE 9
Differences in Change in Blood Pressure (mm Hg)
from Baseline Unadjusted and Adjusted for Average Daily
Dietary Na Intake, by Water Group for Males and Females

Group	Baseline to Weeks 2–4 Unadj.	Adj.	Baseline to Weeks 6–8 Unadj.	Adj.	Baseline to Weeks 10–12 Unadj.	Adj.
MALES						
Systolic						
High	−2.4	−2.2	−2.8	−2.7	−3.6	−3.5
Low+	−3.3	−3.3	−4.0	−4.1	−4.2	−4.3
Low	−2.4	−2.5	−2.8	−2.8	−0.5	−0.6
Diastolic						
High	−3.9	−3.9	−4.6	−4.3	−7.6	−7.3
Low+	−3.9	−4.3	−9.3	−9.5	−3.7	−3.7
Low	−7.2	−7.3	−5.3	−5.3	−2.4	−2.2
FEMALES						
Systolic						
High	−3.6	−3.6	−3.4	−3.4	−3.3	−3.3
Low+	−4.5	−4.5	−5.7	−5.8	−6.0	−6.0
Low	−5.8	−5.7	−6.1	−6.1	−6.8	−6.8
Diastolic						
High	−1.2	−1.1	−4.6	−4.5	−3.0	−2.9
Low+	−2.6	−2.5	−5.6	−5.4	−6.8	−6.7
Low	−6.8	−7.0	−12.2	−12.4	−10.3	−10.5

have been due to differential compliance among the boys, which was not apparent in the compliance questionnaires, or whether the differences have other explanations awaits further research.

ACKNOWLEDGEMENTS

We would like to acknowledge the overall efforts of our research associates Janelle Klar and Thomas Sieger who have been crucial to the success of this project. This research was supported by the Health Effects Research Laboratory of United States Environmental Protection Agency, Cincinnati, Ohio *Grant #R-805612-02.

CHAPTER IV

THE MASSACHUSETTS BLOOD PRESSURE STUDY, PART 4. MODEST SODIUM SUPPLEMENTATION AND BLOOD PRESSURE CHANGE IN BOARDING SCHOOL GIRLS

Robert W. Tuthill and Edward J. Calabrese
Division of Public Health
University of Massachusetts
Amherst, Massachusetts

ABSTRACT

Based upon the results of the earlier work, a sodium supplement study was designed and carried out at a private boarding school. Two hundred and sixteen 9th–12th grade girls were randomly assigned to one of three groups while continuing to eat their regular meals at the dining commons. All participating students took two capsules, under supervision, both mid-morning and subsequent to the evening meal. One group received placebos at both times, one group received 2 G of salt in the morning and a placebo in the evening, and the final group received a placebo in the morning and 2 G of salt in the evening. One week of baseline data and eight weeks of follow-up data were collected twice weekly for BP, pulse, 24-hour urine specimen, and stress of daily events.

Repeated measures analysis of variance failed to detect a significant difference in change in systolic and diastolic BP between groups. Extensive analysis of other variables did not uncover any negative confounding or interaction. Drop out rates were very low and compliance rates very high. The urinalysis clearly demonstrated that the Na excretion in the two supplement groups was similar and significantly elevated over the placebo group, thus documenting the high Na supplement compliance rates.

INTRODUCTION

This paper reports on the most recently completed study on sodium in drinking water and blood pressure in school children conducted at the University of Massachusetts, Amherst. Given the prior results, summarized earlier in this volume, our next study was a sodium supplement investigation at a private boarding school. There was some controversy surrounding the small amount of sodium in the drinking water that was associated with appreciable changes in population blood pressure in our earlier work. For this reason, the study was designed to compare a small sodium supplementation in water and in food against a placebo group. The study was restricted to one sex to reduce sample size needed and females were chosen because they consistently showed an association between blood pressure and drinking water sodium intake in prior studies.

A pretest phase was carried out with twenty graduating seniors to determine the feasibility of various procedures and to find out if such a study was workable on campus. The pretest experience was very helpful in deciding on the most appropriate approaches for the full-scale study and demonstrated that such an effort could be successfully carried out in a teenage female student population.

METHODS

The main study was carried out in two parts, the first being on the West Campus in the fall semester and the second on the East Campus in the Spring semester. Female students in the ninth through twelfth grades were eligible to participate with the signed consent of themselves and their parent/guardian. Participants and their parents each completed background questionnaires. Girls were excluded if one or more of the three consulting physicians (including the campus medical director) considered the student at medical risk if exposed to extra dietary salt. Students were also excluded if they either had a medical condition or took medication which might affect their blood pressure. The blood pressure readings of all the girls were monitored regularly to be alert to any unusual rises which might occur.

Baseline data collected during the first week of the study included blood pressure and 24 hour urine specimens on two different days, two daily stress questionnaires and one major life events questionnaire. Each girl was then randomly allocated to one of three study groups for the eight-week follow-up period. During this time they continued to eat their usual meals at the school dining commons and received a daily sodium supplement and/or placebo in capsule form.

In order to keep the students blind as to their group, the capsules taken by all groups were identical. The capsules were white, contained either 0.5 grams of salt or dextrose and had a slightly salty taste. Capsules were distributed twice daily at midmorning and immediately following the evening meal. On both occasions four capsules were swallowed with water in the presence of a research staff member. The capsules were dispensed from identical boxes each labelled with a participant's name. The staff and students were blind as to the supplement group of each student.

The three supplement groups were designated as placebo, water and food as indicated in Table 1.

TABLE 1
Sodium Supplement Groups

Supplement Group	Mid-Morning	Evening Meal
Placebo	Dextrose	Dextrose
Water	Salt	Dextrose
Food	Dextrose	Salt

Capsule distribution was maintained seven days a week for the eight week period. Provision was made to provide participants with capsules when they were going to be away from school during distribution times. Advanced distribution was limited to valid excuses such as sporting events or week-end passes.

The girls were assigned to a red or blue group such that half of each supplement type (Placebo, Water, Food) was included in each group. The red group was scheduled for blood pressure readings on Monday and Wednesday while the blue group was tested on Tuesdays and Thursdays. This division into color groups was for logistic purposes and spread the work out evenly over four days of the week.

The blood pressure screenings were conducted immediately after dinner. On the days when blood pressure was taken, the evening capsules were swallowed following the blood pressure determination in order to avoid confounding of the measurement due to any immediate effect of the sodium on blood pressure.

Each girl's blood pressure was recorded by two technicians who were blind to each other's readings and to the girls' supplement groupings. Pulse rate was recorded by the first technician. Each girl was always screened by the same team of technicians. An equal proportion of each supplement group was assigned to each team of technicians to avoid any difference between supplement groups which might be caused by team differences. A coordinator at the site controlled the flow of students to the technicians.

The technicians were screened, trained in technique, and validated by a staff member from the MRFIT project in Cambridge, Mass. in the same fashion as in our earlier studies. Immediately after the blood pressure measurement each student completed a checklist of potentially stressful daily events.

Two 24-hour urine specimens were collected weekly from each girl, with the collection period covering midnight to midnight. The blood pressure measurements were taken after dinner on the days covered by the urine specimens. Urine specimens were obtained in snap-top wide-mouthed 20 oz. disposable polystyrene containers. A small crystal of thymol was included in the labelled bottles to minimize bacterial growth and thus improve the accuracy of the creatinine determination. The six containers to be used for the 24-hour collection period were distributed on a regular schedule by a study participant in each dorm who was paid additional compensation for her work. The full containers were collected by the study staff from the dorms early each morning, Tuesday through Friday.

A laboratory for the analysis of the urine specimens was outfitted in the campus health center. Two full-time trained technicians picked up the samples, logged them in, and pooled the sample bottle contents into one container for a volume determination based upon the weight and specific gravity. The sodium and potassium concentration in the pooled samples was determined directly with a IL model 443 flame photometer. In addition, an aliquot of each urine sample was appropriately diluted and stored frozen in a plastic culture tube. Once weekly, the culture tubes were returned to UMass for a creatinine determination using a kinetic method based on the modified Jaffee reaction (Pierce Rapid Stat., Rockford, IL.). The technicians spent Mondays labelling and preparing urine specimen bottles for the rest of the week, and spent Tuesdays through Fridays preparing and analyzing the collected urine samples.

A monetary incentive of sixty dollars was offered to each participant to help maintain high levels of compliance with procedures through the nine-week study. In addition, a bonus incentive of twenty dollars was offered to those participants who missed the fewest capsules, blood pressure measurements, and urine specimens. The payments were made in two stages: first payment of twenty-five dollars and ten dollars of the bonus at the study midpoint; second payment of thirty-five dollars and ten dollars of the bonus at the study conclusion.

FINDINGS

All findings in the study are presented separately for the two campuses because their different experiences during the study precluded combining the results. The participation rates and completion rates are detailed below in Table 2. Although participation rates were less than 50 per cent, the completion rate among the participants was excellent. All tables, figures and data analyses are based upon 107 participants on Campus 1 and 84 participants on Campus 2.

There were factors related to participation in the study probably favoring healthy females who found the $80 incentive attractive and/or who were interested in participating in a scientific study. Once enrolled though, there was little drop-out bias because of the excellent completion rate.

For the blood pressure analysis, the four readings taken each week were combined into a single more stable average (two readings each session, two sessions a week). This decision to combine readings was made, a priori, based

TABLE 2
Recruitment and Completion Rates

Category	Campus 1	Campus 2
Students available	254	294
Volunteers	121 (47.6%)	95 (32.3%)
Medical exclusions	8 (3.1%)	4 (1.3%)
Study participants	113 (44.5%)	91 (31.0%
Drop-outs	4 (3.5%)	3 (3.3%)
Low compliance	2 (1.9%)	4 (4.4%)
Completed	107 (94.6%)	84 (92.3%)

upon the variability in blood pressure readings in the pretest. Due to drop-outs and non-compliance, the number in each supplement group was slightly unequal for the data analysis. Table 3 presents the baseline blood pressure readings for the three supplement groups separately for each campus. None of the groups are statistically different from each other, with the largest discrepancy being 1.4 mm Hg.

Figures 1 and 2 illustrate the change from baseline blood pressure over the eight week study period for the sodium supplement groups on the two campuses. Repeated measures analysis of variance was not significant in any of the four graphs: for campus 1 systolic $p = 0.17$ and $p = 0.48$ while for campus 2 systolic $p = 0.77$ and diastolic $p = 0.31$. Changes in blood pressure were not significantly different between food and water groups or for food and water groups combined versus the placebo group.

Although the treatment groups were not statistically different in baseline blood pressure, a repeated measures analysis of variance was performed controlling for baseline values. The negative results remained unchanged. Since negative confounding might mask an effect, all study variables were examined in this regard using covariance analysis. None of the potential confounders were creating the negative findings.

The steep increase in systolic blood pressure of 3–5 mm Hg on both campuses in the first several weeks of the study was not readily explained by changes in daily stress ratings, the stress of being a new student versus a returnee, athletes versus non-athletes or any of the other potential confounding study variables.

DISCUSSION

There was clearly no significant relationship between sodium supplementation (0.8 grams daily) and change in blood pressure over the eight week period

TABLE 3
Baseline Systolic and Diastolic Blood Pressure by
Treatment Group and Campus

Group	n	Systolic BP (mm Hg) Mean	SD	Diastolic BP (mm Hg) Mean	SD
Campus 1					
Placebo	36	113.5	6.6	71.0	9.2
Food	36	113.9	8.4	71.4	7.9
Water	35	113.4	7.9	70.1	7.0
$p \leq$		0.96		0.79	
Campus 2					
Placebo	29	113.1	6.8	69.7	6.7
Food	28	112.4	6.7	68.9	7.1
Water	27	111.7	7.6	69.3	7.2
$p \leq$		0.76		0.91	

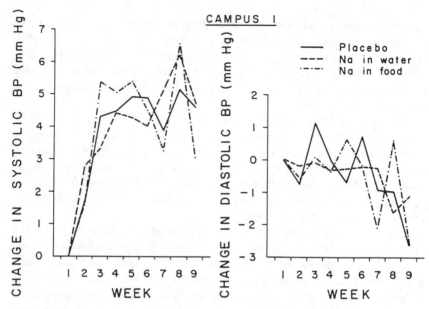

FIGURE 1. Change in systolic and diastolic BP from Baseline to Week Nine by week for Campus 1.

of the study. There are a number of alternative explanations for these negative findings:

1. No association between sodium intake and blood pressure. Although this is a possible explanation, there is sufficient other research to suggest that there is at least a salt-sensitive sub-population. More likely there is a need to consider a variety of other elements besides sodium and potassium such as calcium,

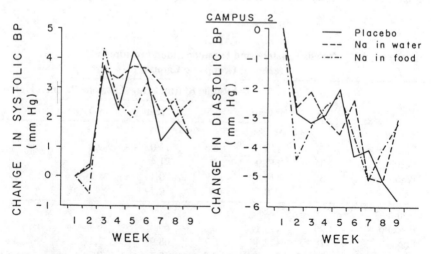

FIGURE 2. Change in systolic and diastolic BP from Baseline to Week Nine by week for Campus 2.

cadmium, barium, zinc, etc. and ratios thereof. Such variables were not included in this study.

2. A lack of compliance with the capsule, blood pressure, and urine specimen regimes. After omitting the seven drop-outs and the six low compliers, the proportion of potential events completed is indicated in Table 4 below.

3. The sodium supplement effect was swamped out by variation in sodium from food sources. Figure 3 below displays the change in the average 24-hour sodium excretion in milligrams per week in the three supplement groups on the two campuses. The two sodium supplement groups were strikingly similar in sodium excretion and quite distinct from the placebo group on both campuses. The desired sodium differential was clearly obtained. As an aside, the rapid rise of sodium excretion evidenced in all groups in the first several weeks appears to coincide with the rapid rise in systolic blood pressure experienced by all groups during the same time period. This higher excretion rate probably reflects a change in diet, and its correspondence with the rise in blood pressure is consistent with a sodium effect on blood pressure. On the other hand, beginning a new semester is in and of itself stressful and could explain the change, although the stress measures used in the study were not related to blood pressure change.

4. The sodium supplement was not large enough and/or maintained long enough for the expected effect on blood pressure to occur. For safety reasons the sodium supplement was limited to only 0.8 grams per day. From clinical research on sodium and blood pressure, it is clear that it is possible to show a decrease in blood pressure with modest reductions in sodium intake whereas it appears to require much larger doses of sodium to effect a short term change in blood pressure.

5. Lack of statistical power. At the onset of the study we anticipated that the data from Campus 1 and Campus 2 would be combined bringing the total sample size to 214 with an average of 71 girls per supplement group. Power and sample size calculations for a repeated measures analysis with three groups indicated that a difference of 1.5 mm Hg in blood pressure would have been detectable at $\alpha = 0.05$ and $\beta = 0.20$. Given the necessity of separating the campuses for analysis, only an average difference of 2.5 mm Hg in blood pressure was detectable under the same conditions. The actual mean blood pressure differences were on the order of 1.4 mm Hg at maximum.

In conclusion, there appears to be no effect on blood pressure of 0.8 grams of sodium extra a day added to the usual dietary intake of healthy teenage girls.

TABLE 4
Compliance With Study Procedures

Category	Campus 1	Campus 2
Capsule Sessions	11 152/11 984 = 93.1%	8 724/9 408 = 92.7%
	Water group = 95.8%	Water group = 94.5%
	Food group = 89.5%	Food group = 96.7%
Blood pressure	1892/1926 = 98.2%	1482/1568 = 94.5%
Urine specimens	1878/1904 = 98.6%	1427/1476 = 96.7%

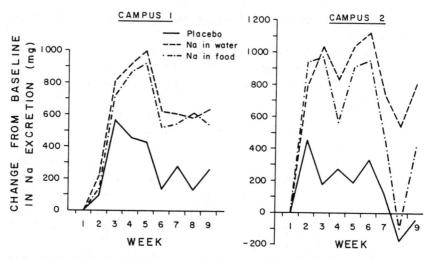

FIGURE 3. Change in urinary Na excretion from Baseline to Week Nine by week for Campus 1 and Campus 2.

Yet, the rapid rise in sodium excretion due to total dietary intake correlates well with the early rise in systolic blood pressure. However, the methodological issues discussed above suggest an interpretation of these data in the context of the other studies on sodium and blood pressure presented at this conference.

ACKNOWLEDGEMENTS

We would like to acknowledge the overall efforts of our research associates Janelle Klar and Thomas Sieger who have been crucial to the success of this project. This research was supported by the Health Effects Research Laboratory of United States Environmental Protection Agency, Cincinnati, Ohio *Grant #R-805612-02.

CHAPTER V

BLOOD PRESSURE AND SODIUM INTAKE: EVIDENCE FROM TWO DUTCH STUDIES

Albert Hofman
Department of Epidemiology
Erasmus University Medical School
Rotterdam, The Netherlands

ABSTRACT

To investigate the relations between sodium intake and blood pressure, two studies were performed in Dutch children.

In the first one, a retrospective follow-up study, the association between sodium concentrations in the drinking water and blood pressure was examined in 348 Dutch children aged 7.7 to 11.7 years. They were born and living in three areas with different levels of sodium in the public drinking water. Sodium content of the water was either long-term low (1.3 mEq/1), long-term high (7.4 mEq/1), or short-term high (7.0 mEq/1 for only one year). Mean values of systolic and diastolic blood pressure were higher in the high sodium areas. After adjustment for dissimilarities in distributions of body weight and height, pulse rate, age, family history of hypertension and time of blood pressure measurement, these differences remained virtually the same, ranging from 1.8 to 4.0 mmHg.

In the second study, a randomized trial, the effect of dietary sodium on blood pressure was investigated in newborn infants, with 245 newborns assigned to a normal-sodium diet and 231 to a low-sodium diet during the first six months of life. The sodium intake of the normal-sodium group was almost three times that of the low-sodium group. After six months systolic pressure was 2.1 mmHg lower in the low-sodium group than in the normal-sodium group. The difference between the groups increased significantly during the first six months of life.

These observations support the hypothesis that sodium intake is casually related to the level of blood pressure. They also are consistent with the view that sodium intake from the drinking water early in life affects blood pressure.

INTRODUCTION

The view that high sodium intake is implicated in the etiology of high blood pressure has protagonists (Freis, 1976) and antagonists (Simpson, 1979). The debate between them is fueled by a lack of evidence concerning the relationship between sodium and blood pressure in humans. We investigated the relationship between sodium intake and blood pressure in two studies: a retrospective follow-up study of drinking water sodium and blood pressure (Hofman et al., 1980) and a randomized trial in newborn infants assigned to a normal-sodium or a low-sodium diet (Hofman et al., 1983).

STUDY 1: DRINKING WATER SODIUM AND BLOOD PRESSURE

Methods. Blood pressure was measured in 348 children, born and still living in three Dutch communities (see Figure 1).

Sodium content of the drinking water was either long-term low (1.3 mEq/1), long-term high (7.4 mEq/1), or short-term high (change from 1.0 to 7.0 mEq/1 because of the introduction of NaOH as an ion-exchanger to soften the water). The three areas are very similar according to demographic characteristics. All children born between 1968 and 1971 and attending the eight largest primary schools in the areas were asked to participate. The response rate was 98% and the age of the children varied from 7.7 to 11.7 years.

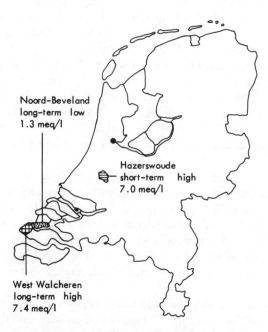

FIGURE 1. Three Dutch areas with different sodium levels in drinking water.

TABLE 1

Mean blood pressure (± SD) values in three areas with different sodium levels in the drinking water.

	Long-term Low	Short-term High	Long-term High
Systolic BP (mm Hg)	100.2 ± 12.3	103.4 ± 9.7	102.9 ± 10.9
Diastolic BO (mm Hg)	57.4 ± 8.6	59.3 ± 9.4	59.5 ± 7.8
Weight (kg)	33.5 ± 6.7	32.0 ± 6.4	32.1 ± 6.2
Height (cm)	143 ± 9	141 ± 10	141 ± 9
Age (years)	10.0 ± 1.2	9.6 ± 1.2	9.7 ± 1.2
No.	110	112	126

Blood pressure was measured with a random-zero sphygmomanometer as described previously (Hofman et al., 1980). The readings were made by one observer, who was not aware of the sodium content of the drinking water. All subjects were studied within a two-week period in September 1979. Weight, height, and pulse rate were recorded. Sodium intake was estimated by measuring 24-hour urinary sodium excretion. Only children exceeding an excretion of 0.16 mMol creatinine/24 hrs/kg body weight were taken into the analysis. A family history of hypertension was assessed by asking the parents whether they or the child's grandparents had ever received any anti-hypertensive medication.

Results. The observations in this study are summarized in Tables 1 and 2.

Average systolic and diastolic blood pressure was lower in the low-sodium area than in the high-sodium areas. The difference ranged from 1.8 to 4.0 mmHg, after adjustment for putative confounders. Mean values of 24-hour sodium excretion was somewhat larger in the low-sodium area than in the other areas; average sodium-creatinine ratios were not different.

STUDY 2: SODIUM INTAKE AND BLOOD PRESSURE IN NEWBORNS

Methods. The study subjects were 476 infants delivered at home or in an outpatient clinic, between January 15 and December 15, 1980, in Zoetermeer, The Netherlands. They were randomly assigned to a group receiving a normal-sodium diet (245) or a group with a low-sodium diet (231) starting immediately after birth. Neither the parents nor the investigators knew which group an infant was assigned to. All participants in the trial received formula milk and solid foods free of charge for six months. The sodium concentration of the low-sodium formula was similar to that of human milk, and it was three times lower than that of the normal-sodium milk (6.3 v 19.2 mMol/1). The sodium concentration of the solid foods ranged, depending on the kind of vegetable, from 2.2 to 13.9 mMol/1 in the low-sodium group and from 22.6 to 76.5 mMol/1 in the normal-sodium group. The sodium-potassium ratio was 0.67 for the low-

TABLE 2
**Differences between mean blood pressure values in mm Hg: long-term high
vs long-term low area, and short-term high vs long-term low areas**

	Long-term high minus long-term low	
	Observed	Adjusted†
Systolic BP	2.7*	3.3***
Diastolic BP	2.1**	1.8*
	Short-term high minus long-term low	
	Observed	Adjusted†
Systolic BP	3.2**	4.0***
Diastolic BP	1.9*	2.3**

†Adjusted for weight, height, pulse rate, family history of hypertension, time of blood pressure
measurement.
* < 0.10
** < 0.05
*** < 0.01 (two-sided t-test)

sodium formula and 0.64 for the normal-sodium milk. The average amount of
sodium (± SD) consumed during the first six months amounted to 0.89 ± 0.26
Mol of Na+ in the low-sodium group and 2.50 ± 0.95 Mol of Na+ in the
normal-sodium group.

We measured the blood pressure of each infant in weeks 1, 5, 9, 13, 17, 21 and
25. Four experienced study nurses, unaware of the diet-group of the babies,
measured systolic pressure. The measurements were performed with a Doppler
ultrasound device connected to a random-zero sphygmomanometer, as described in detail earlier (Hofman et al., 1983a). Weight and length at birth were
obtained from the midwives. The analyses were based on all subjects in whom
blood pressure readings were obtained i.e., infants who deviated from the
protocol were included. We computed the observed difference of mean systolic
pressure between the sodium groups at each occasion of measurement. These
differences were adjusted for slightly different distributions of length and weight
at birth, BP observers, and systolic pressure in the first week, using a model for
multiple linear regression with systolic BP as the outcome variable.

Results. Weight and length at birth, as well as parental blood pressure and
other measured characteristics of the parents, were distributed similarly in the
two groups. Mean values (± ISEM) of systolic blood pressure at various
occasions are given in Figure 2.

Systolic blood pressure increased with age in both groups, but less in the
low-sodium group than in the normal-sodium group. At 25 weeks, systolic
pressure was 2.0 mmHg lower in the low-sodium group (P = .03). The linear
trend of the difference between the groups over time was different from zero (P
= .04). The adjusted differences were slightly larger than the observed ones and
amounted to 2.1 mmHg at 25 weeks (P = .01). The adjusted differences also
increased significantly during first six months (P = .025).

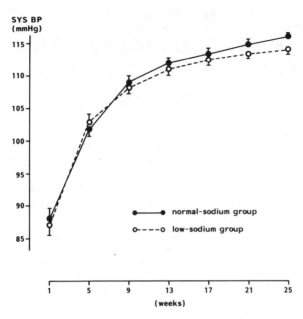

FIGURE 2. Systolic blood pressure in two sodium groups (mean ± 1SEM).

DISCUSSION

Our retrospective follow-up study on drinking water sodium and blood pressure gave evidence that was clearly in conflict with prior views. The observation of higher mean blood pressure in an area with high drinking water sodium was unexpected, as we had designed the study mainly to refute a previous investigation (Tuthill and Calabrese, 1979). Since our confirmative report conflicting findings have been published. Two reviews have been devoted to the subject, also differing in outlook (Willett, 1981; Folson and Prineas, 1982). We have suggested that a Bayesian approach to inference is quite suited to the matter at hand (Hofman, 1983b). If we specify as our hypothesis that high drinking water sodium causes an increase in systolic pressure of 3 - 4 mmHg and take a prior probability of this hypothesis of 0.01, we have calculated that the maximum posterior probability, given our findings, would be 0.10.

The evidence from our study in newborns suggests that sodium intake very early in life is causally related to the level of blood pressure. This may provide a clue to the unexpected finding of higher blood pressure in areas with high sodium concentrations in the drinking water. This observation may reflect the relatively large proportion of their sodium intake that bottle-fed newborns receive from the drinking water when living in a high-sodium area. Therefore, although there is room for scepticism, we conclude that our observations are consistent with the view that sodium intake from the drinking water early in life affects blood pressure.

ACKNOWLEDGEMENTS

These studies were supported by grants from the Netherlands Heart Foundation and the Netherlands Prevention Fund.

REFERENCES

FOLSOM, A.R. and PRINEAS, R.J. (1982) Drinking water consumption and blood pressure: a review of the epidemiology. Am J Epidemiol **115**:818–832.

FREIS, E.D. (1976). Salt, volume and the prevention of hypertension. Circulation **53**:589–595.

HOFMAN, A., VALKENBURG, H.A., and VAANDRAGER, G.J. (1980). Increased blood pressure in school children related to high sodium levels in drinking water. J Epidemiol Commun Health **34**:179–181.

HOFMAN, A., HAZEBROEK, A., and VALKENBURG, H.A. (1983a). A randomized trial of sodium intake and blood pressure in newborn infants. JAMA **250**:370–373.

HOFMAN, A. (1983b). Blood pressure in childhood. Epidemiological probes into the aetiology of high blood pressure. Thesis, Rotterdam, pp. 129–140.

SIMPSON, F.O. (1979). Salt and hypertension: a sceptical review of the evidence. Clin Sci **57** (Suppl 2):463–479.

TUTHILL, R.W., and CALABRESE, E.J. (1979). Elevated sodium levels in the public drinking water as a contributor to elevated blood pressure levels in the community. Arch Envir Health **34**:197–203.

WILLETT, W. (1981). Drinking water sodium and blood pressure: a cautious view of the "second look." Am J Public Health **71**:729–732.

CHAPTER VI

HIGH WATERBORNE SODIUM AND TEENAGE BLOOD PRESSURE

**William H. Hallenbeck, Gary R. Brenniman
and Robert J. Anderson**
*School of Public Health
University of Illinois at Chicago
Chicago, Illinois*

ABSTRACT

The blood pressures of high school juniors and seniors were taken in two communities, LaGrange and Westchester, Illinois. These two communities were well-matched socioeconomically. Drinking water was also similar in minerals which could be related to blood pressure except sodium: LaGrange averaged 405 mg sodium/l and Westchester averaged 4 mg sodium/l. The following covariates were taken into account: salty food intake, cigarette use, height, weight, water softening, and residence time. Of the 386 eligible students in LaGrange, 84% volunteered to have their blood pressures taken. In Westchester, 78% of the 401 eligible students volunteered. Results of the survey indicated that male and female systolic blood pressures in the high sodium community were not significantly higher than those in the low sodium community. Surprisingly, the observed systolic blood pressures of males in the low sodium community were higher than those in the high sodium community. However, the male and female diastolic blood pressures were significantly higher ($p = 0.040$ for males and $p = 0.016$ for females) in the high sodium community. The increases in diastolic blood pressures were approximately 2 mmHg for males and females.

INTRODUCTION

Cardiovascular disease is the leading cause of death in the United States and other industrialized nations, and hypertension is the most important predisposing factor. Several risk factors have been postulated to be associated with the development of primary hypertension: stress, obesity, age, sex, sodium and potassium intake, race or genetic predisposition, acculturation, and water mineralization. Sodium intake is considered to be among the most important of these risk factors (Kaplan, 1980; National Heart, Lung, and Blood, 1977; Page, 1976; Dahl, 1972; Weinsier, 1976). For a more detailed discussion of the relationship between sodium intake and hypertension, the reader is referred to Drinking Water and Health (NAS, 1977).

Sodium intake is usually substantially greater from food than from water. The proportion of waterborne sodium in the total diet is a function of the degree of municipal or home water softening, intake of tap water, and the sodium content of other liquids in the diet. Municipal or home water softening may add several hundred milligrams of sodium per day to the amount normally derived from food, about 4 g/day (Schroeder et al., 1974). Despite the small proportion of sodium in the diet that can be attributed to water intake, it has been reported in a recent study that the blood pressures of a group of high school sophomores exposed to a sodium concentration of 107 mg/liter in municipal drinking water were significantly higher than those of a control group exposed to 8 mg/liter (Tuthill et al., 1979). The present study was undertaken to determine if these results could be repeated in two Illinois communities, LaGrange and Westchester, which are served by drinking water with levels of sodium of 405 mg/liter and 4 mg/liter, respectively.

METHODS

Selection of Test and Control Communities. This survey was designed to compare the blood pressures of students in the third and fourth years of high school (juniors and seniors) from two communities in the Chicago metropolitan area that are separated by a distance of 4.8 km and have similar demographic and socioeconomic characteristics (Hallenbeck et al., 1981). The characteristics are similar to those of the communities studied by Tuthill et al. (1979).

Public drinking water in LaGrange has been softened since 1938 using the lime-soda ash, zeolite, and/or continuous ion exchange methods. These softening processes have caused the sodium concentrations to vary between 300 and 700 mg/liter with a mean concentration (averaged for the years 1972-1978) of 405 mg/liter (Illinois Environmental Protection Agency, 1980). This mean concentration was confirmed during the study period by atomic absorption analyses of water samples. In contrast to LaGrange's very hard ground water supply, Westchester's drinking water is supplied by Chicago (Lake Michigan source) which has a consistently low sodium concentration of about 4 mg/liter (Illinois Environmental Protection Agency, 1980). The only other important differences in mineral quality were high concentrations of chloride, sulfate, and total dissolved solids in LaGrange's treated drinking water (Illinois Environmental Protection Agency, 1980). These three factors have not been associated epidemiologically with mortality from cardiovascular disease (Schroeder et al., 1974).

Selection of Study Populations. Junior and senior students living in LaGrange attend Lyons Township High School, which is located in LaGrange. Junior and senior students living in Westchester attend Proviso West High

School which is located in Hillside. Westchester and Hillside are supplied by drinking water from Chicago.

For the purposes of this study, eligible students were defined as those white, male or female, juniors and seniors living in LaGrange and Westchester who did not consume bottled water or water from the tap that had been treated to remove sodium. Four Westchester students residing in homes with water softeners were excluded from the data analysis because they might be consuming water with elevated sodium. The 42 LaGrange students with home water softeners were not excluded from the data analysis because additional home softening would increase the level of sodium by about 70 mg/liter (Illinois Environmental Protection Agency, 1980). Finally, eligible siblings were randomly removed so that only one junior or senior would be represented per family. As a consequence, familial effects on the blood pressure data were removed. There were 386 eligible students in LaGrange and 401 eligible students in Westchester. Approximately 84 percent of the eligible students from LaGrange (n = 325) and 78 percent of the eligible students from Westchester (n = 313) volunteered.

Collection of Blood Pressure Data. Each student was given a short questionnaire designed to collect data on variables which might affect blood pressure: time of residence, height and weight, intake of salty food, smoking, home water softening, and use of bottled water (Brenniman et al., 1981). Due to budgetary constraints, comprehensive information was not obtained on such dietary habits as type and amount of fluid and solid food intake. However, a small group of 41 LaGrange and 39 Westchester students was evaluated for the intake of tap water and overnight urinary excretion of sodium.

After completing the questionnaire, the height, weight, and blood pressures of each student were taken by a nurse or trained volunteer. All blood pressures were taken with a mercury sphygmomanometer on the left arm of the seated student. The student's arm rested on a table and was at heart level with palm up. The student assumed a relaxed, comfortable position, sitting quietly with legs uncrossed. With the use of a stethoscope, blood pressures were recorded using the first and fifth Korotkoff sounds as the bases for the systolic and diastolic blood pressures, respectively. The rate of descent of the pressure was kept at the recommended 2-3 mmHg per second (National Center for Health Statistics, 1977). Each student had three consecutive blood pressures taken during a five-minute period. Students with blood pressures above normal ($>$ 140 mmHg systolic and/or $>$ 90 mmHg diastolic) were advised to consult their physicians. For data analysis purposes, the second and third blood pressure readings were averaged to obtain the representative value for each student. The first blood pressure was excluded from the data analysis because it is felt that the initial blood pressure is somewhat higher than subsequent readings (National Center for Health Statistics, 1977).

Blood pressure measurements were taken by a staff consisting of registered nurses from the LaGrange Visiting Nurses Association and trained volunteers from the Chicago Heart Association. The same personnel and mercury sphygmomanometers were utilized to carry out the screening in each school. Since each observer took a similar proportion of the readings, it seems reasonable that interobserver biases were minimized. The screening was carried out on January 8-10, 1980 in LaGrange and on February 5-7, 1980 in Westchester.

Urinalysis and Liquid Intake Study. The main purpose of this study was to determine if there was a difference in overall sodium intake from food and water between the test and control communities. Loss of sodium occurs almost exclusively via the urine, and the rate of salt ingestion is balanced by the rate of sodium excretion (Mountcastle, 1974). Hence, overnight urinary sodium excretion was used as a convenient index of overall dietary sodium intake. A secondary purpose was to determine the volume of tap water consumed per student to confirm that LaGrange students were actually exposed to the high sodium municipal water.

A random subsample of those participating in the blood pressure study could not be selected because of general student reluctance to provide urine samples. Hence, a volunteer subgroup of those participating in the blood pressure study was recruited. Therefore, the results of the urinalysis and liquid intake study must be considered preliminary in nature.

Students were asked to collect seven consecutive week-day overnight urine samples and complete a liquid intake diary for each of those seven days (Brenniman et al., 1981). Overnight urine samples were defined as all urine voided during the night and the first urine voided upon awakening in the morning. Five or more urine samples were obtained from 41 LaGrange and 39 Westchester students. Participants were instructed to complete the liquid intake diary by estimating the amount of tap water and tap water based fluids they consumed. Graduated drinking cups were provided. Urinary sodium ion concentrations were determined by flame emission spectrophotometry using an automated Perkin-Elmer 5000 Atomic Absorption Spectrophotometer (Perkin Elmer Corporation, 1976). This instrument was equipped with an automatic sample carousel and computerized data acquisition and processing systems. These features helped to minimize potential observer bias even though urine samples for each community were analyzed in separate groups.

Statistical Analysis. Comparison of the systolic and diastolic blood pressures from the two study groups was done by analysis of covariance using the general linear model procedure of the Statistical Analysis System (Helwig et al., 1979), with separate analyses for males and females. The number of juniors and seniors in each community-sex group was approximately equal. Analysis of covariance allows comparison of group means after adjustment for possible confounding variables. The covariates considered in the present analysis were the salty food index, daily cigarette use, Quetelet index (Laskarzewsi et al., 1980), and months of residence in the community. Intercommunity comparisons of these covariates are presented elsewhere (Hallenbeck et al., 1981). Adjustment was not necessary for the demographic and socioeconomic covariates because of the similarity in these variables between the two communities studied. Only those with complete covariate and blood pressure data were included in this analysis (309 and 303 students from LaGrange and Westchester, respectively).

The salty food index was derived from a questionnaire which elicited information concerning the frequency of consumption of specific food items which can be generally categorized as follows: bacon, other smoked meat, canned foods, canned fish, canned vegetables, hard cheeses, cottage cheese, fruit-flavor geletins, salted nuts, snack crackers, snack foods, pickles, peanut butter, and french fries (Brenniman et al., 1981). The purpose of computing the food index was to detemine if there was a difference between the two communities regarding intake of salty foods.

Daily cigarette use was coded as zero if the individual did not smoke, 1 if less than one-half pack per day was smoked, 2 if one-half to one pack per day was smoked, and 3 if more than one pack a day was smoked.

The Quetelet index calculated as $(weight/height^2) \times 100$ was utilized to describe the obesity of the subjects. Weight was measured in kilograms and height in centimeters.

Elevated blood pressure may be a function of the concentration of sodium in drinking water and the duration of exposure. Therefore residence in months was considered as a possible confounding variable.

The overnight urinary sodium excretion and water intake data were analyzed using a weighted two-way analysis of variance with sex and community as the two factors. Only those individuals who submitted at least five urine samples were included in the statistical analysis of overnight urinary sodium levels. Participants were required to provide at least three days of water intake diaries to be included in the analysis of water consumption. Individual mean urinary sodium and water intake were weighted by the inverse of their respective variances.

RESULTS

Blood Pressure Survey. There were 309 students (172 males and 137 females) from LaGrange and 303 students (142 males and 161 females) from Westchester whose blood pressures were used in data analysis. The mean average systolic and diastolic blood pressures for LaGrange and Westchester males and females are listed in Table 1. These results indicated that male and female systolic blood pressures in the high sodium community were not significantly higher than those in the low sodium community. If a two tailed test were used, the systolic blood pressures of the males in the low sodium community would have been significantly higher than those of the high sodium community. However, the central hypothesis of this study was to determine if exposure to high levels of sodium in municipal drinking water was associated with elevated blood pressure. In contrast, the male and female diastolic blood pressures were significantly higher ($p = 0.040$ for males and $p = 0.016$ for females) in the high sodium community. The significant differences in the unadjusted data were a 1.8 mmHg elevation in mean average diastolic blood pressure among males and a 1.9 mmHg elevation in mean elevation in mean average diastolic blood pressure among females in the high sodium community.

The analysis of covariance of the average systolic and diastolic blood pressures was initially computed utilizing all four covariates: daily cigarette use,

TABLE 1

Mean average systolic and diastolic blood pressures (mmHg)* in the Illinois study

	LaGrange (high sodium drinking water) Mean (SEM)‡		Westchester (low sodium drinking water) Mean (SEM)		Difference between means (p-value)‖	
	Unadjusted	Adjusted§	Unadjusted	Adjusted	Unadjusted	Adjusted
Males	(n = 172)†		(n = 142)†			
Systolic	115.59 (0.79)	115.37 (0.72)	118.81 (0.78)	119.08 (0.80)	-3.22 (0.998)	-3.71 (0.999)
Diastolic	70.11 (0.65)	70.01 (0.69)	68.29 (0.82)	68.41 (0.76)	1.82 (0.040)	1.60 (0.061)
Females	(n = 137)†		(n = 161)†			
Systolic	106.89 (0.74)	106.77 (0.77)	105.65 (0.76)	105.75 (0.71)	1.24 (0.123)	1.02 (0.164)
Diastolic	67.96 (0.61)	68.00 (0.66)	66.02 (0.65)	65.98 (0.61)	1.94 (0.016)	2.02 (0.013)

* Average systolic and diastolic blood pressures were calculated for each student by averaging the second and third blood pressure measurements. The mean average systolic and diastolic blood pressures were calculated by averaging the average blood pressures for each community-sex category.

† Sample size.

‡ Standard errors of the means (SEM) are shown in parentheses.

§ The means were adjusted for one or both of the covariates, cigarettes and Quetelet index, using the models described in the text.

‖ p-values shown in parentheses are those for a one-tailed t-test of the hypothesis: blood pressures in LaGrange are greater than those in Westchester.

54

Quetelet index, months of residence in the community, and salty food index. Standard backward elimination procedures were employed to develop simplified models with only the most important covariates being included in the model (Hallenbeck et al., 1981).

Although the salty food and residence indices were considered as potential covariates in this study, they were found to be not statistically important for explaining the variability of blood pressure in the two communities. The results of the one-way analysis of covariance, which adjusted for Quetelet index and daily cigarette use as given in the models above, are tabulated in Table 1. In comparing the difference between the adjusted means and the unadjusted means in Table 1, it is noted that adjustments had little effect on the mean average blood pressures.

Urinalysis and Liquid Intake Study. The mean overnight urinary sodium excretions for males and females from the high sodium community were not significantly different ($p > 0.05$) when compared to those from the low sodium community (Table 2) (Baukus, 1980). Adjustment for the amount of water ingested did not alter the findings. In addition, the mean water intake values for males and females were not significantly different ($p > 0.05$) in the two communities studied (Table 2) (Baukus, 1980).

DISCUSSION

The results of our Illinois study did not completely corroborate the findings of the Massachusetts study (Tuthill et al., 1979). The main findings of the Massachusetts study were increases of 2.7-5.1 mmHg in the systolic and diastolic blood pressures of both sexes in the high when compared to the low sodium communtiy. In contrast, elevated male and female systolic blood pressures were not observed in the high sodium community of the Illinois study. However, the diastolic blood pressures were elevated approximately 2 mmHg for both males and females in the high sodium community. These elevations were not as large as those observed in the Massachusetts study.

Although the limited demographic and socioeconomic data presented in the Massachusetts study were similar to that of the present study, there were several differences in study design. First, it was reported in the Massachusetts study that systolic and diastolic blood pressure data were based on an average of three readings per individual that were taken by three different nurses. The blood pressure data in the present study were reported as an average of the second and third readings taken by the same nurse. The first blood pressure readings were excluded from the data analysis because other studies have indicated that the initial blood pressure reading is somewhat higher than subsequent readings (National Center for Health Statistics, 1977). Second, height and weight values were self-reported in the Massachusetts study, whereas these values were measured in the Illinois study.

Although a comprehensive assessment of the relationship of diet to blood pressure was not taken in either study, the overall dietary sodium intake (food and water) was assessed in the Illinois study by measuring overnight urinary

TABLE 2

Mean overnight urinary sodium excretion (mg) and mean daily tap water intake (ml) (17) in the Illinois study*

| | LaGrange (high sodium drinking water) | | | | Westchester (low sodium drinking water) | | | | p-value (sodium excretion)§ | p-value (water intake)‖ |
| | Sodium (mg) | | Water (ml) | | Sodium (mg) | | Water (ml) | | | |
	n†	Mean (SEM)‡	n	Mean (SEM)	n	Mean (SEM)	n	Mean (SEM)		
Males	21	586 (76)	19	552 (62)	23	722 (73)	22	428 (52)	0.925	0.132
Females	20	748 (68)	19	327 (39)	16	748 (62)	16	277 (53)	0.500	0.472

* Only those individuals who submitted five or more overnight urine samples were included in the sodium excretion analysis. Only those individuals who submitted three or more days of water intake diaries were included in the water intake analysis. Individual mean overnight urinary sodium excretion and water intake values were weighted by the inverse of their respective variances. Overnight urine samples were defined as all urine voided during the night and the first urine voided upon awakening in the morning.

† Sample size.

‡ The standard errors of the means (SEM) are shown in parentheses.

§ Based on a one-tailed t-test of the hypothesis: overnight urinary sodium excretion in LaGrange is greater than that in Westchester.

‖ Based on a two-tailed t-test of the hypothesis: daily tap water intake in LaGrange is equal to that in Westchester.

sodium excretion, whereas a questionnaire was used in the Massachusetts study. It can be seen in Table 2 that no significant difference in overnight urinary sodium excretion was found between the two groups of students. This implies that there probably was no difference in overall dietary sodium intake between the communities.

There are two final differences between the two studies: 1) socioeconomic data were obtained by use of a questionnaire in the Massachusetts study, whereas these data were obtained indirectly (Hallenbeck et al., 1981) in the Illinois study; 2) 18 covariates were used to adjust blood pressure data in the Massachusetts study, whereas only four covariates were used in the Illinois study. As mentioned previously, in the Illinois study only those covariates were used which were found to be important in explaining the variability of blood pressure. Adjustments for covariates did not change the strength or direction of the findings appreciably in either study.

ACKNOWLEDGEMENTS

Support for this research was provided by the University of Illinois Water Resources Center (Glenn E. Stout, Director) under a grant from the U.S. Department of the Interior's Office of Water Research and Technology. The following organizations and people made important contributions to this study: University of Illinois at the Medical Center, School of Public Health—Alvida Baukus, Marilyn Farber, Marsha Gold, James Melius, Scott Meyer, Alan Cohen and Willa Taylor; Lyons Township High School, LaGrange, Illinois— Arthur Rawers, Josephine Mancuso and Betty Fenstemaker; Proviso West High School, Hillside, Illinois—A. E. Vallicelli, Shirley Jayne, Bernie Skul, Myrtle Gould and Mary Vaccaro; Visiting Nurses Association of LaGrange— Dennis Minnice, Sharon McVickers, Donna Nighswander and Beatrice Nelligan; Chicago Heart Association—Barbara Gale; University of Illinois at Chicago Circle Computer Center—Patricia Harrison; Illinois Environmental Protection Agency—Dorothy Bennett.

REFERENCES

BAUKUS, A.T. (1980). Urinary sodium excretion levels in two communities with different municipal water supplies. Chicago: University of Illinois Medical Center School of Public Health.

BRENNIMAN, G.R., HALLENBECK, W.H., ANDERSON, R.A., and BAUKUS, A.T. (1981). The relationship between high sodium levels in municipally softened drinking water and elevated blood pressures. Urbana: Water Resources Center, University of Illinois.

DAHL, L.K. (1971). Salt and hypertension. Am. J. Clin. Nutr. 25:231–244.

HALLENBECK, W.H., BRENNIMAN, G.R., and ANDERSON, R.J. (1981). High sodium in drinking water and its effect on blood pressure. Am. J. Epid. 114:817–826.

HELWIG, J.T. and COUNCIL, K.A., eds. (1979). SAS users guide, Raleigh: SAS Institute.

ILLINOIS ENVIRONMENTAL PROTECTION AGENCY. (1980). Division of Water Supplies. Springfield.

KAPLAN, N.M. (1980). The control of hypertension: a therapeutic breakthrough. Am. Sci. **68**:537–545.

LASKARZEWSKI, P., MORRISON, S.A., MELLIES, M.J., KELLY, K., GARTSIDE, P.S., KHOURY, P., and GLUECK, C.J. (1980). Relationships of measurements of body mass to plasma lipoproteins in school children and adults. Am. J. Epid. **111**:395–406.

MOUNTCASTLE, V.B., ed. (1974). Medical Physiology. Vol. 2, 13th ed. St. Louis: C.V. Mosby.

NATIONAL ACADEMY OF SCIENCE. (1977). Drinking Water and Health. Washington, D.C.

NATIONAL CENTER FOR HEALTH STATISTICS. (1977). Blood pressure levels of persons 6-74 years, U.S. 1971–74. Hyattsville, MD: National Center for Health Statistics. (Vital and Health Statistics, Series 11: Data from the National Health Survey, no. 203) (DHEW publication (HRA) 78-1648).

NATIONAL HEART, LUNG, AND BLOOD INSTITUTE'S TASK FORCE ON BLOOD PRESSURE CONTROL IN CHILDREN. (1977). Report of the task force on blood pressure control in children. Pediatrics (supplement, part 2) **59**:797–820.

PAGE, L.B. (1976). Epidemiologic evidence on the etiology of human hypertension and its prevention. Am. Heart J. **91**:527–534.

PERKIN-ELMER CORPORATION. (1976). Analytical methods for atomic absorption spectrophotometry. Norwalk, CT.

SCHROEDER, H.A. and KRAEMER, L.A. (1974). Cardiovascular mortality, municipal water, and corrosion. Arch. Environ. Health. **28**:303–311.

TUTHILL, R.W. and CALABRESE, E.J. (1979). Elevated sodium levels in the public drinking water as a contributor to elevated blood pressure levels in the community. Arch. Environ. Health. **34**:197–203.

WEINSIER, R.L. (1976). Salt and the development of essential hypertension. Prev. Med. **5**:7–14.

CHAPTER VII

SOFTENED WATER USAGE AND BLOOD PRESSURE

Paul R. Pomrehn
Department of Preventive Medicine and Environmental Health,
College of Medicine, University of Iowa,
Iowa City, Iowa

ABSTRACT

In a survey of 2152 school children, we collected data on medical history, source of drinking water and demographic information and measured blood pressure, heart rate, height, weight and skinfold thickness. Over 40% of children surveyed came from homes with water softeners. In homes where samples were taken, water softeners added approximately 140 mg/liter of sodium and lowered calcium carbonate 270 mg/liter. Softened water was being used for cooking or drinking in 70% of homes that had water softeners. Those children consuming softened water at home did not have higher mean blood pressure than children who were not consuming softened water.

In a subsample of 218 children and their parents, we collected additional dietary and fluid consumption data and repeated blood pressure measurements in the home. Adult men and women who consumed softened water had mean blood pressures which were equivalent to mean blood pressures of those not having water softeners. Children's blood pressures were 2.0 mm of Hg and 2.5 mm of Hg higher for systolic and diastolic in the group consuming softened water. These differences were not significant after adjustment for covariates.

The meaning of associations between drinking water hardness and cardiovascular disease mortality has been controversial (Heyden, 1976). Studies in progress may elucidate the nature of the association (Pocock et al., 1980). If future work substantiates a causal relationship between some constituent of drinking water and cardiovascular disease, hypertension will likely be considered an intermediate in the association.

Literature relating blood pressure to various drinking water constitutents has recently been reviewed (Folsom et al., 1982). High sodium (DHEW, 1979) and low calcium (McCarron et al., 1982) intake have been implicated as factors in the development of high blood pressure. Drinking water is a source of both of these minerals, although the contribution to total dietary intake is quite small (Folsom et al., 1982).

Home water softeners increase the concentration of sodium while decreasing the calcium content of drinking water. The high prevalence of home softener usage in communities where our blood pressure survey was conducted (Pomrehn et al., 1983) allowed us to compare blood pressure levels of groups of children and a subset of parents according to their consumption of softened water.

METHODS

Study Design. This cross-sectional study was designed to detect associations between drinking water mineral content and blood pressure levels in children and their parents. Our investigation was conducted in two parts: an initial school survey of 2152 children in eight communities followed by a more detailed study of 218 children and their parents in four communities. Data collection was completed in the summer of 1981.

Community selection. Eight Iowa communities, population 2,000-7,000, were selected for inclusion on the basis of drinking water mineral content. All eight communities use ground water from wells which are deeper than 150 feet. These communities have used the same source of water for over a decade.

Municipal water softening is practiced in two of these communities. One (Rockwell City) softens using zeolite ion exchange, a process which substantially increases sodium level while decreasing hardness. Another (Sac City) softens with lime (calcium carbonate) precipitation, which lowers hardness but only slightly increases sodium levels. None of the other communities uses any treatment process which alters the sodium and hardness levels found in untreated water. Records maintained by the University of Iowa Hygienic Laboratory indicate that the mineral content of the drinking water from these communities has not varied significantly over time.

Water samples were taken in each community at the time the school survey was conducted. Samples from the drinking fountains at the schools were analyzed using the standard procedures recommended by the Environmental Protection Agency (APHA, 1975). The results of these analyses are displayed in Table 1.

School Survey. Elementary school children in grades 3-5 were chosen to participate in the school survey. In the four smaller school districts, we included second grade children to increase the sample of children from those communities. The entire sample of over 2000 children in eight communities was selected anticipating that 30 percent of the children would be from rural homes with private wells and one-third of homes would have water softeners. This sample size would provide the statistical power to detect a 4 mm of Hg difference between groups with over ninety-five percent probability.

The children took consent forms and questionnaires home to be completed by their parents. The questionnaires asked for demographic information about the children and their families, occupational and educational level of parents,

TABLE 1
Water Mineral Content of the Eight Iowa Communities Surveyed

	Mineral Content (mg/liter)				
	Sodium	Potassium	Calcium	Magnesium	Total Hardness
Community					
Anamosa	78	13	65	33	298
Lake City	44	5	140	44	536
Manchester	5	1	71	19	158
Manson	340	2	17	1	49
Mt. Pleasant	250	22	103	42	433
Rockwell City[1]	390	25	41	18	178
Sac City[2]	24	5	21	9	91
Washington	217	20	100	49	456

[1]softening of municipal water is by zeolite ion exchange
[2]softening of municipal water is by lime precipitation

family histories of high blood pressure and medical histories of participating children. Questions were also asked about the household's source of water, the presence of a home water softener, usage of softened water for cooking or drinking and length of time the family had resided in the community.

Prior to commencing the study, the survey team completed an 80-hour training course with particular emphasis on proper technique of blood pressure measurement. Techniques were demonstrated and practiced using tape-timer simulation. These demonstrations were followed with several days of practicing on adults and children. Team members were tested using written materials on blood pressure measurement technique (Prineas, 1977). Validation of observer measurements was made before the survey, and a pilot study was conducted using a class of 23 second-grade students.

In the morning on survey days, children with signed consent forms had height, weight and skinfold measured in class. Small groups of children were taken to a quiet room where their blood pressure was measured twice using random-zero sphygmomanometers. Systolic and diastolic fourth and fifth phase pressures were recorded. Heart rate was counted between blood pressure measurements by palpating the brachial artery. Two additional blood pressure measurements and a heart rate determination were made in the same manner during the afternoon of the same day. All children were sitting quietly for five minutes prior to measurement of blood pressure. Schedules were planned to insure children had not eaten within an hour nor exercised within one-half hour of the time of measurement.

The study protocol allowed measurement of approximately 50 children per day. The school survey was conducted during a ten-week period in the fall of 1980.

Family Study. A subsample of children from the school survey was selected and these children and their parents were asked to participate in a more detailed investigation. The Family Study was designed to compare blood pressures of adults and children with different patterns of consumption of softened water. We chose to include only four communities: Washington, Mt. Pleasant, Anamosa, and Manchester.

From a listing of children whose homes were serviced by the municipal water system, we created a randomly ordered listing of children by home-softener usage as determined by the school survey questionnaire. We solicited participation of equal numbers of families with and without softeners from each of the four communities.

The participants in the family study were asked to complete a questionnaire which included family medical history, medication usage, and a dietary history of high sodium foods and fluid intake. A series of questions on source of drinking water were also included. The parents and index child each had height, weight, skinfold, heart rate and two blood pressures measured in their home. Measurements were made by two members of the school survey team.

We collected drinking water samples from the homes of a subsample of families. Water samples were analyzed for content of sodium, potassium, magnesium, calcium, and total hardness. Those homes with water softeners had paired samples taken, one from a tap with treated water and a second from a tap which bypassed the softener. Softened water contained 141 mg/liter more sodium and 6.8 mg/liter, 66.4 mg/liter, 27.0 mg/liter, and 270 mg/liter less potassium, calcium, magnesium and calcium carbonate respectively than the unsoftened bypass samples. How water analysis results varied by commuity and the presence of a water softener is illustrated in Table 2.

Pattern of Water Usage. From the question "Do you receive water from the municipal water system?" we determined that 62% (1,337) of children participating in the school survey came from homes receiving water from the municipal supply. This remainder of children (813) were from homes (mostly farms) with private wells.

From the question "Do you have a water softener in your home?" we determined that 41% (880) of children's homes had water softeners in them. Fifty-three percent of children from homes with private water sources had softeners in the home. Only 33% of children from homes with municipal sources had softeners in the home. The difference between the prevalence of water softeners in homes on municipal supplies and those on private supplies was due to the small number of children (17/500) in Manson, Rockwell City, and Sac City with softeners in their home. These towns have soft water.

When asked "Do you use softened water for cooking or drinking purposes?", 71% of families with softeners reported that they used softened water for these purposes.

Analytic and Statistical Methods. In the school screen four random zero blood pressures were obtained on each child: two in the morning and two in the afternoon. All analyses reported in this paper are for the average of the four blood pressures. Separate analyses were performed on the average of the two morning blood pressures and the average of the two afternoon blood pressures. The results for these agreed with those based on the average of the four so they are not reported.

TABLE 2
Mineral Content of Home Water Samples
by Community and Softener Usage - Family Survey

	Washington		Manchester		Anamosa		Mt. Pleasant	
	x*	c.v.**	x	c.v.	x	c.v.	x	c.v.
No Softener (n)	7		10		8		8	
Sodium	207.0	5	7.2	27	73.8	6	238.0	9
Potassium	20.9	5	3.2	58	14.8	5	23.4	8
Calcium	100.0	6	68.9	8	64.3	12	103.0	9
Magnesium	43.7	3	22.2	7	38.6	45	41.5	9
Total Hardness	435.0	3	265.0	7	278.0	19	428.0	8
Softened (n)	13		11		15		9	
Sodium	394.0	19	127.0	24	188.0	27	434.0	16
Potassium	9.4	64	.2	124	7.9	60	10.6	74
Calcium	19.5	175	6.4	156	13.4	157	13.0	155
Magnesium	7.9	186	2.2	171	6.3	176	7.9	216
Total Hardness	82.0	178	39.0	209	60.0	162	65.0	187
Bypass (unsoftened)	4		10		8		5	
Sodium	205.0	3	12.1	104	70.3	4	242.0	6
Potassium	20.3	2	3.0	89	14.3	4	23.8	2
Calcium	102.5	5	64.2	18	62.1	8	106.0	8
Magnesium	43.3	3	21.0	14	33.0	5	42.2	6
Total Hardness	432.0	3	247.0	17	292.0	4	440.0	5

* x = mean in milligram per liter
** c.v. = coefficient of variation = standard deviation/mean x 100

In the family study two random zero blood pressures were obtained on each participant: mother, father and child. Analyses were based on the average of these duplicate readings.

In order to assure that any observed differences in blood pressure means between groups were not due to differences in age, sex, body size variables or family history of hypertension, it was necessary to adjust for these concomitants. The list of possible confounding variables included the following variables: age, sex, height, weight, heart rate, Quetelet Index (weight/height^2), triceps skinfold, education of parents, socioeconomic status, family history of hypertension, observer, and room temperature. Stepwise regression was used to develop regression equations which would relate systolic and fourth phase diastolic blood pressures to these covariates. For both systolic and diastolic blood pressures the best-fitting models included weight, heart rate, family history of hypertension in the parents, and sex. No other variables contributed significantly to variability explained once these variables were in the model.

Similar equations were developed for men and women for the family study data. For adults, Quetelet Index, heart rate and family history of hypertension were the variables that were significant at the 5 percent level. These covariables were used to adjust the parent means.

The SAS statistical package (SAS, 1979) was used in the analyses. The procedure GLM was used to compare means. Unadjusted means were compared using one-way analysis of variance and analysis of covariance was used to compare adjusted means. The adjusted means are the least-squares means provided by GLM. These means are the usual adjusted means from analysis of covariance. Only those variables found to be significant in the stepwise regressions were used in the adjustment.

The school survey data allow us to compare blood pressures of groups of children with variable levels of softened water consumption. We categorized children into: 1) those from homes without home water softeners, 2) those from homes with home water softeners where softened water is not used for cooking or drinking, and 3) those from homes with home water softeners where softened water is used for cooking or drinking. The mean blood pressures of children so categorized can be compared as an indication of the effect of softened water consumption on blood pressure.

Lake City, Manson, Rockwell City, and Sac City are clustered in a two county area in northwestern Iowa. Lake City has a deep well with hard water and low sodium (Table 1). Manson has a deep well with high sodium and relatively low hardness. Rockwell City employs zeolite ion exchange to soften water to resultant high sodium and moderate hardness. Sac City softens using lime precipitation which results in low sodium and moderate hardness. Because of the diversity of drinking water quality in these otherwise similar communities, we compared blood pressures of children living in these towns if they reported receiving municipal water. In Lake City, those children with water softeners in their homes were eliminated from consideration in the comparison of these four communities.

Using the same groupings of softened water consumption, we categorized Family Study participants according to their pattern of softened water consumption. In a separate analysis for men, women, and children, we compared blood pressure means of these three groups.

RESULTS

Home Water Softener Usage and Blood Pressure - School Survey. We classified children into three categories of potential exposure to softened water: no softener in home, softener in home but softened water reportedly *not* used for cooking or drinking, and softener in home with softened water reported to be used for cooking or drinking. For all study participants, there was no difference in the blood pressures of these three groups (Table 3). Adjustment for covariates previously described does not alter these findings.

The number of homes having water softeners is quite low in three communities with soft water (Sac City, Rockwell City and Manson). Using the same softened water usage categories, we analyzed data from children in the other five communities. We also excluded data from children whose homes are supplied by non-municipal water sources. No significant relationship was found between softener usage in these communities individually or in the aggregate. Only in

TABLE 3
Mean Blood Pressure of Children by Water Softener Usage

	n	Systolic	Diastolic
No softener in home	1277	98.9	62.6
Softener in home not used for cooking or drinking	259	98.9	63.7
Softener in home used for cooking or drinking	602	99.0	62.5

Manchester was there a suggestion that blood pressure levels were increased in those consuming softened water (Table 4).

A similar analysis was done on data for children living in rural homes with private wells (Table 5). Mean blood pressures in these children do not suggest that exposure to softened water is associated with increased blood pressure. Adjustment for covariates previously discussed does not alter these results.

Community Softening and Blood Pressure. Another approach to investigating the influence of water softening on blood pressure is to compare communities with varying softening processes. Rockwell City softens its drinking water at the wellhead using ion exchange similar to the process of home softeners. Sac

TABLE 4
Blood Pressure Means of Children* in Five Communities by Softened Wate Usage

		n	Systolic	Diastolic
WASHINGTON	No softener	119	98.6	64.0
	S⁺, no C or D	28	98.4	65.1
	S⁺, C or D	102	97.2	63.0
MANCHESTER	No softener	126	.99.7	64.2
	S⁺, no C or D	26	96.9	63.9
	S⁺, C or D	35	101.0	64.9
LAKE CITY	No softener	40	97.9	60.8
	S⁺, no C or D	23	97.8	63.8
	S⁺, C or D	32	98.6	61.9
ANAMOSA	No softener	75	100.2	61.5
	S⁺, no C or D	20	96.8	61.9
	S⁺, C or D	43	99.6	60.8
MT. PLEASANT	No softener	156	99.4	62.2
	S⁺, no C or D	16	96.4	61.0
	S⁺, C or D	77	97.1	60.0
All 5 Towns combined	No softener	516	99.3	62.9
	S⁺, no C or D	113	97.4	63.4
	S⁺, C or D	289	98.2	62.0

S^+= softener in home
C or D = cooking or drinking soft water
*Limited to children from homes on municipal distribution system

TABLE 5
Relationship of Softener Usage to Blood Pressure in Rural Children*

	n	Systolic	Diastolic
No softener in home	379	99.2	63.2
Softener in home not used for cooking or drinking	137	100.2	64.4
Softener in home used for cooking or drinking	286	99.6	62.9

*homes with private water supplies

City softens with lime, a process that adds little if any sodium in the process. Manson has naturally soft water from a deep well. Table 6 compares the blood pressure of children from these towns who live in homes on municipal water systems. Included also are the means of children from Lake City, who live in town in homes without home softeners. Children from the high sodium communities with the highest sodium levels in the water have slightly higher blood pressure means than children from Lake City (unsoftened) and Sac City. This difference is significant only for diastolic pressure. Adjustment for weight, sex, family history, and heart rates does not change the results.

Home Water Softener Usage and Blood Pressure - Family Survey. With softener usage categories described previously, we evaluated the association between consumption of softened water and blood pressure. Water softener usage was not associated with increased mean blood pressures in men, women or children (Table 7) except for diastolic pressure in children. Children from homes with softeners where softened water was used for cooking or drinking had blood pressure 2.5 ml higher than children from homes without water softeners ($p < .05$). After adjustment for covariates age, sex, and weight the difference was not statistically significant.

We collected overnight urines from a 50% sample of Family Survey participants to measure sodium excretion. The estimated 24 hour sodium excretion presented in Table 8 showed no consistent relationship between softened water consumption and sodium excretion. Adjustment for weight does not alter these small and statistically insignificant differences. Softener usage was not related to consumption of high sodium foods in men, women, or children.

TABLE 6
Comparison of Blood Pressure of Children from Communities With Various Sources of Softened Water

	Softening Method	n	Systolic	Diastolic
Rockwell City	Zeolite	148	98.6	61.7
Sac City	Lime	201	97.1	60.3*
Manson	Natural	151	98.3	62.6
Lake City	None	40	97.9	60.8

*Different from Manson, $p < .05$ after adjusting for multiple comparisons

TABLE 7
Comparison of Blood Pressure by Water Softener Usage Group Family Survey

	n	Systolic	Diastolic
Fathers			
No softener in home	100	122.7	75.2
Softener not used for cooking and drinking	34	121.2	74.7
Softener used for cooking and drinking	67	123.2	75.9
Mothers			
No softener in home	101	111.0	69.8
Softener not used for cooking and drinking	35	111.7	68.3
Softener used for cooking and drinking	68	110.9	69.4
Children			
No softener in home	105	101.4	62.4
Softener not used for cooking and drinking	37	100.4	63.0
Softener used for cooking and drinking	76	103.4	64.9*

* $p < .05$

DISCUSSION

The survey results described here do not lend any consistent support to the hypothesis that the consumption of softened water leads to relative increases in blood pressure levels in children or adults. We concur with Armstrong et al. (1982) and Folsom et al. (1982) who have argued that the contribution of drinking water to total daily mineral intake is very small and, consequently, the lack of an association would be expected. Our sodium excretion data and fluid intake history indicate consumption of softened water contributes very little to total sodium consumption.

The communities surveyed by us all had deep wells and some towns use very hard water by national standards. Home water softeners are used in these communities to prevent excessive corrosion of pipes. Home softeners are

TABLE 8
Urinary Sodium Excretion by Usage of Softened Water Family Survey

	No Softener	Softener Present	
		Consumed	Not consumed
Fathers	50	29	20
Mg/24 hrs.	3730	3599	3412
Mg/Kg/24 hrs.	44.4	41.3	31.7
Mothers	53	32	17
Mg/24 hrs.	2160	2192	2509
Mg/Kg/24 hrs.	31.6	34.9	40.9
Children	53	32	23
Mg/24 hrs.	1731	1712	1990
Mg/Kg/24 hrs.	46.4	45.3	55.6

effective in removing calcium and other cations which are replaced by sodium. The amount of sodium added varies directly with the amount of hardness removed. Consequently the water sodium and calcium content in the water from those homes with water softeners differs substantially from levels in water from homes without softeners in the communities we surveyed. Given the size of this difference in mineral concentration and the statistical power we had to detect a small difference in blood pressure, we could have expected to find a relationship if it existed in our study population.

Aside from the suggestion that the children from homes using softened water in the Family Survey had slightly elevated blood pressure, we found no evidence that home softeners increased blood pressure. Even these small differences were statistically nonsignificant after adjustment for covariates. Regardless of the absence of a consistent association and given the plausibility of the dietary sodium and blood pressure relationship, it seems prudent to recommend that drinking water sodium levels be kept down. One way to accomplish this is to recommend that kitchen taps that bypass home softeners be installed in homes with softeners.

ACKNOWLEDGEMENT

This study was supported by the U.S.E.P.A. Grant R807217-01.

REFERENCES

AMERICAN PUBLIC HEALTH ASSOCIATION. Standard methods for the examination of water and wastewater. 14th edition, APHA, 1975.

ARMSTRONG, B.K., MASGETTS, B.M., MC CALL, M.G., BINNS, C.W., CAMPBELL, N.A. and MASAREI, J.R.L. (1982). Water sodium and blood pressure in rural children. Archives of Environmental Health 37:236–245.

DHEW. (1979). Report of the Hypertension Task Force. NIH Publication No. 79-1630, Volume 8.

FOLSOM, A.R. and PRINEAS, R.J. (1982). Drinking water composition and blood pressure. A review of the epidemiology. Am J Epidemiol 115:818–831.

HEYDEN, S. (1976). The hard facts behind the hard-water theory and ischemic heart disease. J Chron Dis. 29:149–157.

MC CARRON, D.A., MORRIS, C.D., and COLE, C. (1982). Dietary calcium in human hypertension. Science 217:267–269.

POCOCK, S.J., SHAPER, A.G., COOK, D.G., PACKHAM, R.F., LACEY R.F., POWELL, P.P. and RUSSELL, P.F. (1980). British Regional Heart Study: geographic variations in cardiovascular mortality, and the role of water quality. British Med J. 1243–1249.

POMREHN, P.F., CLARKE, W.R., SOWERS, M.F., WALLACE, R.B., and LAUER, R.M. (1983). Community differences in blood pressure levels and drinking water sodium. Am J Epidemiol 118:60–71.

PRINEAS, R.J. Blood Pressure Sounds: Their Measurement and Meaning. Gamma Medical Products Corporation, 1977.

SAS INSTITUTE. SAS Users' Guide. 1979 edition, SAS Institute, Inc.

CHAPTER VIII

WATER SODIUM, BLOOD PRESSURE AND CARDIOVASCULAR MORTALITY IN WESTERN AUSTRALIA

Barrie M. Margetts and Bruce K. Armstrong

NH & MRC Research Unit in Epidemiology and Preventive Medicine, Department of Medicine, University of Western Australia, Nedlands, Western Australia

ABSTRACT

Blood pressures were measured in 326 boys and 309 girls, aged 12 to 14 years, who attended schools in two towns from each of three levels of water sodium (1.8, 4.8, 9.3 mmol/1). Differences between mean blood pressure levels in children living in the three groups of towns did not appear to result from differences in water sodium levels. Differences in the towns' water sodium levels were reflected in the relative contribution made by water to the total sodium intake (2%, 5%, 8%). There was good agreement between estimated total sodium intake and urinary sodium excretion. No effect of water sodium on urinary sodium was evident. While blood pressures were significantly related to various anthropometric measurements, controlling for these variables in a covariance analysis did not uncover any relationship between water sodium and blood pressure.

Age standardised mortality rates for various categories of cardiovascular disease (CVD) were calculated for adult populations in each of the three areas defined by water sodium level used in the childhood study. There was no consistent relationship evident between CVD mortality and level of sodium in water.

INTRODUCTION

Studies in both children (Tuthill and Calabrese, 1979; Hofman et al., 1980) and adults (Steinbach et al., 1974; World Health Organization, 1979) have suggested a positive relationship between the level of sodium in water and blood pressure. More recently, however, Pomrehn et al. (1983) found no such relationship in children from eight Iowa communities. If there is a relationship at the level suggested by Tuthill and Calabrese (1979), it implies a high degree of sensitivity of blood pressure to changes in sodium intake. Small changes in blood pressure, if applied at a community level, can have a significant impact on

69

overall mortality (Hypertension Detection and Follow-up Program Committee Group, 1979).

This study was undertaken to determine whether or not a relationship between water sodium and blood pressure existed in Western Australia and also to determine what effect varying levels of long term exposure to water sodium may have had on cardiovascular mortality.

Water Sodium and Blood Pressure in Rural Children

Methods. The methods used in this study have been described in detail elsewhere (Armstrong et al., 1982; Margetts et al., 1983). In summary all children in their first year of high school in two towns in each of three strata of water sodium were included in the study. Towns were selected on the basis of proximity to Perth, school size and having a single main water supply provided by the State Government Water Board. The towns were basically rural centres servicing surrounding farming areas.

Children were asked to complete a self administered questionnaire dealing with diet, fluid intake and lifestyle. In addition they were asked to keep a 24-hour diet record. Subsequently they had their height, weight, triceps skinfold thickness, mid-upper-arm circumference, pulse rate and sitting and standing blood pressures measured. Standardised techniques were used throughout by the same study team using the same equipment. Diet records were checked using household measures and food models. Boys were asked to make two consecutive 24-hour collections of their urine in which sodium and potassium were measured by flame photometry.

Six samples of the water supply in each town were taken for measurement of concentrations of sodium, potassium, calcium, magnesium, total dissolved solids and lead and cadmium (Table 1) by use of standard techniques in the W.A. Government Chemical Laboratory.

Lead and cadmium levels in each town were below the level of detection of the method used (0.05 and 0.01 μmol/l respectively).

TABLE 1
Analysis of water contents in each study town

Town	Sodium (mmol/l)	Potassium (mmol/l)	Chloride (mmol/l)	Calcium (mmol/l)	Magnesium (mmol/l)	TDS (mg/l)
Manjimup	1.46)	0.03 L	1.48	0.16	0.80	141.7
Pinjarra	2.22)	0.06	2.58	0.27	0.29	216.6
Northam	4.73)	0.05 M	6.06	0.36	0.66	451.6
Merredin	4.80)	0.06	6.35	0.35	0.71	450.0
Narrogin	8.93)	0.05 H	13.34	0.72	1.98	920.0
Katanning	9.69)	0.08	13.90	0.96	2.93	985.0

Results and Discussion. Of 792 children eligible for the survey 635 (80.2%—309 girls and 326 boys) participated. Analysis presented here are confined to 288 girls and 308 boys of caucasian origin born in Australia, New Zealand or Britain.

Blood Pressure. In neither boys nor girls whose homes were supplied with water from the town reticulation was there any clear tendency for either sitting or standing mean blood pressures to increase with water sodium levels. Within towns there was also no consistent tendency for children drinking low sodium water to have lower blood pressure than children drinking the main water supply. Table 2 presents the mean blood pressures for girls and boys combined from each of the three strata of water sodium. Means were adjusted for differences in the sex distributions between the three water sodium strata.

Urinary Excretion. Presumably complete 24-hour urine samples were obtained from 274 of 308 boys. Results were not included if urine volume was below 500 ml or known to be incomplete. Mean 24-hour urinary excretion of sodium and potassium and the urinary sodium to potassium ratio are shown according to water sodium strata in those boys whose homes were supplied from the town reticulation (Table 3). While sodium excretion was highest in the high water sodium group, the lowest urinary sodium was in the intermediate group. There was highly significant between group heterogeneity ($p < 0.0001$).

Within each town there were no statistically significant differences in urinary excretion of sodium, potassium or sodium/potassium ratios between boys with home supplies of low sodium concentration and boys whose homes were connected to the town supply.

Sodium Intake. Children were asked to record both the type and amount of drinks they had over a usual week. From this the number of cups of fluid consumed per day were estimated together with a breakdown of the sources of the fluid (Table 4). In each water sodium stratum about 28% of all fluid intake was derived from non-local sources. The sodium intake of fluid from non-local sources was estimated to be about 4.5 mmol/litre, the sodium content of water used by the major soft drink manufacturers supplying most rural centres. All children drank about one and a half litres of fluid a day.

From the above estimates the mean sodium intake from fluids was calculated and added to the dietary sodium intake derived from the analyses of diet records

TABLE 2

Mean blood pressure levels (with standard deviations) in boys and girls together whose homes were supplied from the main town reticulation

TOWN WATER SODIUM	No. of Subjects	BLOOD PRESSURES (mmHg)			
		Sitting		Standing	
		Systolic	Diastolic	Systolic	Diastolic
Low	122	97.5 (13.2)	50.1 (10.7)	106.2 (17.7)	66.6 (12.8)
Medium	192	99.2 (9.3)	47.9 (11.1)	108.1 (11.0)	66.1 (11.8)
High	142	97.5 (10.4)	47.7 (10.2)	107.1 (11.4)	66.9 (10.4)

TABLE 3
Mean urinary excretion of sodium and potassium according to town water sodium level in boys whose homes were reticulated from the town water supply

TOWN WATER SODIUM	24-HOUR URINARY EXCRETION (mmoles)		
	Sodium	Potassium	Sodium/Potassium Ratio
Low	123.1 (45.9)	42.2 (15.0)	3.1 (1.3)
Medium	104.1 (36.6)	33.6 (13.3)	3.5 (1.7)
High	138.6 (48.3)	64.6 (18.8)	3.4 (1.3)

(Table 5). Differences in the town water sodium levels were reflected in the percent contribution made to total sodium intake. There was good agreement between estimated sodium intake and urinary excretion of sodium, with urinary sodium as a percent of dietary sodium ranging from 80.1% up to 101.6%.

The analysis of the estimated dietary intake and urinary excretion of sodium would suggest that the methods used in this study have given a valid indication of the actual intake. That blood pressure was not apparently related to these estimates of sodium intake tends to support the more recent study of Pomrehn et al. (1983).

Other factors potentially confounding the relationship beween water sodium and blood pressure were assessed. There were strongly positive pooled within group correlation coefficients between blood pressures and pulse rate, Quetelet's index, mid-upper-arm circumference and skinfold thickness. There were no consistent relationships between blood pressure and the main relevant nutrients. Nutrient intakes and several body measures were analysed by water sodium stratum (Table 6). There were no differences apparent between water sodium stratum when the sexes were combined and the means adjusted for differences in the sex distributions.

Levels of physical activity were assessed in each school. For girls, but not boys, there was significant heterogeneity in mean sitting and standing diastolic blood pressures between categories of activity with a gradient towards lower pressures in those who were most active. There were no statistically significant differences in distributions of physical activity scores between strata of water sodium.

TABLE 4
Percent Distribution of source of fluid intake and usual daily fluid intake in each water sodium stratum

TOWN WATER SODIUM	CUPS PER DAY	PERCENT DISTRIBUTION OF SOURCES		
		Non-Local	Local	
			Home	School
Low	7.3	28	44	28
Medium	7.7	28	46	26
High	7.4	29	38	33

TABLE 5
Estimates of mean sodium intake from diet records and questionnaires in children whose homes were supplied from the town reticulation

TOWN WATER SODIUM	INTAKES Sodium			Percent contribution to total sodium from fluid
	Food	Water	Total	
Low	121.3 (58.3)	2.7 (1.4)	125.7 (58.2)	2.1
Medium	122.6 (62.6)	6.5 (2.8)	129.9 (72.7)	5.0
High	125.4 (53.6)	11.3 (3.9)	136.4 (54.0)	8.3

Covariance Analysis. Analysis of covariance was done for each blood pressure measurement, with school as the factor and the possible explanatory variables such as body measurements, nutrient intakes, physical activity and urinary excretion as the covariates. The pattern of differences between the adjusted means was not appreciably different from that between the unadjusted means (Table 2).

Water Sodium and Cardiovascular Mortality

Methods. Age standardised mortality rates for various categories of cardiovascular disease (CVD) were calculated for adult populations from local government areas in each of the three strata of water sodium used in the childhood study. Local government areas were included provided that there was reliable information on the long term supply of water to the main towns in the area. Mortality data were available from 1969 to 1981. The five year mortality around the 1971 and 1976 Household Census and the three year mortality around the 1981 Household Census were divided by 5, 5 and 3 respectively to give average annual numbers of deaths. By use of the populations from each Census, average annual age and sex specific mortality rates were derived for the periods 1969-73, 1974-78, 1979-81 in each stratum of water sodium. Age standardised rates were calculated by use of the total 1976 Census population of the three water sodium strata as the standard population.

Results and Discussion. Table 7 presents the age standardised mortality rates

TABLE 6
Estimated mean intakes of fat and energy and mean body measurements in children whose homes were supplied with water from the town reticulation

TOWN WATER SODIUM	Intake		WEIGHT/ HEIGHT^2 (gm/cm^2)	Arm circum- ference (cm)	Skinfold thickness (mm)
	Fat (gm)	Energy (KJ)			
Low	95.7 (31.5)	9414 (2823)	1.89 (.26)	22.9 (2.4)	10.3 (4.0)
Medium	100.6 (31.6)	9879 (2748)	1.85 (.26)	22.5 (2.6)	10.3 (4.2)
High	95.1 (37.6)	8936 (2656)	1.88 (.25)	22.4 (2.5)	10.0 (3.4)

TABLE 7
Age standardised mortality from cardiovascular disease
for each stratum of water sodium by sex and census year

TOWN WATER SODIUM	1971	1976	1981
Males			
Low	95.6 (12.2)	88.1 (11.1)	77.0 (9.6)
Medium	118.2 (16.0)	111.4 (15.4)	106.4 (14.6)
High	101.0 (14.0)	85.1 (12.5)	81.2 (12.9)
Females			
Low	76.0 (11.1)	60.5 (9.2)	52.5 (7.8)
Medium	89.5 (14.4)	70.3 (12.7)	56.3 (10.6)
High	69.8 (11.3)	49.9 (9.3)	35.8 (7.4)

for all cardiovascular diseases distributed by sex, Census year and water sodium strata.

Mortality was highest in the intermediate stratum of water sodium. Within each stratum of water sodium, CVD mortality fell over the three periods. In each water sodium stratum, water sodium levels have remained fairly constant, suggesting therefore that the fall in mortality was due to factors other than water sodium. Similar patterns were seen for separate categories of CVD—specifically hypertensive heart disease (ICD9 rubrics 4000 to 4059), ischaemic heart disease (ICD9 rubrics 4100 to 4149) and cerebrovascular disease (ICD9 rubrics 4300 to 4389). The CVD mortality rates in the stratum were compared with levels of blood pressure from the childhood study. Amongst boys, there was a consistent relationship between mean blood pressure and cardiovascular mortality; the intermediate water sodium area with the highest CVD mortality also recorded the highest mean blood pressures, and the area with the lowest blood pressures recorded the lowest CVD mortality.

CONCLUSIONS

Despite substantial differences in water sodium levels and after adjusting for possible confounding factors, this study, like that of Pomrehn et al. (1983) and unlike those of Tuthill and Calabrese (1979) and Hofman et al. (1980), found no relationship between water sodium and blood pressure.

The lack of relationship between water sodium and blood pressure seen in children was reflected in a similar lack of relationship for cardiovascular disease mortality in adults. Robertson et al. (1979) found no evidence of increased mortality from hypertension and related vascular diseases in English towns with water supplies containing more than 3 mmol sodium per litre. Our study does not support evidence from Russia (WHO, 1979) and Romania (Steinbach et al., 1974) suggesting a relationship between water sodium and hypertensive disease in adults.

Differences in methods and composition of the population may account for some of the variation in the studies, although it is difficult to see how these factors would explain the differences in results. The most likely reason for a falsely positive (or negative) result is the existence of some unmeasured confounding factor.

If there is a positive relationship between water sodium and blood pressure it would suggest a high degree of sensitivity of blood pressure to change in sodium (e.g., 1 mmol/l rise in water sodium per 1 mmHg rise in blood pressure). Studies by Kestleloot et al. (1980) and Cooper et al. (1980) would suggest a much lower sensitivity—between 17-50 mmol of sodium per 1 mm rise in blood pressure.

ACKNOWLEDGEMENTS

We gratefully acknowledge the cooperation of the staff and students from schools involved; the members of the survey team; the Education Department and staff of the Department of Clinical Biochemistry. We would particularly like to thank Nicholas de Klerk and Toni Berry for assistance with cardiovascular mortality. The research was supported by a grant from the TVW Telethon Foundation.

REFERENCES

ARMSTRONG, B.K., MARGETTS, B.M., McCALL, M.G., BINNS, C.W., CAMPBELL, N.A., and MASAREI, J.R.L. (1982). Water sodium and Blood Pressure in Rural School Children. Archives of Environmental Health 37:236–245.

COOPER, R., SOLTERS, I., LIU, K., BERKSON, D., LEVINSON, S., and STAMLER, J. (1980). The association between urinary sodium excretion and blood pressure in children. Circulation 62:97–104.

HOFMAN, A., VALKENBURG, A., and VAANDRAGER, F.J. (1980). Increased blood pressure in school children related to high sodium levels in drinking water. Journal of Epidemiology and Community Health 34:179–181.

HYPERTENSION DETECTION AND FOLLOW-UP PROGRAM COMMITTEE GROUP (1979). Five-year findings of the Hypertension Detection and Follow-up Program. I. Reduction in mortality of persons with high blood pressure including mild hypertension. Journal of the American Medical Association 242:2562–2571.

KESTLELOOT, H., PARK, B.C., LEE, C.S., BREMS–HEYNS, E., CLAESSENS, J., and JOOSSENS, J.V. (1980). A comparative study of blood pressure and sodium intake in Belgium and in Korea. European Journal of Cardiology 11:169–182.

MARGETTS, B., ARMSTRONG, B., BINNS, C., MASAREI, J., and McCALL, M. (1983). Prevalence of some risk factors for cardiovascular disease in rural Western Australian Community Health Studies VII:256–265.

POMREHN, P.R., CLARKE, W.R., FRAN SOWERS, M., WALLACE, R.B., and LAUER, R.M. (1983). Community differences in blood pressure levels and drinking water sodium. American Journal of Epidemiology 118:60–71.

ROBERTSON, J.S., SLATTERY, J.A., and PARKER, V. (1979). Water sodium, hypertension and mortality. Community Medicine 1:295–300.

STEINBACH, M., CONSTANTINEANU, M., HARNAGEA, P., TOEDORINI, S.,

CRETESCU, G.R., MANICATIDE, M., NICOLAESCU, V., SUCIU, A., VLA-
DESCU, G., VOICULESCU, M., and GEORGESCU, A. (1974). The ecology of
arterial hypertension. Reviews of Roumanian Medicine 12:3–6.

TUTHILL, R.W. and CALABRESE, E.J. (1979). Elevated sodium levels in the public
drinking water as a contributor to elevated blood pressure levels in the community.
Archives of Environmental Health 34:197–202.

WORLD HEALTH ORGANIZATION. (1979). Sodium, Chlorides and Conductivity
in Drinking–Water. Euro Reports and Studies 2. World Health Organization,
Copenhagen.

CHAPTER IX

DRINKING WATER SODIUM AND BLOOD PRESSURE: A CRITIQUE

Graham A. Colditz* and Walter C. Willett†
*Channing Laboratory, Department of Medicine
Brigham and Women's Hospital and Harvard Medical School

†Department of Epidemiology, Harvard School of Public Health

ABSTRACT

We review the observational studies conducted to quantify the association between drinking water sodium and blood pressure. The methods used to measure sodium intake, including urinary excretion, are reviewed, as are other factors that may explain the initial observation of an association between community water sodium content and blood pressure. The possible causal nature of this association is addressed with particular reference to the reproducibility of the findings, and the biologic plausibility of the results. The need to quantify any association between small to moderate changes in total sodium intake and change in blood pressure is emphasized. We highlight the need for further research to refine methods for the measurement of individual sodium intake.

INTRODUCTION

The potential interest in drinking water sodium as a modifier of blood pressure emerges from a far larger literature that has focused on the association between sodium intake and blood pressure. At the extremes of intake, sodium does have an impact on blood pressure (Pickering, 1980). Epidemiologic evidence supporting this association includes interpopulation studies of primitive tribes (Prior et al., 1968; Page et al., 1974; Oliver et al., 1975; Maddocks, 1967) and their comparison with other industrialized populations (Gleibermann, 1973; Porter, 1983; McCarron et al., 1982). Experimental evidence from studies on volunteers shows that extremely high intakes of sodium up to 30g/day) will induce elevations in blood pressure (Murray et al., 1978; Luft et al., 1979). Against this background of comparisons between extremes of intake, attempts have been made to study the impact of sodium intake on blood pressure within populations. One such area of study is that of drinking water sodium and blood pressure.

Tuthill and Calabrese focused attention on this area with their reports that blood pressures in children and adolescents in a community with high drinking water sodium (108mg/1) were 3-5 mmHg higher than those of children living in a contiguous community with low drinking water sodium (8mg/1) (Calabrese and Tuthill, 1977; Tuthill and Calabrese, 1981). Methodologic problems with these studies have previously been addressed (Willett, 1981). Many of these issues apply not only to the initial studies, but more generally to subsequent studies addressing this possible association (Hofman et al., 1980; Hallenbeck et al., 1981; Armstrong et al., 1981; Faust, 1982; Pomrehn et al., 1983). Of these more recent studies, only that by Hofman has supported the original findings.

We would emphasize at the outset, that in this type of study design, the exposure (drinking water sodium) is a characteristic of the community, and there is only one unit in each exposure group. As a consequence, any difference in community characteristic such as ions other than sodium in the drinking water, or difference in dietary sodium intake, physical activity, ambient temperature etc., is associated with observed blood pressure differences just as strongly as is the drinking water sodium concentration. There is no possibility for control of the potential confounding effects of characteristics that apply to the community as a whole in the analysis.

The average American has a total daily intake of sodium ranging from 4 to 5.8 grams with about one third occurring naturally in food, one third added during food processing, and one third added by the consumer (Fregly, 1983). Drinking water contributes less than 10% of total daily sodium intake and may be measured quite accurately. All studies of drinking water sodium and blood pressure discussed in this paper attempted to measure total daily sodium intake in order that it could be controlled in the analysis (see Table 1).

Despite these attempts to measure sodium intake, wide daily variation in intake means that 24-hour diet recall histories and single 24-hour urine collections are poor measures of individual intake. They may, however, provide a reasonable measurement of mean values for the community. Similarly, food frequency questionnaires are limited by the assignment of standard values for

TABLE 1
Estimation of Sodium Intake

Author	Food	Urine
Tuthill (1979	eating habits regarding salty items	
Hofman (1980)		24-h urine - One
Faust (1982)	food frequency questionnaire plus 24-h recall	24-h overnight = three 9-h collections
Hallenbeck (1981)	salty food index using 14 items	overnight - seven
Armstrong (1982)	diet diary salty food index: frequency of 39 foods use of table salt	24-h urine - two
Pomrehn (1983)		timed overnight urine on subsample of 25 in each of four communities.

sodium content to a class of food after first allocating a standard portion size.

Imprecise measures such as these may be adequate if comparisons are being made between populations with wide differences in sodium intake. However, the variation being addressed in the current intrapopulation studies is small, and more precise measures are needed. Accordingly, repeated urinary excretion values were measured in several of the studies. Since sodium is not retained in the body, the 24-hour intake is accurately reflected by the 24-hour excretion. Unfortunately, the day to day intraindividual variation in sodium intake means that a single 24-hour urine collection is a poor measure of an individual's average intake. Thus Liu et al. (1979), after studying variability in a Chicago business community, concluded that 10 specimens would be needed to rank their study population into highest and lowest tertiles of sodium intake with a probability of misclassification less than 0.01. The number of measurements required is a consequence of the intraindividual variation, and must be calculated for each unique study population. As a consequence of this variability, the use of one or two 24-hour urine collections is most likely to severely diminish the correlation between urinary concentration and another variable. Addressing this same problem, Luft et al. (1982) estimated that with controlled random variation around a mean daily intake of 150meq sodium, one would need nine collections to accurately estimate sodium intake. Furthermore, in this study, these authors show that 24-hour urines are much more effective as estimates of sodium intake than are overnight samples. In the early studies that justified the use of overnight urines as a means of estimating 24-hour urine sodium excretion, spuriously high correlation coefficients were obtained by comparing the overnight specimen with the 24-hour specimen that included the overnight sample (Pietinen et al., 1976; Langford and Watson, 1973).

Due to the day to day variability of individual sodium intake, it is not surprising that the majority of studies using 24-hour urines have found no association between sodium excretion and blood pressure (Dawber et al., 1967; Ljungman et al., 1981; Schlierf et al., 1980; Simpson et al., 1978; Staessen et al., 1983). In addition, several of the studies of drinking water sodium have detected higher urinary sodium values from towns with lower drinking water sodium (Hofman et al., 1980; Hallenbeck et al., 1981; Pomrehn et al., 1983). This renders interpretation of an association between drinking water sodium and elevated blood pressure nearly impossible.

Methodologic problems in the measurement of individual sodium intake probably affect the estimation of sodium more seriously than most dietary variables. Such problems have been invoked to explain the failure to find a relation between individual sodium intake and blood pressure in many studies (Dahl, 1972; Watt and Foy, 1982).

If the measurement of individual sodium intake is very inaccurate, as suggested by the evidence above, it is inappropriate to use this measurement as a covariate in a multivariate analysis, and then interpret the effect of drinking water sodium as having been "adjusted" for dietary sodium intake. Adjustment for a poorly measured confounding variable does not adjust for the confounding effects of that variable (Greenland, 1980). Thus, data on drinking water sodium in the original reports by Calabrese and Tuthill (1977), remained confounded by dietary sodium. Their study therefore relates overall sodium intake to blood pressure, with drinking water accounting for only a small part of the difference. Similarly, though Faust (1982) found no association between drinking water sodium and blood pressure in either children or adults, he obtained a statistically significant relationship between dietary intake and diastolic blood pressure in children, and between 24-hour urine sodium excretion and mean blood pressure for both adults and children.

All studies measured a number of variables other than drinking water sodium intake and included these in a multivariate analysis. Several of these analyses included the use of stepwise programs that delete from a model a potential confounder based on tests of significance (Schlesselman, 1982). Such procedures do not distinguish between associations that are causal, non causal, or artificial. In addition these procedures emphasize formal tests of significance, which are dependent on the sample size of the study. Although a reduced model will give a more precise estimate, it may at the same time be more biased. In two of the current studies, the salty food index was deleted by such procedures (Hallenbeck et al., 1981; Armstrong et al., 1982) when in fact we might reason that this contribution of sodium intake should be controlled for, despite its apparent statistically nonsignificant contribution to the model as a whole. The exclusion of this covariate implies a commitment to its coefficient taking a value of zero, that is to say it has no impact on the outcome variable.

The outcome measure in these studies, blood pressure, would appear to be one of the more easily measured variables. However, it is evident that even here bias may have entered into at least one of the studies (Willett, 1981). Unless a study of blood pressure can be performed with the recorder blinded to the hypothesis under investigation, the only way to avoid the possibility of systematically recording higher (or lower) values at a given location is to use a mechanical recording device. Such devices do offer the investigator the potential to record blood pressures and interpret them in a manner that will ensure that the interpretation is made while blinded to the exposure status of individuals.

Armstrong et al. (1982) have emphasized the importance of ambient temperature as a modifier of blood pressure, since they observed a higher mean systolic blood pressure as temperature decreased. At the same time there was a rise in standing diastolic blood pressure (but not sitting), as ambient temperature increased. When only small differences in blood pressure are being investigated, bias such as this may exert an important influence on the results that are obtained. Thus all means available to the investigator must be used to minimize their effect.

Several additional criteria must be considered (Hill, 1971) when interpreting data relating drinking water sodium and blood pressure. Support for an observed relationship being causal is enhanced if the observations are consistent with others made in different populations. Despite the early reports of a significant association between drinking water sodium and mean community blood pressure the more recent studies have failed to reproduce these same results, leaving us without strong evidence of consistency. Secondly, we can consider the results in terms of the biologic plausibility of the hypothesis. Here we must assume that the drinking water sodium is contributing to the difference in sodium intake between communities, proportional to the differences in water sodium concentration. Based on this assumption, the original reports estimated one fourth of the 2.5 to 4.0 mmHg to be due to the drinking water.

From the perspective of total sodium intake, the effect reported by Tuthill and Calabrese (1981) (2.4–4.0 mmHg for a difference of 400mg of sodium daily) is equivalent to 6–10 mmHg/gram of daily sodium intake. This reported effect is extremely large in view of the variability of sodium intake in the typical American diet (3 to 6 grams). Although Gleibermann (1973) in her review of sodium intake in different populations estimated a 0.1 mmHg rise in blood · pressure per mmol of sodium intake (4.3 mmHg/gram sodium) which, given the smaller functional mass of the children studied by Tuthill and Calabrese, is comparable with their observed effect, other data suggest that the effect of salt on blood pressure is much less. Other observatonal studies among normotensive human subjects have not detected any significant effect. Comparing highest and lowest quartiles from the Heidelberg study Schleirf et al. (1980) show a rise of 0.5 mmHg/g sodium. Studying men in Finland, Karvonen and Punsor (1977) observed a negative correlation between sodium excretion and blood pressure, as did Ellison et al. (1980) when studying normal adolescents in the Boston area. In a study of some 5,000 adults in Connecticut, Holden et al. (1983) failed to detect a significant relationship between a salt use index and blood pressure, although a 2 mmHg elevation in blood pressure was observed for both males and females when comparing those in the highest percentile of salt use with those in the lowest percentile. For diastolic blood pressure, the difference was negative for men (–0.7 mmHg), but remained for women (1.8 mmHg). Unfortunately, no quantification of the relative intake of salt was made, thus limiting the ability to determine an association between blood pressure and sodium intake. Experimental interventions on humans have shown small effects of sodium intake on blood pressure 0.28 mmHg/gram sodium (Fitzgibbon et al., 1982) and 0.48 mmHg/gram sodium (Luft et al., 1979). In view of this small response, it is not surprising that many studies with few subjects have had inadequate power to detect this apparently small effect. Cooper et al. (1980) also reported a significant correlation between mean individual sodium excretion and blood pressure, but a subsequent attempt to reproduce this result using the same study methods failed to substantiate their initial findings (Cooper et al., 1982). Thus, the magnitude of the effect of drinking water sodium originally reported is biologically implausible, which adds additional doubt regarding the reported association.

Data on the dose-response relation of sodium intake to blood pressure among children and normotensive adults remains inconclusive and inadequate. As the effects of drinking water sodium or moderate changes in dietary sodium are likely to be small, objective and uniform measurements of blood pressure and potential confounding variables such as dietary sources of sodium and other electrolytes, must be made in future studies. There is thus a need for research to refine the methods for measurement of daily sodium intake within a population.

From the public health perspective, the benefits of reducing sodium intake need to be quantified. Although an effect of 1-2 mmHg elevation in blood pressure is not likely to be thought of as clinically significant from the standpoint of the individual, evidence from the Hypertension Detection and Follow-up Program indicates that an aggregate reduction of 5-6 mmHg was associated with a 17 percent decrease in overall mortality (Hypertension Detection and Follow-up Program, 1979). Although small changes in blood pressure may be important, the public health priority of reducing sodium intake at a community level must still be weighed against other interventions such as smoking cessation and increased physical activity. With reliable data on the benefits of change, this data may be analyzed against the respective costs so that policy may ultimately be focused on the areas where the greatest benefit can be achieved for the population as a whole.

REFERENCES

ARMSTRONG, B.K., CAMPBELL, N.A., MARGETTS, B.M., McCALL, M.G., MASAREI, J.R.L., and BINNS, C.W. (1982). Archives of Environmental Health 32:236–245.

CALABRESE, E.J., and TUTHILL, R.W. (1977). Elevated blood pressure and high sodium levels in public drinking water. Archives of Environmental Health 32:200–202.

COOPER, R., SOLTERO, I., LIU, K., BERKSON, D., LEVINSON, S., and STAMLER, J. (1980). The association between urinary sodium excretion and blood pressure in children. Circulation 62:97–104.

COOPER, R., LIU, K., TREVISAN, M., MILLER, W., and STAMLER, J. (1983). Urinary sodium excretion and blood pressure in children: Absence of a reproducible association. Hypertension 5:135–139.

DAWBER, T.R., KANNEL, W.B., KAGAN, A., DONABEDIAN, R.K., McNAMARA, P.N., and PEARSON, G. (1967). Environmental factors in hypertension. In: Stamler, J, Stamler, R., Pullman, T.N., eds. The epidemiology of hypertension, New York. Grune and Stratton. 1976. 255–288.

ELLISON, R.C., SOSENKO, J.M., HARPER, G.P., GIBBONS, L., PRATTER, F.E., and MIETTINEN, O.S. (1980). Obesity, sodium intake, and blood pressure in adolescents. Hypertension 2 (suppl 1):I-78-I82.

DAHL, L.K. (1982). Salt and hypertension. American Journal of Clinical Nutrition 25:231–244.

FAUST, H.S. (1982). Effects of drinking water and total sodium intake on blood pressure. American Journal of Epidemiology 35:1459–1467.

FITZGIBBON, W.R., MORGAN, T.O., and MYERS, J.B. (1982). 'Salt sensitivity' of normotensives: Interactions between changes in red blood cell ^{22}Na efflux rate constant, dietary sodium intake and changes in blood pressure. Clinical Experimental Pharmacology and Physiology 9:291–295.

FREGLY, M.L. (1983). Estimates of sodium and potassium intake. Annals of Internal Medicine 98:792–799.

GLEIBERMANN, L. (1973). Blood pressure and dietary salt in human populations.

Ecology of Food and Nutrition 2:143–156.

GREENLAND, S. Effect on blood pressure. American Journal of Epidemiology 114:817–826.

HALLENBECK, W.H., BRENNIMAN, G.R., and ANDERSON, R.J. (1981). High sodium in drinking water and its effect on blood pressure. American Journal of Epidemiology 114:817–826.

HOFMAN, A., VALKENBURG, H.A., and VAANDRAGER, G.J. (1980). Increased blood pressure in schoolchildren related to high sodium levels in drinking water. Journal of Epidemiology and Community Health 34:179–181.

HILL, A.B. (1971). Principles of medical statistics. 9th ed. New York, Oxford University Press. Chap 24, pp 309–323.

HOLDEN, R.A., OSTFELD, A.M., FRIEMAN, D.H., HELLENBRAND, K.G., and D'ATRI, D.A. (1983) Dietary salt intake and blood pressure. Journal of the American Medical Association 250:365–369.

HYPERTENSION DETECTION AND FOLLOW-UP PROGRAM. (1979). Five year findings of the Hypertension Detention and Follow-up Program. 1. Reduction in mortality of persons with high blood pressure including mild hypertension. Journal of the American Medical Association 242:2562–2571.

KARVONEN, M.J., and PUNSAR, S. (1977). Sodium excretion and blood pressure of West and East Finns. Acta Medica Scandinavica 202:501–507.

LANGFORD, H.G., and WATSON, R.L. (1973). Electrolytes, environment and blood pressure. Clinical Science and Molecular Medicine 45:1115–1135.

LIU, K., COOPER, R., MC KEEVER, J., MC KEEVER, P., BYINGTON, R., SOLTERO, I., STAMLER, R., GOSCH, F., STEVENS, E., and STAMLER, J. (1979). Assessment of the association between habitual salt intake and high blood pressure: Methodological problems. American Journal of Epidemiology 110:219–226.

LJUNGMAN, S., AURELL, M., HARTFORD, M., WIKSTRAND, J., WILHELMSEN, L., and BERGLUND, G. (1981). Sodium excretion and blood pressure. Hypertension 3:318–326.

LUFT, F.C., FINEBERG, N.S., and SLOAN, R.S. (1982). Estimating dietary sodium intake in individuals receiving a randomly fluctuating intake. Hypertension 4:805–808.

LUFT, F.C., RANKIN, L.I., HENRY, D.P., BLOCH, R., GRIM, C.E., WYEMAN, A.E., MURRAY, R.H., and WEINBERGER, M.H. (1979). Plasma and urinary norepinephrine values at extremes of sodium intake in normal man. Hypertension 1:261–266.

MADDOCKS, I. 91967). Blood pressure in melanesians. Medical Journal of Australia 1:1123–1126.

MC CARRON, D.A., HENRY, H.J., and MORRU, C.D. (1982). Human nutrition and blood pressure regulation, an integrated approach. Hypertension 4(suppl III):2–13.

MURRAY, R.H., LUFT, F.R., BLOCH, R., and WEYMAN, A.E. (1978). Blood pressure responses to extremes of sodium intake in noraml man. Proceedings of the society for experimental biology and medicine 159:432–436.

MYERS, J., MORGAN, T., WAGA, S., and MANLEY, K. (1982). The effect of sodium intake on blood pressure related to the age of the patients. Clinical and Experimental Pharmacology and Physiology 9:287–289.

OLVIER, W.J. COHEN, E.L., and NEEL, J.V. (1975). Blood pressure, sodium intake and sodium related hormones in Yanomamo Indians, a 'no-salt' culture. Circulation 52:146.

PAGE, L.B., DANION, A., and MOELLERING, R.C. (1974). Antecedents of cardiovascular disease in six solomon Island societies. Circulation **49**:1132–1148.

PICKERING, G. (1980). Salt intake and essential hypertension. Cardiovascular Reviews and Reports **1**:13–17.

PIETINEN, P.I., FINDLEY, T.W., CLAUSEN, J.D., FINNERTY, F.A., and ALT-SCHUL, A.M. (1976). Studies in community nutrition, estimation of sodium output. Preventive Medicine **5**:400–407.

POMREHN, P.R., CLARKE, W.R., SOWERS, M.F., WALLACE, R.B., and LAUER, R.M. (1983). Community differences in blood pressure levels and drinking water sodium. American Journal of Epidemiology **118**:60–71.

PORTER, G.A. (1983). Chronology of the sodium hypothesis in hypertension. Annals of Internal Medicine **98**:720–723.

PRIOR, I.A.M., EVANS, J.G., HARVEY, H.P.B., DAVIDSON, F., and LINDSAY, M. (1968). Sodium intake and blood pressure in two Polynesian populations. New England Journal of Medicine **279**:515–520.

SCHLESSELMAN, J.J. (1982). Case-control studies. Design, Conduct, Analysis. Oxford. New York. 253–254.

SCHLIERF, G., ARAB, L., SCHELLENBERG, B., OSTER, P., MORDASINI, R., SCHMIDT-GAYK, H., and VOGEL, G. (1980). Salt and hypertension: Data from the "Heidelberg Study." American Journal of Clinical Nutrition **33**:872–875.

SIMPSON, F.O., WAAL-MANNING, H.J., BOLLI, P., PHELAN, E.L., and SPEARS, G.F.S. (1978). Relationship of blood pressure to sodium excretion in a population survey. Clinical Science and Molecular Medicine **55**:373s–375s.

STAESSEN, J., BULPITT, C., FAGARD, R., JOOSSENS, J.V., LIGNEN, P., and AMERY, A. (1983). Four urinary cations and blood pressure. A population study in two Belgian towns. American Journal of Epidemiology **117**:676–687.

TUTHILL, R.W. and CALABRESE, E.J. (1979). Elevated sodium levels in the public drinking water as a contributor to elevated blood pressure levels in the community. Archives of Environmental Health **34**:179–202.

TUTHILL, R.W. and CALABRESE, E.J. (1981). Drinking water sodium and blood pressure in children: a second look. American Journal of Public Health **71**:722–729.

WATT, G.C.M. and FOY, C.J.W. (1982). Dietary sodium and arterial pressure: problems of studies within a single population. Journal of Epidemiology and Community Health **36**:197–201.

WILLETT, W.C. (1981). Drinking water sodium and blood pressure: a cautious view of the "second look." American Journal of Public Health **71**:729–732.

CHAPTER X

HEALTH IMPLICATIONS OF A 5 MM HG INCREASE IN BLOOD PRESSURE

John R. Wilkins III* and Edward J. Calabrese†
*Department of Preventive Medicine
College of Medicine
The Ohio State University
Columbus, Ohio 43210

†Division of Public Health
School of Health Sciences
University of Massachusetts
Amherst, Massachusetts 01003

ABSTRACT

The health implications of a mean increase in blood pressure on the order of 5 mm Hg among young persons are explored primarily from a public health point of view. After an overview of the epidemiologic behavior of human blood pressure is provided, the phenomenon of "tracking" of blood pressure is examined as is the possible relationship between the rate of blood pressure change over time and the initial value. In the last part of the paper, the community benefits of lowering the average blood pressure 5 mm Hg (in terms of number of heart attacks prevented) are estimated under several simplifying assumptions.

INTRODUCTION

Several epidemiologic studies have reported an association between sodium (Na) in drinking water and the level of blood pressure among elementary and secondary school students (Folsom and Prineas, 1982). More specifically, studies in Massachusetts have demonstrated a 3-5 mm Hg increase in blood pressure among school children living in a community with more than 100 milligrams of Na per liter of drinking water, as compared to a group of peers living in a referent community served water having a Na concentration less than 10 milligrams per liter (Calabrese and Tuthill, 1977; Calabrese and Tuthill, 1978; Tuthill and Calabrese, 1979; Tuthill and Calabrese, 1981). While the "associational" nature of the findings has been stressed, the question naturally arises as to what the public health significance is of a mean increase in blood pressure on the order of 3-5 mm Hg in a population of young persons.

The following paper will explore this matter, by first reviewing briefly relevant aspects of the epidemiologic behavior of blood pressure in human populations, and then addressing the question of the ability of blood pressure levels in the young to be predictive of blood pressure levels in adults. The last part of the paper is an attempt to estimate the potential impact on public health of a shift in the average blood pressure of a population on the order of 5 mm Hg.

In order to put into context differences in blood pressure in the range of 3-5 mm Hg, it should be helpful to first review briefly the relevant descriptive epidemiology.

The epidemiologic behavior of human blood pressure is distinguished by the fact that there are notable age, race, and sex differences. In modern, industrialized societies, blood pressure, both systolic and diastolic, increases with age. This has been shown by numerous studies, including the first Health and Nutrition Examination Survey of the U.S. population conducted by the National Center for Health Statistics (Roberts and Maurer, 1977). In this particular study, single systolic and diastolic blood pressure readings were made on nearly 18,000 persons ranging in age from 6-74 years. Persons were selected for study from a national probability sample and were examined sometime between April of 1971 and June of 1974.

A portion of the data obtained from this survey is displayed in Figure 1. What is shown is a plot of the mean arterial blood pressure for white males and white females separately, by age. Among white children ranging in age from 6-11 years and among adolescents ranging in age from 12-17 years, there is a steady increase in the systolic pressure with age. The mean systolic pressure of white males increases from 94.2 mm Hg at 6 years to 120.1 mm Hg at 17 years of age - an absolute increase of nearly 26 mm Hg. This represents an average rate of increase of 2.2 mm Hg per year. Mean systolic pressure for white females was found to be 96.5 mm Hg at 6 years of age and 112 mm Hg at 17 years of age - an absolute increase of 15.5 mm Hg and an average rate of increase of 1.6 mm Hg per year. These rates of change are the highest achieved at any point along the age span. There are no statistically significant mean differences in systolic pressure between white males and females until the ages of 16 and 17 are reached, although the progressive divergence of male and female systolic pressures seen in these data begins around the age of 14.

With respect to the diastolic blood pressures of white children and adolescents, there are no statistically significant differences between the age-specific means, males compared to females, although once the teen years are reached diastolic pressures for males were found to be slightly higher than those for females. Among white males, diastolic pressures were found to average 59.4 mm Hg at 6 years of age, and they increase monotonically at an average rate of 1.1 mm Hg per year, reaching a level of nearly 74 mm Hg by the age of 17. At 6 years of age, diastolic pressures for white females are slightly higher than diastolic pressures for males, averaging 62.1 mm Hg, but rise at a slightly lower rate, 0.9 mm Hg per year, reaching a level of 71.1 mm Hg by the age of 17. The

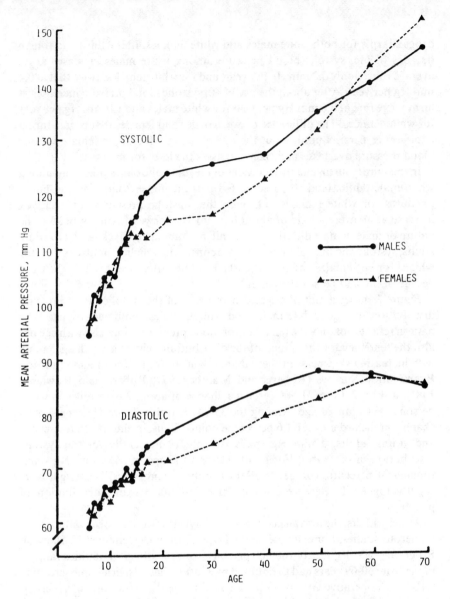

FIGURE 1. Mean systolic and diastolic blood pressure of U.S. white males and females 7-74 years of age, by age, 1971–1974 (Roberts and Maurer, 1977).

divergence seen between male and female systolic pressures is also evident for diastolic pressures.

The overall pattern for white children and adolescents seen in these data is similar for blacks, with respect to both systolic and diastolic pressures. There are also no consistent black-white differences, for either males or females, in this age range.

Once adult stature is reached, the rate of change in systolic blood pressure drops sharply for both white males and white females. In the third and fourth decades of life, systolic blood pressure among white males increases at an average rate of only 0.2 mm Hg per year, and for white females, twice that at 0.4 mm Hg per year. After about the age of 40, systolic blood pressure increases at an average rate of 0.6 mm Hg per year for white males and 1.0 mm Hg per year for white females. The difference between males and females that began during adolescence persists until about the age of 60, at which time female systolic blood pressure overtakes and then surpasses the level for males.

In the third, fourth, and fifth decades of life, diastolic blood pressures among white male adults tend to be some 6-8 percent higher than diastolic blood pressures for white females, although the diastolic pressures for each sex increase at an average rate of about 0.5 mm Hg per year. Among blacks, the nature of male/female differences is similar. Comparing black adults to white adults, systolic and diastolic pressures are consistently higher for blacks than for whites, for both males and females. Black/white differences begin in the third decade of life and persist thereafter.

Figure 2 shows a plot of selected percentiles of the systolic blood pressure distribution for U.S. white males and white females combined, by age. The pattern reflects not only the tendency for blood pressure to increase with age but also the tendency for the spread of the distribution to increase with age, along with increasing skewness. In these data, taken from the Health and Nutrition Examination Surveys (Roberts and Maurer, 1977; Roberts and Rowland, 1981), a shift of 1 mm Hg represents a change of about 2 percentiles in white persons 7-34 years of age. Among the 35-74 year olds, 1 mm Hg represents a change on the order of 1.1-1.6 percentile points. Thus, in children, adolescents, and young adults, 5 mm Hg spans roughly 10 percentiles of the systolic distribution of pressures. For adults beyond the age of 34, 5 mm Hg spans roughly 6-8 percentiles of the systolic distribution of pressures. These figures are slightly higher if reference is being made to the diastolic distribution of pressures.

Among adults, the prevalence of essential hypertension has been estimated in numerous studies. For example, in the Hypertension Detection and Follow-up Program (HDFP), nearly 160,000 persons from 14 U.S. communities ranging in age from 30-69 years had their blood pressures measured in a home screening (HDFP Cooperative Group, 1977). Depending on the definition of "hypertension," prevalence estimates range from 1.4 percent to 25.3 percent. In the Health and Nutrition Examination Survey, for both sexes and all races combined, among persons 18-74 years of age, the prevalence of "definite" hypertension—defined as either systolic pressure of 160 mm Hg or more or diastolic pressure of 95 mm Hg or more—was found to be 18.1 percent (Roberts and Maurer, 1977). Among whites, the overall prevalence was found to be 17 percent and among blacks the overall prevalence was found to be 28.2 percent. Among whites, the prevalence of definite hypertension is greater in males than in females, as Figure 3 indicates, for all ages, until the fifth decade of life, where the prevalence reaches a maximum and ranges from about 25-35 percent. Among blacks, prevalence of definite hypertension also increases with age and

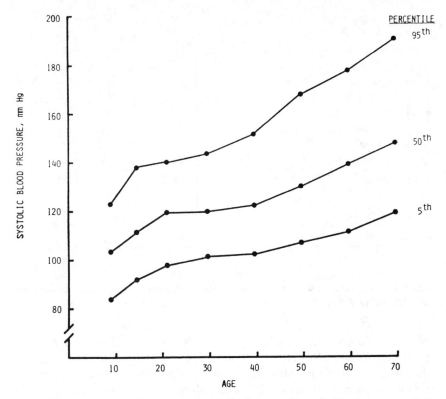

FIGURE 2. Selected percentiles from the distribution of systolic blood pressures, U.S. whites 7-74 years of age, by age, 1971–1975 (Roberts and Maurer, 1977; Roberts and Rowland, 1981).

reaches a maximum in the sixth and seventh decades of life, at values on the order of 50 percent or more. Prevalence of hypertension in blacks is generally greater than that for whites at every age.

By contrast, essential hypertension among children is thought to be rare, although reported estimates of the prevalence of pediatric hypertension do range from 0.9 percent to 13.4 percent (Kilcoyne et al., 1974; Levine et al., 1979). In addition, hypertension in the young was at one time thought, in most cases, to have identifiable causes; this is not generally believed today (Lieberman, 1980; Lieberman, 1982). In spite of such uncertainties regarding the prevalence and causes of hypertension in young persons, one thing is clear: blood pressure levels among children, adolescents, and young adults are not associated (in the early years of life) with the forms of cardiovascular morbidity and mortality seen in older persons. Data are, however, available that suggest that the pathophysiologic consequences of elevated blood pressure manifested in adults are actually the end-stage of a long gradual process that began very early in life, possibly during childhood (Szklo, 1979). It follows therefore that the earlier in life preventive strategies are employed, the more likely such strategies are to be

89

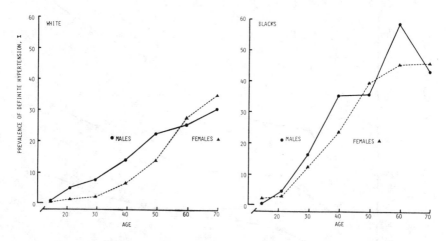

FIGURE 3. Prevalence of definite hypertension among U.S. whites and blacks, by age and sex, 1971-1975 (Roberts and Maurer, 1977; Roberts and Rowland, 1981).

effective. Indeed, it appears that a person's relative ranking in the blood pressure distribution of his or her peers is "fixed" or "set" relatively early in life, thus suggesting the possibility that the monitoring of blood pressure in young persons might be used to identify individuals prone to become hypertensive in later life. If the phenomenon of "tracking" of blood pressure in children and adolescents does occur, and there is no intervention, then children and adolescents with relatively high blood pressure will become adults with relatively high blood pressure.

The evidence supporting the notion that blood pressures begin to track early in life comes primarily from several longitudinal studies of children (Zinner et al., 1974; Beaglehole et al., 1977; Rosner et al., 1977; Rames et al., 1978; Clarke et al., 1978; Zinner et al., 1978; Voors et al., 1979; Voors et al., 1980). These studies have addressed the tracking hypothesis from basically two angles. One approach involves regressing the blood pressure measured at some follow-up point in time against the initial blood pressure, and then computing either the correlation or regression coefficient, either quantity sometimes referred to as the "tracking" coefficient. For example, several hundred children from Boston ranging in age from 2-14 years had their blood pressures measured initially and then 4 years later, and than 4 years after the first follow-up (Zinner et al., 1974; Zinner et al., 1978). Follow-up and initial systolic and diastolic blood pressures were found to be related at both follow-up intervals, since the estimated regression coefficients were all statistically significant. In this particular study, the correlation between initial and follow-up blood pressures was stronger after 8 years than after 4 years. This result contrasts with the results of a study of Welsh children that found a weaker correlation between initial and follow-up

90

blood pressures with a longer follow-up period (Rosner et al., 1977). In the study of the Welsh subjects, after 15 years of follow-up, it was found that the tracking (correlation) coefficient tended to increase with time, from about 0.25 for systolic blood pressure among subjects initially 5-9 years of age, to at least twice that level, ranging from about 0.5 to 0.7 by the time adult stature was reached. Other studies taking this simple regression approach have reported roughly the same results: once adult stature is reached, the correlation of follow-up blood pressure to initial blood pressure will be on the order of 0.6 for systolic blood pressure and 0.4 for diastolic blood pressure (Szklo, 1979). In general, lower values are found for children than for adults, possibly because of the greater variability of blood pressures in the young, a reflection of rapid growth and development up to the point when adult stature is reached.

The other basic approach to the tracking hypothesis involves first ranking subjects in terms of their initial blood pressures and then comparing their initial relative position in the blood pressure distribution to their relative position at the time of follow-up. For example, in the study of children from Boston, among 58 children with initial systolic blood pressures greater than or equal to 1 standard deviation above the mean, 18 of them, or 31 percent, retained this relative position in the distribution 8 years later (Zinner et al., 1978). In the Muscatine (Iowa) Study, among children starting out in the highest quintile of systolic blood pressures, the probability of remaining there 6 years later was only 17 percent, for diastolic pressures only 9 percent (Clarke et al., 1978). In the Bogalusa (Louisiana) Heart Study, among children initially in the top decile for systolic blood pressure, 33 percent of them were there 3 years later, although among children in the highest decile after 3 consecutive years of examinations, nearly 60 percent of them were found to be in the highest decile in the fourth year (Voors et al., 1980).

Overall then, the results of tracking studies in children, it could be argued, are not particularly compelling. However, both methods of examining the tracking hypothesis are deficient in that they do not in general take into account regression-to-the-mean, a phenomenon resulting from random errors in blood pressure measurement. In essence, this phenomenon can be expected to spuriously reduce the regression coefficient that relates the rate of blood pressure change to the initial value. In other words, as a result of regression-to-the-mean, the magnitude of the *observed* regression coefficient relating change to initial value will be less than the magnitude of the *true* regression coefficient. Further discussion (plus in-depth mathematical treatments) may be found in Gardner and Heady (1973), Blomqvist (1977), Svardsudd and Blomqvist (1978), and Wu et al. (1980). When regression-to-the-mean is taken into account, as in the Bogalusa Heart Study, considerably stronger evidence in favor of the tracking hypothesis emerges (Voors et al., 1979). The extent to which environmental factors, for example Na intake, influence a person's "track" is unknown.

While tracking studies deal with the relative position of young persons in their age-, race-, and sex-specific blood pressure distributions, the results of such studies tell us very little about the absolute value of blood pressures attained in later life, which brings us to a potentially very important aspect of temporal trends in blood pressure. Certain data suggest that the level of blood pressure among young adults—the "initial" pressure—determines the rate at which blood pressure changes over time (Blomqvist, 1977; Blomqvist and Svardsudd, 1978; Svardsudd and Tibblin, 1980; Wu et al., 1980). Young persons with the highest pressures may therefore attain, in later life, the highest levels of blood pressure—and they would accomplish this in less time than peers having lower initial pressures.

A small number of longitudinal studies of blood pressure have involved attempts to quantitate the relation between the rate of blood pressure change over time and the initial level. Although a variety of approaches have been taken, they all reduce to regressing individual rates of blood pressure change over time against the individual initial values, and then fitting a linear model to the data. As suggested by Wu et al. (1980), a person's expected rate of change in blood pressure over time can be estimated from the following equation:

$$\hat{b}_i = \hat{\beta} + \hat{\theta}\,(m_i - \hat{\mu})$$

Here, the b_i are the expected rates of change in blood pressure, expressed in terms of mm Hg per unit time; $\hat{\beta}$ is the mean rate of increase for the group; and $\hat{\mu}$ is the mean initial pressure for the group. The estimated linear regression coefficient, $\hat{\theta}$, is expressed in terms of mm Hg per unit time per mm Hg. The m_i represent the individual initial values.

In the context of the question at hand, it should therefore be of interest to predict what a difference in blood pressure of 5 mm Hg in early life may mean in terms of pressure levels in later life. The available data that provide a means for speculation on this are unfortunately sparse and do not address the question of rate of blood pressure change over time and initial value in children per se. It is possible, however, to make some calculations on the assumption that a 5 mm Hg difference in blood pressure exists at the age of 35, the youngest age for which relevant data are available. For example, based on data from the Health and Nutrition Examination Surveys referred to previously, the average U.S. white male will have a systolic blood pressure of 126.2 millimeters of mercury at the age of 35. From this starting point, his rate of change in systolic pressure can be modeled as a function of the initial value, using the data and methods published by Wu et al. in their 1980 paper in the *Journal of Chronic Diseases*. Accordingly, the average 35 year old U.S. white male with a mean initial systolic pressure of 126.2 mm Hg will reach a systolic pressure of 142.6 mm Hg 30 years later at the age of 65—an absolute increase of 16.4 mm Hg. This estimated systolic blood pressure of 142.6 mm Hg at 65 years of age based on longitudinal data compares well with the cross-sectional Health and Nutrition Examination Survey data showing a mean systolic blood pressure of 143.3 mm Hg among 65 year old U.S. white males. On the other hand, a 35 year old white male whose initial systolic pressure is 5 mm Hg higher, that is, his starting point is 131.2 mm Hg, will attain a systolic pressure of 151.8 mm Hg by the time he reaches 65 years of age—an absolute increase of 20.6 mm Hg. Thus, a difference in systolic

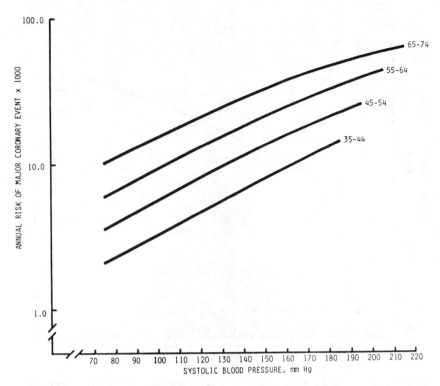

FIGURE 4. Annual risk of a Major Coronary Event among U.S. white males, by age and systolic blood pressure (The Pooling Project Research Group, 1978).

blood pressure of 5 mm Hg in early adulthood may translate into a difference greater than 9 mm Hg at the age of 65. If the relation between rate of change and initial value begins even earlier in life—which is yet to be shown—then larger differences would be expected in the older age groups. (It should be noted that in a recent study by Hofman and Valkenburg (1983), no evidence of a relationship between rate of change in blood pressure and initial value was found among 596 Dutch children ranging in age from 5-19 years.) With respect to risk of cardiovascular morbidity, a difference in blood pressure of 5 mm Hg has virtually no short-term clinical implications among persons 35 years of age or younger, except that a difference of 5 mm Hg may become a difference of nearly 10 mm Hg at 65 years of age. And at this age—say among 65-74 year old U.S. white males—a difference in systolic blood pressure of 10 mm Hg represents a difference in the average risk of a heart attack on the order of 14 percent.

To explore the public health implications of a 3-5 mm Hg difference in blood pressure from another perspective, it will be helpful to first examine the relation between risk of cardiovascular disease and blood pressure. Figure 4 shows the annual risk of a "Major Coronary Event" plotted as a function of systolic blood pressure, for 35-44, 45-54, 55-64, and 65-74 year old U.S. white males.

The risk estimates are derived from the final report of the Pooling Project, a cooperative effort where the results of 5 prospective studies of risk factors for

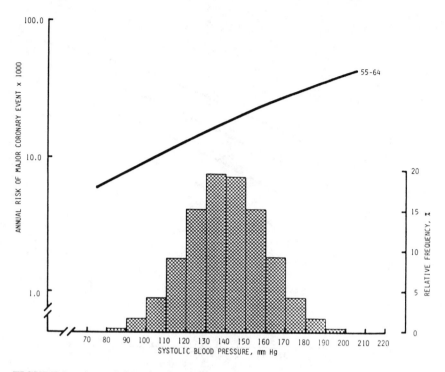

FIGURE 5. Annual risk of a Major Coronary Event and relative frequency of specified systolic blood pressure level among 55-64 year old U.S. white males.

coronary heart disease among white males were pooled, resulting in more than 8400 person-years of experience (Pooling Project Research Group, 1978). The end-point studied, and the one used here for purposes of illustration, is designated the Major Coronary Event, defined as a fatal or non-fatal myocardial infarction or a sudden coronary heart disease death. In addition to systolic and diastolic blood pressure, the effect of serum cholesterol, smoking, relative weight, and ECG abnormalities on the risk of a Major Coronary Event was also estimated. All risk factors were examined separately and in combination by standard logistic regression analyses. The risk estimates used here are derived directly from the bivariate logistic regression results relating the annual risk of a Major Coronary Event to age and systolic blood pressure.

As Figure 4 indicates, the age-specific risk among U.S. white males of having a Major Coronary Event increases steadily over all levels of systolic blood pressure. A similar pattern is seen if the diastolic blood pressure is used to predict risk. Using the lowest class of systolic blood pressures as the reference category (70-80 mm Hg), the "relative risk" of a Major Coronary Event, that is, the risk of a Major Coronary Event at any systolic blood pressure relative to the lowest level of risk, also climbs steadily in each age group, reaching a maximum value of about 7 for each age group. However, looking only at the relative risks can be misleading, as Geoffrey Rose (1981) has pointed out, and as Figure 5

TABLE 1

Expected number of Major Coronary Events (based on Pooling Project risk estimates), by age and systolic blood pressure (SBP) class, U.S. white males.

Age	Mean SBP	No. USWM*	SBP Class	% of USWM	Major Coronary Events No./yr	%
35-44	127.2	10,005,000	<140	82.6	41,669	75.5
			140–160	16.6	12,689	23.0
			>160	0.8	845	1.5
				100.0	55,203	100.0
45-54	134.5	10,112,000	<140	62.2	53,754	50.1
			140–160	30.0	39,441	36.7
			>160	7.8	14,125	13.2
				100.0	107,320	100.0
55-64	140.1	7,974,000	<140	50.0	56,644	37.8
			140–160	34.4	57,523.	38.3
			>160	15.6	35,817	23.9
				100.0	149,984	100.0
65-74	146.8	4,925,000	<140	37.4	42,248	27.1
			140–160	36.1	57,437	36.8
			>160	26.4	56,437	36.1
				99.9	156,122	100.0

*1970 U.S. Census data

illustrates. In this figure, the annual risk of a Major Coronary Event is plotted against systolic blood pressure, for U.S. white males 55-64 years of age. Superimposed on this plot is a histogram showing the approximate percentage of U.S. white males 55-64 years of age with a given level of systolic blood pressure, the relative frequency scaled along the ordinate on the right-hand side of the figure. Although the absolute and the relative risk of a Major Coronary Event increases with increasing blood pressure, the number of persons—in this case the number of U.S. white males—exposed to a given degree of risk varies considerably. Clearly, the very highest risks, and the very lowest risks, apply to the fewest persons. Certainly from a clinical point of view, it is highly undesirable for a person to have a systolic blood pressure greater than 200 mm Hg. Fortunately, among U.S. white males 55-64 years of age, approximately less than 1 tenth of 1 percent of them have systolic pressures this high. From the community point of view, in contrast to the clinical perspective, a different picture emerges when one considers simultaneously the absolute risk level and the number of people "exposed" to a given level of risk.

To illustrate the point, the absolute risk estimates for a Major Coronary Event from the Pooling Project and the blood pressure distribution data from the Health and Nutrition Examination Surveys (Roberts and Maurer, 1977; Roberts and Rowland, 1981) were used to demonstrate the community impact

95

of different levels of systolic blood pressure. For example, the age-specific number of Major Coronary Events expected to occur among U.S. white males was estimated for each category of systolic pressure—each interval having a width of 10 mm Hg. This was done by first taking the reported mean and standard deviation of the systolic blood pressures and constructing a standard normal distribution for each age group. The age-specific number of U.S. white males falling into each category of systolic pressure was estimated from 1970 Census figures (U.S. Bureau of the Census, 1982). The age- and pressure-specific number of Major Coronary Events were thus estimated by multiplying the annual risk of a Major Coronary Event by the estimated number of U.S. white males.

Table 1 summarizes the results of these calculations. For each age group, the mean systolic blood pressure and the estimated total number of U.S. white males from the 1970 Census data are shown. For each of 3 classes of systolic blood pressure, less than 140 mm Hg, 140-160 mm Hg, and greater than 160 mm Hg, the estimated percentages of U.S. white males falling into each category are shown along with the number of men expected to suffer a Major Coronary Event per year, by each level of systolic pressure. As can be seen, the age-specific total number of Major Coronary Events expected to occur in 1 year increases with age, from over 55,000 events per year in the 10 million 35-44 year olds to over 156,000 events per year in the 5 million 65-74 year olds. For each age group, the majority of cases arise from those men with systolic blood pressures less than the 160 mm Hg cut-point. Even in the 65-74 year old men, those men with the highest pressures and therefore the greatest cardiovascular risks, nearly two-thirds of all the estimated Major Coronary Events result from systolic blood pressures less than 160 mm Hg. The percentage of Major Coronary Events stemming from systolic blood pressures considered "borderline" (140-160) range from 23 percent to over 38 percent.

What we might do next is ask: What if these men had reached mean systolic blood pressures 5 mm Hg less than the ones observed? In other words, what if the 35-44 year old U.S. white males had attained, not a mean systolic blood pressure of 127.2 mm Hg, but rather a mean systolic blood pressure of 122.2 mm Hg. By assuming normality of blood pressure distributions as before, the age-specific number of Major Coronary Events can again be estimated by applying the absolute risk estimates. Table 2 summarizes the impact that such a reduction in the mean systolic blood pressure might be expected to have on the "hypothetical" 33 million U.S. white males. Take for instance the 35-44 year olds. At a mean systolic blood pressure of 127.2 mm Hg, 55,203 Major Coronary Events would be anticipated. A mean systolic blood pressure 5 mm Hg lower than that in this age group translates into 49,552 Major Coronary Events, an absolute difference of 5,651 events—a 10.2 percent reduction. Note that although the percent reduction in the number of Major Coronary Events declines with increasing age, the absolute number of cases averted per year increases with increasing age, and then drops slightly. Totalled over all 4 age groups, 5 mm Hg at each age might be expected to reduce the number of Major Coronary Events in such a population by approximately 35,000 Major Coronary Events per year.

TABLE 2

Hypothesized public health impact of "lowering" the mean systolic blood pressure (SBP) 5 mm Hg among U.S. white males, by age and SBP class.

Age	SBP class	Major Coronary Events No./Yr	%	Hypothetical Major Coronary Events No./yr	%	Cases prevented/yr.	% reduction
35-44	<140	41,669	75.5	42,237	85.2		
	140–160	12,689	23.0	7,032	14.2		
	>160	845	1.5	283	0.6		
		55,203	100.0	49,552	100.00	5,651	10.2
45-54	<140	53,754	50.1	60,401	61.3		
	140–160	39,441	36.7	30,204	30.6		
	>160	14,125	13.2	8,000	8.1		
		107,320	100.0	98,605	100.00	8,715	8.1
55-64	<140	56,644	37.8	65,930	47.5		
	140–160	57,523	38.3	49,469	35.6		
	>160	35,817	23.9	23,525	16.9		
		149,984	100.0	138,924	100.00	11,060	.7.4
65-74	<140	42,248	27.1	51,229	35.1		
	140–160	57,437	36.8	54,409	37.2		
	>160	56,437	36.1	40,521	27.2		
		156,122	100.0	146,159	100.00	9,963	6.4

It should be emphasized that the results of this simple exercise—an exercise inspired by the writings of Geoffrey Rose (1981)—illustrate an important principle of primary prevention: that the exposure of many persons to a small risk is likely to result in more cases of disease than the exposure of relatively few people to a large risk. This concept certainly underlies the large effort put forth in previous years in seeking an understanding of the true nature of the relationship between hardness of water and risk of cardiovascular disease. The public health benefits of many persons lowering their blood pressure a few mm Hg by safe non-pharmacologic means is therefore likely to be equal to or greater than the public health benefits resulting from the so-called "high-risk strategy": the identification and treatment of the relatively few persons with exceptionally high pressures. Although the individual gains very little as a result of a mass public health intervention, the community as a whole stands to gain a lot. The mass approach is appealing since the level of a cardiovascular risk factor as important as blood pressure might be lowered by altering some aspect of the environment that affects most if not all of a population—and moreover, individual compliance is not a prerequisite.

With specific reference to Na in drinking water, it is true that the contribution of waterborne Na to the total daily intake is relatively small, ranging from less than 1 percent to about 9 percent (Safe Drinking Water Committee, 1977). It is also true that the exact nature of the relationship between Na intake and level of blood pressure is not fully understood, although it is probably safe to say that large changes in Na intake will affect blood pressure, at least in Na-sensitive persons. It does not therefore seem unreasonable to imagine that small differentials in Na intake due to drinking water could possibly have a small effect on blood pressure. It follows that one of the most important questions to pursue in future studies is that of the relation between rate of change in blood pressure and the initial value among young persons.

What relevance do these findings have for the U.S.E.P.A.? If it can be established that a specific contaminant or group of contaminants in drinking water increases blood pressure a quantifiable amount, the agency could use the approach just illustrated, or a variation thereof, to assess the public health implications of intervention strategies. Part of the significance of such an analysis is that it allows one to assess the benefit if only a specific region of the blood pressure distribution curve is affected. Clearly, the greatest impact would occur if the entire blood pressure distribution was affected, as was apparently the case in the studies of Na in water and blood pressure conducted in Massachusetts. The general approach may then become a powerful tool for regulatory agencies in the decision-making process when public health risks need to be factored into an overall cost-benefit assessment.

ACKNOWLEDGEMENT

The authors gratefully acknowledge the assistance of Mrs. Patricia Price for manuscript preparation.

REFERENCES

BEAGLEHOLE, R., SALMOND, C.E. and EYLES, E.F. (1977). A longitudinal study of blood pressure in Polynesian children. American Journal of Epidemiology 105:87–89.

BLOMQVIST, N., and SVARDSUDD, K. (1978). A new method for investigating the relation between change and initial value in longitudinal blood pressure data. Scandinavian Journal of Social Medicine 6:125–129.

CALABRESE, E.J. and TUTHILL, R.W. (1977). Elevated blood pressure and high sodium levels in public drinking water. Archives of Environmental Health 32: 200–202.

CALABRESE, E.J. and TUTHILL, R.W. (1978). Elevated blood pressure levels and community drinking water characteristics. Journal of Environmental Science and Health A1310:718–802.

CLARKE, W.R., SCHROTT, H.G., LEAVERTON, P.E., CONNOR, W.E. and LAUER, R.M. (1978). Tracking of blood lipids and blood pressures in school age children: The Muscatine Study. Circulation 58:626–634.

FOLSOM, A.R. and PRINEAS, R.J. (1982). Drinking water composition and blood pressure: A review of the epidemiology. American Journal of Epidemiology 115:818–831.

GARDNER, M.J. and HEADY, J.A. (1973). Some effects of within-person variability in epidemiological studies. Journal of Chronic Diseases **26**:781–795.

HOFMAN, A. and VALKENBURG, H.A. (1983) Determinants of change in blood pressure during childhood. American Journal of Epidemiology **117**:735–743.

HYPERTENSION DETECTION AND FOLLOW-UP PROGRAM COOPERA-TIVE GROUP. (1977). The Hypertension Detection and Follow-up Program: A progress report. Circulation Research (Supplement I) **40**:1106–1109.

KILCOYNE, M.M., RICHTER, R.W. and ALSUP, P.A. (1974). Adolescent hypertension. I. Detection and prevalence. Circulation **50**:758–764.

LEVINE, R.S., HENNEKENS, C.H., KLEIN, B. and FERRER, P.L. (1979). A longitudinal evaluation of blood pressure in children. American Journal of Public Health **69**:1175–1177.

LIEBERMAN, E. (1980). Pediatric hypertension. In Hunt, J.C. (1980), *Hypertension Update,* Health Learning Systems, Inc., Bloomfield, N.J., pp. 95–106.

LIEBERMAN, E. (1982). Hypertension in childhood and adolescence. In Kaplan, N.M., *Clinical Hypertension,* Williams and Wilkins, Baltimore, pp. 411–435.

RAMES, L.K., CLARKE, W.R., CONNOR, W.E., REITER, M.A. and LAUER, R.M. (1978). Normal blood pressures and the evaluation of sustained blood pressure elevation in childhood: The Muscatine Study. Pediatrics **61**:245–251.

ROBERTS, J. and MAURER, K. (1977). Blood pressure levels of persons 6-74 years, United States, 1971-1974. Vital and Health Statistics: Series 11 - Number 203, DHEW Publication number (HRA) 78–1648.

ROBERTS, J. and ROWLAND, M. (1981). Hypertension in adults 25-74 years of age, United States, 1971-1975. Vital and Health Statistics: Series 11 - Number 221, DHHS publication number (PHS) 81–1671.

ROSE, G. (1981). Strategy of prevention: Lessons from cardiovascular disease. British Medical Journal **282**:1847–1851.

ROSNER, B., HENNEKENS, C.H., KASS, E.H. and MIALL, W.E. (1977). Age-specific correlation analysis of longitudinal blood pressure data. American Journal of Epidemiology **106**:306–313.

SAFE DRINKING WATER COMMITTEE. (1977). *Drinking Water and Health.* National Academy of Sciences, Washington, D.C., pp 402.

SVARDSUDD, K. and BLOMQVIST, N. (1978). A new method for investigating the relation between change and initial value in longitudinal blood pressure data. Scandinavian Journal of Social Medicine **6**:85–95.

SVARDSUDD, K. and TIBBLIN, G. (1980). A longitudinal blood pressure study. Change of blood pressure during 10 yr. in relation to initial values. The study of men born in 1913. Journal of Chronic Diseases **33**:627–636.

SZKLO, M. (1979). Epidemiologic patterns of blood pressure in children. Epidemiologic Reviews **1**:143–169.

THE POOLING PROJECT RESEARCH GROUP. (1978). Relationship of blood pressure, serum cholesterol, smoking habit, relative weight and ECG abnormalities to incidence of major coronary events: Final report of the Pooling Project. Journal of Chronic Diseases **31**:201–306.

TUTHILL, R.W. and CALABRESE, E.J. (1979). Elevated sodium levels in the public drinking water as a contributor to elevated blood pressure levels in the community. Archives of Environmental Health **71**:722–729.

U.S. BUREAU OF THE CENSUS. (1982). *Statistical Abstract of the United States: 1982-83.* U.S. Government Printing Office, Washington, D.C., pp. 27.

VOORS, A.W., WEBBER, L.S. and BERENSON, G.S. (1979). Time course studies of blood pressure in children—The Bogalusa Heart Study. American Journal of

Epidemiology **109**:320–334.

VOORS, A.W., WEBBER, L.S. and BERENSON, G.S. (1980). Time course study of blood pressure in children over a three-year period. Bogalusa Heart Study. Hypertension. 2 (Supplement I). I102–I108.

WU, M., WARE, J.H. and FEINLEIB, M. (1980). On the relation between blood pressure change and initial value. Journal of Chronic Diseases **33**:637–64.

ZINNER, S.H., MARTIN, L.F., SACKS, F., ROSNER, B. and KASS, E.H. (1974). A longitudinal study of blood pressure in childhood. American Journal of Epidemiology **100**:437–442.

ZINNER, S.H., MARGOLIUS, H.S., ROSNER, B. and KASS, E.H. (1978). Stability of blood pressure rank and urinary kallikrein concentration in childhood: An eight-year follow-up. Circulation. **58**:908–915.

DISCUSSION I

Calabrese: There remain a lot of unresolved issues, at least from a research perspective, with regard to the relationship of sodium in drinking water—as well as in foods—to blood pressure. The research progression that I have seen that is most encouraging is the attempt to go from cross-sectional association efforts to an intervention form. The intervention approach offers the best opportunity to assess whether modest decreases or increases in sodium intake can be reflected in changes in the blood pressure. I think that in terms of the paper that Bob Tuthill presented today, one thing that always stands out is what would have happened if we had been able to carry that study out not over 8 or 9 weeks, but over a considerably longer period of time. While the answer to that question remains to be determined, it is quite evident that over 8 or 9 weeks, it didn't emerge. In the bottled water study, we observed a decrease in the females relatively rapidly, even though it wasn't sustained in the males. What I am wondering about, which we really haven't addressed—and maybe future studies may—is whether one can lower blood pressure more significantly and quickly by removing sodium as compared to increasing blood pressure by adding it to the water and diet. Our studies suggested that if the causal relationships are real that we presented, then decreasing sodium may have a more immediate effect. But, that still doesn't necessarily prove that the sodium caused the increase in blood pressure in the first place.

Tuthill: There are a few things that have occured to me. I agree with Ed Calabrese that the most significant progress will probably be made with some kind of intervention. Current tests are primarily reducing sodium and seeing its effect on blood pressure, but unfortunately, as Ed Calabrese said, that doesn't prove that raising sodium will raise the blood pressure. We have ethical problems when we try to do the latter. I think that one of the most critical things in the field is a need for some kind of biochemical or biological or simple diagnostic test to determine people's sensitivity to sodium. If we had this as the control variable, I think we could sort out a lot better what else is going on. Where such a marker will come from is another question. Let's hope that somebody does come up with that kind of technique. If they do, we are, I think, epidemiologically way ahead of the game when we try to sort out these other factors. Because, that is the big variability that we cannot get a handle on and it can certainly swamp out other effects that we are trying to look at. The business that Ed Calabrese mentioned on diet, I have now—in almost final stage—a diet intake history—this is a recall in the last three months how often have you eaten such and what portion size you ate. This diet intake history for sodium, potassium or calcium is based on the Hanes II survey in terms of the frequency with which the item was consumed as well as its content of sodium, potassium or calcium, taking a list of about 120 items that covers the major sources of sodium, potassium and calcium and covers 95% or better of the sources of all those nutrients from the 24-hour diet records that are recorded in Hanes II survey. This is current, up-to-date information on what Americans are actually consuming and what the major sources actually are. The plans are to enter this into the micro-computer so that you can do a micro-computerized interview. It then ties into our nutrient databank here at UMASS, whereby in 5 minutes after you put data in, you have your answers back because it is all coded to that database. It allows a very quick survey, but it can also be done by hand since it is only 120 items. But the point is, if you do it on the micro-computer, then you can save the data and send it right over to the nutrient databank and quickly get back your results. You don't have these hours and hours of calculations—looking it up in books and so forth. I would like to—in fact, I have already planned to—do a study looking at dietary intake of these sources using this particular instrument coupled with sampling of the hair, coupled with urine and with blood serum samples, looking at sodium, potassium and calcium and relating that to hypertension. The purpose is to see which particular modes of biological sampling have the best correlation with hypertension. I think that is going to be interesting. And it also applies very much to future studies—for anybody looking into sodium in the diet and/or water as it relates to hypertension. One other thing that Dr. Calabrese and I had talked about before came up when we went back to Reading and Stoneham and looked at the 4th and 8th graders. We always screened Stoneham first and Reading second. This time we screened Reading first and Stoneham second and we got a reversal in the difference in blood pressure. So, at this point, I think it would be very interesting for all of the investigators that have done their studies to indicate the order in which the groups were studied and see if there was a downward progression of blood pressure. This is tentative from our own data, but I think if everybody else had the same experience—if you look at the order in which your groups were done and blood pressure goes down as you go through that order, then I think there is some kind of effect of the interviewers in doing the blood pressure. It is not a bias in terms of them knowing the hypothesis, but rather when you do screening like this in large numbers, the systolic and diastolic blood pressures that they get tend to get lower and lower as perhaps they develop greater skill or whatever in detecting the sounds. I think that is a very important hypothesis. That is all I have to say at this point.

Hofman: Thank you very much. The first thing I want to say is that I enjoyed both the papers and the discussion immensely. It is nice to encounter the American spirit. Secondly, what I would like to do now is present to you three observations. The first refers to Dr. Wilkins who discussed the matter of whether there is "tracking" and "horseracing" of blood pressure in childhood. We have some data on that and I will be able to show you those. Second, there is the question of the etiologic relation of sodium intake and blood pressure. And third, what are the implications of our combined findings for the question of whether sodium in drinking water is related to blood pressure in childhood?

As far as the first question is concerned whether there is "tracking" or "horseracing," Dr. Wilkins was talking about the concept that people who have a high initial level of blood pressure may be the big increasers of blood pressure over time. This implies that people are not characterized by a certain level of blood pressure, but by a certain rate of increase in blood pressure. The general reasoning is that it might be very good to look at the rate of increase of blood pressure over time. It might be the key issue in determining which people will be hypertensive later on in life. The main features of a model like this are: (1) that you start out with approximately the same blood pressure level, say during conception or birth; (2) that you have a fixed rate of increase of blood pressure that is typical for you as an individual. The model predicts that those who have the highest blood pressure at a certain initial time A, have the biggest increase after that initial time A. The highest level is related to the biggest increase. This is referred to as "horseracing." It is a term that I believe was used for the first time by Mr. Richard Peto. It has been first analyzed in the context of pulmonary function decrease over time. In adults two data sets (from Framingham and Gotenburg) have—after a proper correction for regression towards the mean—suggested indeed that there is a positive relation between the initial level of blood pressure and the subsequent increase. Does the model also hold in children? We analyzed 600 Dutch children, ages 5 to 19. We measured blood pressure each year for at least 6 years. And we computed an initial blood pressure level, a rate of increase— that is the linear slope of blood pressure regressed on time—and then we corrected for regression towards the mean, using the method of Blomquist. The regression coefficients of blood pressure slope on the initial level were negative, and not as you would expect from the model, positive. It applied to systolic as well as diastolic pressure. This was not, by the way, the first analysis of this kind in young people. This particular problem was analyzed before in 1934 by Dr. Rachel Jenss, a biostatistition from Johns Hopkins University and she addressed this question and came to the same conclusions. After analyzing these data she said: "Perhaps there is some sort of biological adjustment in the earlier age periods which tends to bring the pressure of an individual—which is either too high or too low—to a more normal level." It seems very much that this is what we have observed in childhood, and I propose that one might call this phenomenon the Jenss phenomenon: children who jump out of the distribution of blood pressure in one way or another, are by one mechanism or another forced back into the mainstream of that particular distribution. Whether you are too high or too low, Nature takes care of you. It might be that in adulthood, this particular physiological phenomenon disfunctions. In fact, one might speculate that it is the result of atherosclerosis affecting aortic baro-receptors. If that is the case then it is not so that you get atherosclerosis because of high blood pressure, but it is the other way around: you get high blood pressure because you have athero-sclerosis at your aorta.

What about my second question, the general relationship between sodium intake and blood pressure? This question has not really been very much addressed in this meeting. I think that our newborns study addresses this particular question. I would believe—not only looking at these data, but also at other data sets and published reports—that indeed there is a case to be made for the contention that sodium intake is etiologically related to blood pressure.

However, as to the third question concerning drinking water sodium and blood pressure, I really wonder whether we should not start off with the statement: Let's forget about it! Because it seems to me that the amount of sodium consumed early in life, even if it is a high proportion, is not really so much that you would expect a big impact on blood pressure later on in life. You might be able to show an effect in children, but this effect of sodium in drinking water on blood pressure tends to be overrated when you get into adulthood. So, given the equivocal evidence, I think we should not try to make too much out of it. I am saying this particularly because it seems that the initial studies in Massachusetts and our study from The Nether-lands are the only ones that really support the view of an early impact of sodium in drinking water on blood pressure and I believe that Dr. Hallenbeck's study that suggested that there might be an an effect on diastolic blood pressure is the only other data set that has something of an effect. That particular finding bothers me some-what because of the very strong correlation between systolic and diastolic blood pressure and their physiological interrelation. I have the feeling that perhaps the drinking water/sodium issue should not be played up too high. Perhaps what one should do is try to avoid the suggestion that people get large amounts of sodium in their drinking water because of, for example, the use of sodium hydrox-ide as an ion exchanger in the softening process. But, to spend much time, energy and even dollars or guilders on reducing sodium levels, I wonder whether that would be a very good idea. Thank you very much.

Pomrehn: Well, first of all I think we're all here for a purpose. My speciality is preventive medicine, and I think we're talking about the number one cause of death in this country and that's heart disease. So I think all of these investigations are important because we're looking at ways to prevent hypertension which leads to heart disease. Now, I was really hoping when I first heard Bob Tuthill talk in Iowa City about his study, and I put in a grant proposal and it was accepted, that there was something different about sodium and water. And that it was going to explain a little bit of that variance about the development of hypertension. And I don't honestly believe that I can say that it does. I do feel, and I think Dr. Hofman's study is one good bit of evidence, that sodium is a bad actor in the whole, and I think it is related to blood pressure, and again we don't know how much of hypertension is caused by high sodium in our diet, and I think we can be prudent and say cut down on your sodium and if that means getting a by-pass around your softener and not making your Campbell's soup with softened water, then I think that is worth recommending, particularly for those who need to be on low sodium diets. I think these efforts are worthwhile. I guess I'm not going to be sitting on the side of advocating anything to be done necessarily about drinking water sodium. I guess that's about all.

Margetts: I think the second thing that I've learned today is that there are a lot of methodological problems involved in all of the studies that we have done and everybody else has done that make it very difficult to speak, and make it very difficult to interpret those results. I think I can only paraphrase what Dr. Hofman and Dr. Pomrehn have said about the relationship between dietary sodium and water sodium and blood pressure. It would have to be some remarkably unique characteristic of sodium in water for such a small amount of it to have such a marked effect on blood pressure at least as far as I and the group that I've come from would believe.

Colditz: I really don't know that there is very much more to say than we have so far. I suppose one thing I didn't place all that much emphasis on, when discussing the precision of measurement, was the outcome measure—blood pressure. I have placed more emphasis on the exposures (drinking water sodium and total sodium intake) than on this outcome measure. However, I think everyone would agree that we've heard that blinding or non-blinding of those reading the blood pressures may really be the major determinant behind some of the problems in the interpretation of the results. Again this highlights for me the emphasis that has to be placed on the precision of that measurement.

Wilkins: At this time I have several comments to make. One, I'd like to express my gratitude to Dr. Hofman for elaborating somewhat on the rate-of-change and initial value relationship and pointing out that it does not apparently exist in children. On the other hand, there is evidence in two studies that he referred to, showing a relation between rate of change in blood pressure and initial value among adults. Now, there is still a decade or two of life in between the older adults and the children. I think the question still remains whether or not there is a relationship between rate-of-change and the initial value. And I think that's potentially a very promising area to pursue in future studies. The second comment I have is really an elaboration on the model that I alluded to in my presentation. I'm sure you are all aware that that was really taking a cross-sectional view of what might happen in a population if the mean blood pressure was reduced 5mm of mercury. I think that this has actually stimulated quite a bit of thought on my part and also for some folks that I work with, and we now plan to not take a cross-sectional view, but try to mathematically model what might happen in a free-living population by taking a longitudinal view and simultaneously attempting to take into account competing risks. You can imagine a population starting out at the age of say, 35 years, for example, and as they age there will of course be competing risks to consider. We are also thinking of adding another level of complexity to the model and that would be looking at what would happen if not only blood pressure was modified to some extent, but some other highly prevalent risk factor for cardiovascular disease as well.

CHAPTER XI

OVERVIEW

L. J. McCabe

U.S. Environmental Protection Agency
Health Effects Research Laboratory
Toxicology and Microbiology Division

It has been twenty-one years since I first presented a paper on the area covered by this conference (McCabe, 1963) and we do not seem to be ready for a public health program to prevent cardiovascular disease by adjusting drinking water quality. Possibly a few people did not buy water softeners after reading some of the popular press accounts of the research, but we still have the dilemma—is there something good for us in hard water or something bad in soft water?

Most of us gathered here four and a half years ago and exchanged ideas, but were not able to provide advice to the water supply utilities on what they should do about drinking water quality. Calabrese summarized that drinking water can be a contributing factor in the development of cardiovascular disease (Calabrese and Moore, 1980).

Results of the four major epidemiological studies were presented and all agreed that these were not definitive. Fortunately, work has continued and updates on three of the studies will be presented tomorrow. In the intervening years, studies have been reported from two other countries. Sonneborn's (1983) studies of cardiovascular disease in the Federal Republic of Germany found that no statistically confirmed relationship between either the calcium concentration or the magnesium concentration in drinking water and the cumulative mortality rates for cardiovascular diseases or for ischemic heart disease exists. One was an ecological correlation study with the problem of knowing the quality of water consumed in each of the areas. The problem was controlled by only using vital statistical areas where at least 75% of the population of the area was served by the community water supply. A second study had 40 morbidity parameters that were related to 35 mineral and trace elements in drinking water supplies with a random pattern of positive and negative correlations. These ecological studies do not help us to be more specific about which one of the elements dissolved in water is causatively related to cardiovascular disease but when no associations are observed with a water factor in a particular country we know that we cannot generalize. More definitive studies are being conducted but the results cannot apply to all countries' probability because of the effects of risk factors other than water. A report of a study from China (National Research Collaborating Group, 1983) is more difficult to consider as I have only been able to read the abstract. Multiple regression methods were used on ecological data from 37 cities and positive correlations found for hardness, calcium and magnesium and coronary heart disease and hypertensive heart disease. In some countries the more important determinants of cardiovascular disease may overwhelm the minor effect of a water factor. In some countries the water factor association has been repeatedly demonstrated and I hope at the end of the conference we can conclude that there is a more specific relationship than some vague, unknown effect. It is possible that because of the great geographical and social differences covered in these studies, a universal model will not apply.

Toxicological studies have also continued, and I understand that they have found some unexpected results that should require another iteration of the epidemiological studies to see if the same effects also occur in man. Epidemiologists have done a lot of studies relating chlorination to cancer but not to heart disease. Price in his book, "Coronaries, Cholesterol and Chlorine" (Price, 1969), considers chlorination of drinking water to be a necessary and sufficient cause of coronary heart disease and strokes. Most feel that this overstates the evidence—that there are multiple causative factors. Hewitt, in the panel discussions at the last conference, made much of the High Density Lipid hypothesis as being more important than any water factor mentioned (Sharrett 1980). Dr. Revis may be able to tell us that all these factors may be related and working together.

An aside comment on the design of experiments may be of interest. We spend much time in developing protocols, but when an investigator is on a limited budget and decides to use up a batch of animal feed he has on hand, we may get a serendipitous result, especially when the diet is deficient in calcium.

At the last conference, I discussed research priorities and pointed out then that we needed some data within the next few months, and I am happy to report that we will have four papers on barium at this conference.

Toxicological research on these problems seems to be picking up, as *Science* had two papers in recent months, one on chloride and another on magnesium. But today we will explore another subset of the problem using epidemiological approaches. I understand that when you look in some places you find an effect of sodium but in other places it is not there. I hope the speakers will be prepared for the discussion when we try and find out why these opposite results occur, and how we can provide guidance to the water utilities.

ACKNOWLEDGEMENT

The research described in this paper has been subject to the Agency's review and it has been approved for publication. Mention of trade names or commercial products does not constitute endorsement or recommendation for use.

REFERENCES

CALABRESE, E.J. and MOORE, G.S. (1980). Conference on Cardiovascular Disease and Drinking Water Factors—Principal Findings and Future Research Needs. J. of Environ. Path. and Tox. **4-2,3**:323–326.

McCABE, L.J. (1963). The Correlation of Drinking Water Quality and Vascular Disease. Presented at the Conference of Cardiovascular Disease Epidemiology, Chicago.

NATIONAL RESEARCH COLLABORATING GROUP. (1983). Relationship Between Hardness of Drinking Water and Mortality of Cardiovascular Disease. Chinese J. of Prevent Med. **17(3)**:129–133.

PRICE, J.M. (1969). Coronaries, Cholesterol and Chlorine. Pyramid Publications, New York.

SHARRETT, R. (1980). Panel Discussion: The Relationship of Hard Water and Soft Water in CVD and Health. J. of Environ. Path. and Tox. **4-2,3**:113–141.

SONNEBORN, M., MANDELKOW, J., SCHON, D. and HOFFMEISTER, H. (1983). Health Effects of Inorganic Drinking Water Constituents, Including Hardness, Iodiele, and Fluoride. CRC Critical Review on Env. Control **13(1)**:1–22.

CHAPTER XII

THE BRITISH REGIONAL HEART STUDY: CARDIOVASCULAR DISEASE AND WATER QUALITY

S.J. Pocock,* A.G. Shaper* and P. Powell†

*Department of Clinical Epidemiology and General Practice,
Royal Free Hospital School of Medicine, London, England*

† *Water Research Centre,
Medmenham, Marlow, England*

ABSTRACT

The Regional Heart Study aims to explain the marked regional variations in ischaemic heart disease and stroke in Great Britain and to provide fundamental information about the causes of cardiovascular disease. The role of water quality has received particular attention.

In Phase 1 cardiovascular mortality for 1969-73 in 234 British towns was related to water quality and a wide range of other environmental and socio-economic factors. The negative association between cardiovascular mortality and water hardness was considerably reduced after allowance for climate and socio-economic factors. A study of changes in water hardness and cardiovascular mortality between 1961 and 1971 in 76 county boroughs of England and Wales has shown results consistent with the Phase I findings.

Phase 2 is a clinical study of 7735 middle aged men in 24 towns which has identified certain personal risk factors, cigarette smoking and blood pressure, as being contributors to the geographic variations in ischaemic heart disease. Phase 2 has also enabled more intensive study of trace elements and bulk minerals in domestic drinking water. Ischaemic heart disease mortality and prevalence in the 24 towns were both significantly associated with the following water factors:—alkalinity, calcium, lead, potassium, silicon and total hardness.

Overall, current information indicates that water hardness makes a small, independent contribution to regional variations in cardiovascular disease in Great Britain. The practical implications of this finding are discussed.

INTRODUCTION

In Great Britain there exist marked regional variations in cardiovascular disease (ischaemic heart disease and stroke). Figure 1 shows the standardized

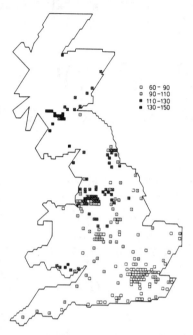

FIGURE 1. Standardized mortality ratios for cardiovascular disease in men and women aged 35–74 in 253 British towns.

mortality ratio for cardiovascular disease in 253 British towns in 1969-73. Towns indicated by black squares have at least a 30% excess mortality from cardiovascular disease and these are to be found in the west of Scotland, north west England and south Wales. Conversely, towns with a lower than average mortality are predominantly in the south east of England. The highest mortality is in two towns near Glasgow which have double the death rate of certain affluent London suburbs.

The British Regional Heart Study is a large-scale epidemiological survey to investigate the aetiology of ischaemic heart disease and stroke with an emphasis on identifying those personal and environmental factors which are responsible for these marked geographic variations in cardiovascular disease. The role of water quality has received particular attention.

In section 2 of this paper, we review findings from Phase 1 of the study, relating the mortality rates in Figure 1 to social and environmental factors, including water hardness. In section 3 we summarize recent findings relating changes in water hardness in some areas to changes in cardiovascular mortality. Sections 4 and 5 present the methods and results from Phase 2, the main field survey of the Regional Heart Study, relating ischaemic heart disease prevalence and mortality in 24 British towns to risk factors and tap water quality parameters obtained from individual middle aged men. Section 6 provides an overall discussion of the practical implications of research into water hardness and cardiovascular disease.

PHASE I: CARDIOVASCULAR MORTALITY
IN 234 TOWNS

Figure 2 shows the negative association between cardiovascular mortality in 1969-73 and water hardness in 234 British towns (r = −.67). Such a tendency for soft water areas in Britain to have greater cardiovascular mortality has been shown for earlier years (Morris et al., 1961; Crawford et al., 1968).

However, one needs to avoid leaping to the conclusion that water hardness is a major risk factor. In particular, it is important to consider other influences on cardiovascular mortality that may follow a similar geographic pattern. For instance, it is well recognized that the south of England tends to be more affluent and has less manufacturing industry than further north. Also, the north and west tend to be colder and wetter than the south and east.

Stepwise multiple regression techniques have been used to assess the contributions of water quality, social factors and climate to cardiovascular mortality rates in the 234 British towns. From the wide range of variables, described in more detail by Pocock et al. (1980), were identified five principal factors each making an independent and highly significant statistical contribution to explaining the geographic variation in cardiovascular mortality:

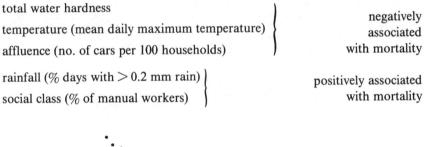

total water hardness	
temperature (mean daily maximum temperature)	negatively associated
affluence (no. of cars per 100 households)	with mortality
rainfall (% days with > 0.2 mm rain)	positively associated
social class (% of manual workers)	with mortality

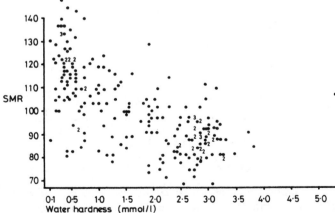

FIGURE 2. Water hardness plotted against the standardized mortality ratio for cardiovascular disease in 234 British towns.

Here we will focus on describing the water hardness association and how it is affected by adjustment for the other factors. The continuous line in Figure 3 shows the mean standardized mortality ratio for towns grouped into equally spaced intervals of water hardness. Adjustment for the other four factors (using analysis of covariance) greatly reduces this negative association, as indicated by the dotted line in Figure 3. This adjusted curve shows a continuous fall of around 10% in moving from very soft to medium hard waters, but no substantial further reduction in mortality in moving from medium to very hard waters. That is, there appears to be a non-linearity in the water hardness/CV mortality association.

Pocock et al. (1982) describe a method of extending multiple regression to allow for these problems of weighting and spatial correlation. Applying this method to these data led to an anticipated reduction in the statistical significance of each of the five factors and also reduced the evidence of non-linearity in the water hardness association. However, the overall conclusions were confirmed.

It is useful to quantify the results of this weighted spatial model. It is estimated that an area of soft water (0.5 mmol/l) has a 7.8% excess CV mortality relative to a hard water area (3.0 mmol/l) after allowance for social and climatic factors. The 95% confidence limits for this reduction are 3.7% and 12.0%.

The above methods of analysis have also been adopted in studying geographic variations in mortality from *stroke* and *ischaemic heart disease* separately. The association of water hardness was similar for both diseases, as were the climatic and socio-economic effects, so that their combination under an overall

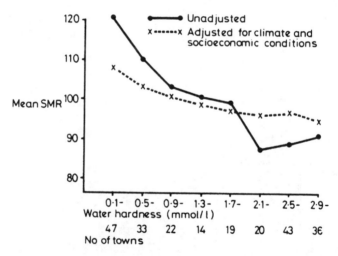

FIGURE 3. Geometric means of the standardized mortality ratio for cardiovascular disease (men and women aged 35–74) for towns grouped according to water hardness. It should be noted that conventional use of multiple regression in this context makes no allowance for:

a) towns being of unequal population size and,
b) towns close to one another having similar mortality.

heading of cardiovascular disease seems appropriate. Furthermore, there was no evidence of any association of water hardness with non-cardiovascular mortality. We have also studied cardiovascular mortality for *men and women separately* and found similar associations with water hardness. While we have so far restricted attention to total water hardness, it is important to recognize that total hardness is closely related to carbonate hardness (alkalinity), calcium, electrical conductivity and several trace elements. Also, softer water supplies tend to come from upland reservoirs. Hence, it is impossible in geographic mortality studies of this kind to separate out which of these closely interrelated water parameters is the causative agent, if indeed a causal relationship exists at all. Hence, we wish to emphasize that water hardness is merely a useful global measure in studying the water quality/cardiovascular mortality relationship.

More extensive description of these findings from Phase 1 of the Regional Heart Study is given by Pocock et al. (1980, 1982), Shaper et al. (1980) and Packham et al. (1982).

CHANGES IN WATER HARDNESS

It is always difficult to make valid inferences from cross-sectional geographic studies in view of the many confounding factors that might be involved. Additional useful insight can be obtained from studies relating changes in water hardness in specific towns to subsequent changes in cardiovascular mortality. Lacey and Shaper (1984) and Lacey (1981) describe results from one such study which we will now summarize. Between 1961 and 1971, substantial changes in water hardness occurred in 14 of the 76 county boroughs of England and Wales. These changes in hardness are indicated on the horizontal axis of Figure 4; 5 boroughs had a reduction in hardness, 9 had increased hardness while the remaining 62 boroughs had no notable changes in hardness. Since results in section 2 suggest the effect of water hardness is only evident up to 1.7 mmol/l, changes above this level have not been included. On the vertical axis of Figure 4 is plotted the ratio:

$$\frac{\text{Male CV death rate for ages 55–74 in 1969-73}}{\text{Male CV death rate for ages 45–64 in 1958-64}}$$

This enables the increases in cardiovascular mortality over the 10 year period for approximately the same population of men (who have of course aged 10 years during this period) to be related to the changes in hardness.

From the data in Figure 4 there is a significant association ($P = .01$) such that there is an estimated 8.1% reduction in mortality (standard error 3.1%) for an increase in hardness of 1.0 mmol/l. However, the equivalent results for females, shown in Figure 5, indicate no association between changes in hardness in the range up to 1.7 mmol/l and changes in cardiovascular mortality.

These conclusions were confirmed when allowance was made for changes in two socio-economic factors (% manual workers and % unemployed). Whilst the

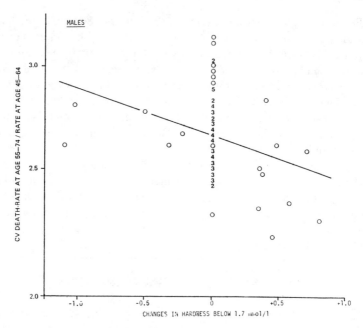

FIGURE 4. Changes in cardiovascular death rates and water hardness (1961–1971) for male cohorts in 76 county boroughs in England and Wales.

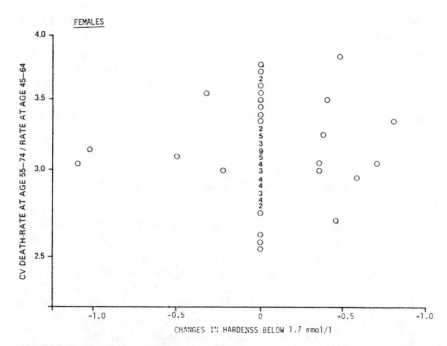

FIGURE 5. Changes in cardiovascular death rates and water hardness (1961–1971) for female cohorts in 76 county boroughs in England and Wales.

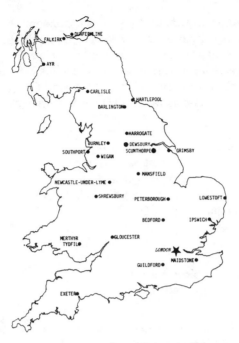

FIGURE 6. The 24 towns in Phase 2, the field study of 7735 men aged 40–59.

size of the water hardness association in men agrees with the results of Phase 1, the result for women does not. Overall, however, the results from this 'natural experiment' are consistent with the possibility of a weak negative association between water hardness and cardiovascular mortality.

PHASE 2: A FIELD SURVEY
IN 24 TOWNS—METHODS

In order to properly understand the causes of regional variations in cardiovascular disease it is important to have information on the geographic variation in established personal risk factors (e.g., smoking, blood pressure and blood lipids) as well as social and environmental factors. Accordingly, Phase 2 of the Regional Heart Study is a large scale field survey of individuals in different regions of Britain. *Men aged 40–59 were randomly selected from representative general practices in 24 British towns, a total of 7735 men in all.* Shaper et al. (1981) provide full details of the selection of towns, general practices and the methods of screening, so only a brief summary of methods will be provided.

Figure 6 shows the 24 towns which were chosen to represent the variations in cardiovascular mortality and water hardness previously shown in Figure 2. Towns were mostly of size 50–100,000 population and large conurbations were excluded. Every effort was made to ensure that the chosen group general practice in each town would adequately represent the social structure of the

117

town. Around 400–450 men aged 40–59 were randomly selected from each practice's age-sex register and overall 78% of men attended for screening. Thus, the 7735 men screened provide an average of 320 men per town which should be sufficient to characterize the variations in risk factors between towns.

The survey took place during 1978–80. A team of three nurses spent two weeks in each town obtaining the following *information from each man*:

> questionnaire including medical history
> > chest pain symptoms
> > employment history
> > smoking, alcohol, diet, exercise
>
> three-lead computerized ECG
> blood pressure
> height and weight
> lung function
> blood samples for biochemistry/haematology
> Bortner attitude questionnaire

Necessary quality control procedures were undertaken to ensure reliable collection and measurement of each item.

In addition, a survey team from the Water Research Centre undertook to collect *samples of water from the kitchen tap in the homes of 40 representative men in each town* (i.e., around 12% of each town's sample of screened men, a total of 960 men in all).

This cross-sectional study of a large representative sample of British middle-aged men has provided valuable information on a variety of topics including:

> prevalence of ischaemic heart disease, Shaper et al. (1984)
> unemployment and health, Cook et al. (1982)
> lead in blood and drinking water, Pocock et al. (1983)
> alcohol and smoking, Cummins et al. (1983)
> blood pressure and its determinants, Shaper et al. (1981)
> blood lipids and their determinants, Thelle et al. (1983)

In addition, *Phase 3* of the Regional Heart Study is a *prospective study* in which all 7735 men are being followed for cardiovascular events (both fatal and non-fatal). Preliminary results relating personal risk factors to subsequent major ischaemic heart disease will appear shortly. Thus, in a sense the Regional Heart Study is a British equivalent of the Framingham study, except that it is studying men from 24 communities rather than the single-community approach that characterizes most prospective studies of cardiovascular disease.

This geographical component of the study forms the basis for the following new results relating *between-town differences in the prevalence and mortality from ischaemic heart disease (IHD) to between-town differences in water quality and personal risk factors*. The focus is now ischaemic heart disease since for men under age 65 this is by far the most common form of cardiovascular disease.

First, we need to define the town measures of disease, water quality and risk factors to be employed.

IHD mortality. For each of the 24 towns we have used the number of deaths from IHD (ICD code 410–414) for men aged 35–64 for the years 1979-1982 and population at the 1981 census, both in 10-year age groups. We have compared these data with national age-specific death rates for IHD in order to derive a Standardised Mortality Ratio (SMR) for IHD in men aged 35–64 in each town. These SMRs range from 71 in Ipswich to 135 in Ayr. These mortality data are based on reorganized local authority areas some of which are substantially larger than the original towns selected for the Phase 2 field study. However, such expansion into contiguous areas is unlikely to distort the SMRs.

Prevalence of IHD. Each man in the survey was declared to have evidence of IHD prevalence if he had either:

1. ECG evidence of myocardial infarction or ischaemia or
2. questionnaire evidence of severe chest pain (possible myocardial infarction) or chest pain on exertion (angina).

Shaper et al. (1984) give further details of these definitions. We here use the percentage of men in each town thus defined as having prevalent IHD, which ranges from 17% in Lowestoft to 31% in Merthyr Tydfil.

Thus, IHD mortality relates to the whole population of middle-aged men in each town whereas IHD prevalence is derived from the 300 or so men screened in the field survey.

Water quality measures. The tap water samples from the 40 men in each town have been used to provide arithmetic means for the 34 water measurements listed in Table 1. We have used the *"first draw"* water samples collected first thing in the morning. Similar results were also obtained for random daytime and flushed samples, except for values of lead, zinc and copper which tended to be higher in first draw samples. However, it was thought the use of first draw samples would give a more reliable estimate of between-town differences in these trace elements.

Risk factors. It was decided to concentrate on those risk factors which are

TABLE 1
Tap Water Measurements Recorded for 40 Men in Each Town

Alkalinity	Conductivity	Potassium
Aluminium	Copper	Silicon
Barium	Iron	Silver
Berrylium	Lead	Sodium
Bismuth	Lithium	Strontium
Boron	Magnesium	Sulphate
Cadmium	Manganese	Titanium
Calcium	Molybdenum	Total hardness
Chloride	Nickel	Total organic carbon
Chromium	Nitrate	Vanadium
Cobalt	pH	Zinc
		Zirconium

well-established as being associated with individual risk of IHD. Accordingly, for the 300 or so men in each town *means* of the following *quantitative risk factors* were calculated:

> systolic blood pressure
> diastolic blood pressure
> serum total cholesterol
> HDL-cholesterol
> body mass index (weight/height^2)

Qualitative risk factors were included by calculating the *percentage of men* in each town with each of the following characteristics:

> smoking—% currently smoking cigarettes
> social class—% employed in manual occupations.

PHASE 2: A FIELD SURVEY
IN 24 TOWNS—RESULTS

Ischaemic Heart Disease and Water Hardness. The association between *IHD mortality (1979-82)* and *water hardness* is shown in Figure 7. For these 24 towns the negative association remains highly significant ($r = -.51$, $P < .001$), though it is somewhat weaker than 10 years before. However, this is largely attributable to the fact that Hartlepool, the town with the hardest water supply, has an increased SMR compared with 10 years previously. With this exception, it can be seen that towns with the SMR for IHD above 120 have very soft water supplies.

The association between IHD prevalence and water hardness is shown in Figure 8. Again a highly significant negative association exists, $r = -.46$. This is not unexpected since the two IHD measures, the SMR and the % prevalence, are two different attempts to characterize the underlying risk of IHD for men in each town, which are highly correlated ($r = +.72$) but each subject to random fluctuations.

Ischaemic Heart Disease and Other Water Parameters. Of the 34 water parameters listed in Table 1, six have significant associations with IHD mortality and prevalence as indicated by the correlation coefficients in Table 2.

Alkalinity and water *calcium* are so highly correlated with total hardness that their potential contributions to IHD mortality are statistically inseparable. In fact, water calcium has a slightly higher negative correlation with IHD mortality ($r = -.60$) which is explained by magnesium's lack of correlation with IHD mortality, $r = -.03$. In this respect, the British situation seems to differ from that in North America where some studies, e.g., Neri and Johansen (1978) in Canada, have found magnesium to be more strongly associated with cardiovascular mortality than calcium.

The positive association of water *lead* with IHD mortality and prevalence can be examined further since we also have blood lead measured on all 300 or so men in each town. The correlations of mean blood lead with IHD mortality and prevalence are $+.32$ and $+.37$ respectively. Thus, the correlation is not improved by using this more direct measure of lead exposure on the larger

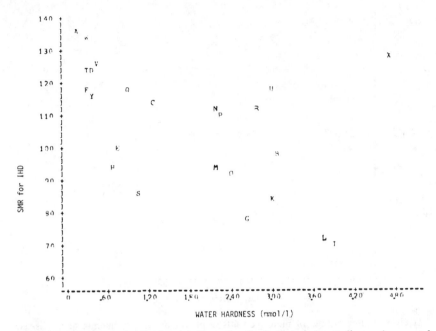

FIGURE 7. The standardized mortality ratios for ischaemic heart disease (men aged 35–64) plotted against mean water hardness in 24 towns.

A = Ayr	I = Ipswich	Q = Darlington
B = Bedford	K = Maidstone	R = Grimsby
C = Carlisle	L = Lowestoft	S = Shrewsbury
D = Dewsbury	M = Mansfield	T = Merthyr Tydfil
E = Exeter	N = Newcastle-	U = Scunthorpe
F = Falkirk	under-Lyme	V = Dunfermline
G = Guildford	O = Gloucester	W = Wigan
H = Harrogate	P = Southport	X = Hartlepool
		Y = Burnley

group of men per town. This suggests that the water lead association may not be causal. However, more powerful data will eventually be available from studies of blood lead in individual cases of IHD in the prospective phase of the Regional Heart Study.

Water *potassium* concentrations had the strongest negative association with IHD mortality and prevalence. However, water potassium is highly correlated with water hardness ($r = +.81$) and water potassium intake is only a small fraction of the total dietary potassium. Also, water sodium had no significant association with IHD mortality and prevalence ($r = -.14$ and $-.24$ respectively). Thus, there is no real evidence here of a role for the potassium/sodium ratio in the aetiology of IHD.

Negative associations also exist between water *silicon* concentrations and IHD mortality and prevalence. As with potassium, water silicon and water hardness are also highly correlated ($r = +.68$). This potential role of water

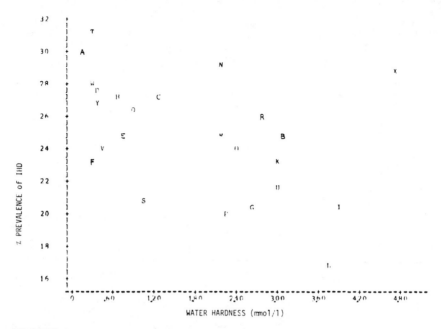

FIGURE 8. Percentage of men aged 40–59 prevalent with ischaemic heart disease plotted against mean water hardness in 24 towns.

silicon is supported by studies in the United States, Schroeder (1966), and Finland, Schwarz et al. (1977). Again, however, water silicon contributes little to the total dietary intake.

Overall, there are no particularly convincing biological explanations for any single factor in Table 2 to be claimed as the causative agent in water quality associations with IHD. Because of their high degree of correlation with water hardness, it may be more sensible to consider these five factors as being different manifestations of an underlying relationship between IHD mortality and water hardness.

TABLE 2
Correlations of several water parameters with IHD
mortality, IHD prevalence and water hardness (24 towns)

	IHD mortality	IHD prevalence	mean water hardness
mean alkalinity	− .48	− .44	+ .97
calcium	− .60	− .54	+ .96
lead	+ .43	+ .39	− .37
potassium	− .67	− .52	+ .81
silicon	− .64	− .55	+ .68
hardness	− .51	− .46	

Ischaemic Heart Disease and Risk Factors. It is well established that certain risk factors (e.g., cigarette smoking, high blood pressure, raised serum total cholesterol) are strongly associated with the risk of IHD in individual men. From this evidence in individuals, it is sensible to investigate whether these same risk factors are associated with the geographic variation in IHD mortality and prevalence. Accordingly, Table 3 shows the correlations of IHD mortality and prevalence with several risk factors (each summarized on a town basis by either means or percentages in 300 or so men).

Evidently, IHD mortality and prevalence both tend to be higher in towns with a higher percentage of cigarette smokers, a higher mean blood pressure (systolic and diastolic), and a higher percentage of manual workers. Serum total cholesterol, though a very powerful risk factor in individual men, is not associated with geographic variations in IHD mortality and prevalence. This may be because the British diet does not exhibit any radical differences between areas, particularly as regards the contribution and composition of fat in the diet. Indeed, some would argue that the British diet is uniformly lethal in all areas of the country! Similarly, HDL-cholesterol and body mass index do not appear to contribute to geographic variations in IHD. The curious positive association of HDL-cholesterol and IHD prevalence, where a negative association might have been expected, may be due to the fact that areas of high IHD (i.e., Scotland and the north of England) tend to have a higher alcohol consumption which would elevate HDL-cholesterol.

In order to explore further the key findings in Table 3, scatter plots of IHD mortality by percentage cigarette smokers, mean systolic blood pressure and percentage manual workers are shown in Figures 9, 10 and 11. Each of these factors shows a marked geographic variation, which not surprisingly is followed by an increasing trend in IHD mortality.

Table 3 also shows the correlation of each risk factor with water hardness. The three key factors smoking, systolic blood pressure and % manual workers are only weakly associated with water hardness. Nevertheless, it is sensible to see if the association of water hardness with IHD mortality and prevalence shown in Figures 7 and 8 is reduced after allowance for these three factors. In fact, the

TABLE 3
Correlations of risk factors with IHD mortality,
IHD prevalence and water hardness in 24 towns

	IHD mortality	IHD prevalence	water hardness
% smoking cigarettes	+ .59	+ .42	− .22
% manual workers	+ .54	+ .35	.00
mean systolic blood pressure	+ .60	+ .47	− .13
mean diastolic blood pressure	+ .53	+ .49	− .17
mean serum total cholesterol	− .22	− .07	− .33
mean HDL-cholesterol	+ .06	+ .42	− .44
mean body mass index	+ .14	+ .18	.00

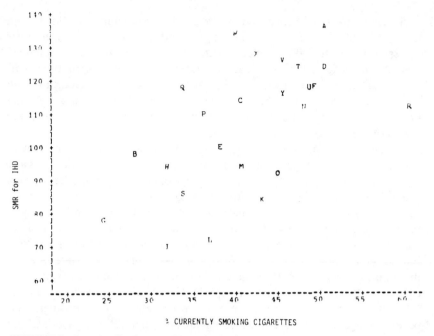

FIGURE 9. Standardized mortality ratio for ischaemic heart disease plotted against percentage of men currently smoking cigarettes in 24 towns.

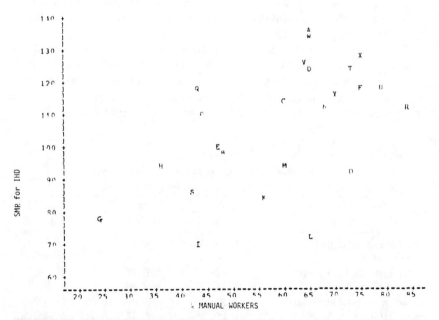

FIGURE 10. Standardized mortality ratio for ischaemic heart disease plotted against mean systolic blood pressure for men in 24 towns.

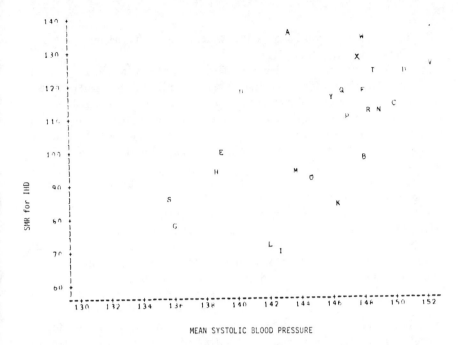

FIGURE 11. Standardized mortality ratio for ischaemic heart disease plotted against percentage of manual workers in 24 towns.

partial correlation of water hardness with IHD mortality and prevalence (adjusting for these three factors) are −.57 and −.41 which are similar to the crude correlations in Table 2. Hence, *the association of water hardness with IHD appears to be largely independent of the geographic variation in personal risk factors*, at least in this British study of 7735 middle-aged men in 24 towns.

DISCUSSION AND PRACTICAL IMPLICATIONS

The association of cardiovascular disease with water hardness and other water quality parameters has received considerable attention in Britain over the past 25 years. A recent review of the British "water story" is provided by Shaper (1984). Also Packham et al. (1982) provide a fuller discussion of the practical implications of recent research.

The findings from the British Regional Heart Study presented in this paper have shown that the 'water story' cannot be explained away by other confounding factors whether these be environmental, social or personal risk factors.

Perhaps the most important practical contribution has been to estimate the magnitude of the water hardness/CV mortality association. From results in section 2 it appears that very soft water areas may have a cardiovascular mortality excess of the order of 10% after allowance for climatic and social factors. Since personal risk factors are not substantially associated with water hardness (section 5) this estimate from Phase 1 remains the most valid attempt to quantify the impact of soft water on cardiovascular mortality. The results of

IHD prevalence in section 5 suggest that water hardness has a similar strength of association with non-fatal IHD.

In assessing the practical relevance of water hardness in the aetiology of cardiovascular disease it is important to recognize that certain personal risk factors exert a far greater influence on risk. For instance, cigarette smokers have about three times the risk (i.e., a 200% excess risk) of myocardial infarction compared with non-smokers. Also, middle-aged men with moderate elevations in blood pressure (e.g., systolic hypertension over 160 mm Hg) have at least double the risk (i.e., a 100% excess risk) of myocardial infarction, compared with men having lower blood pressures. This impact of high blood pressure is even greater for cerebrovascular disease.

Thus, although the 'water story' appears to be a genuine phenomenon, at least in Great Britain, it appears to have assumed a greater importance than it merits. As regards prevention policy for cardiovascular disease, far greater rewards could be achieved by changes in the smoking behaviour of the population, better control of high blood pressure and the adoption of a prudent diet.

However, one could argue that soft water is a rather different kind of potential risk factor in that it affects whole communities and cannot be declared the responsibility of the individual. Hence, even though it is not making a major impact on cardiovascular disease, do we still have a community responsibility to act?

Though the costs of hardening water supplies are substantial (Packham et al., 1982) the main argument put forward for not undertaking artificial hardening of soft water supplies is that it is still far from clear whether soft water actually *causes* an increase in cardiovascular disease. The statistical evidence inevitably rests on "ecological studies" which are well known as being a weak epidemiological method which cannot by itself provide sound evidence of a causal mechanism. Hence it would be unwise to invest in large-scale water hardening programs, the full health consequences of which are poorly understood. At the same time it would seem prudent not to undertake artificial softening of drinking water supplies below certain levels. In the European community this may well be secured by a proposed directive setting a limit of 1.5 mmol/l below which municipal supplies may not be softened.

ACKNOWLEDGEMENTS

The British Regional Heart Study is supported by a programme grant from the Medical Research Council. Work carried out by the Water Research Centre is supported by the Department of the Environment. We are grateful to Dr. Deborah Ashby and Mrs. Mary Walker for their valuable contributions in data analysis and preparation.

REFERENCES

COOK, D.G., BARTLEY, M.J., and CUMMINS, R.O. (1982). Health of unemployed middle-aged men in Great Britain. Lancet I:1290-4.

CRAWFORD, M.D., GARDNER, M.J., and MORRIS, J.N. (1968). Mortality and hardness of local water supplies. Lancet I:827.

CUMMINS, R.O., SHAPER, A.G., WALKER, M., and WALE, C.J. (1981). Smoking and drinking by middle-aged British men: effects of social class and town of residence. Br Med J 283:1497–1502.

LACEY, R.F. (1981). Changes in water hardness and cardiovascular death-rates. Water Research Centre Technical Report TR171.

LACEY, R.F., and SHAPER, A.G. (1984). Changes in water hardness and cardiovascular death rates. Int J Epidemiology 134:18–24.

MORRIS, J.N., CRAWFORD, M.D., and HEADY, J.A. (1961). Hardness of local water supplies and mortality from cardiovascular disease. Lancet I:860.

NERI, L.C., and JOHANSEN, H.L. (1978). Water hardness and cardiovascular mortality. Ann. NY Acad. Sci. 304:203–19.

PACKHAM, R.F., LACEY, R.F., POWELL, P., SHAPER, A.G., and POCOCK, S.J. (1982). Drinking water quality and cardiovascular disease-practical implications of recent research. Water Bulletin. 34:Nov 19 (Supplement).

POCOCK, S.J., SHAPER A.G., COOK, D.G., PACKHAM, R.F., LACEY, R.F., POWELL, P., and RUSSELL, P.F. (1980). British Regional Heart Study: geographic variations in cardiovascular mortality and the role of water quality. Br. Med. J 280:1243–9.

POCOCK, S.J., COOK, D.G., and SHAPER, A.G. (1982). Analysing geographic variation in cardiovascular mortality: methods and results. J. Roy. Statist. Soc. A 145:313–41.

POCOCK, S.J., SHAPER, A.G., WALKER, M., WALE, C.J., CLAYTON, B., DELVES, T., LACEY, R.F., PACKHAM, R.F., and POWELL, P. (1983). Effects of tap water lead, water hardness, alcohol, and cigarettes on blood lead concentrations. J. Epid. and Comm. Health 37:1–7.

POWELL, P., PACKHAM, R.F., LACEY, R.F., RUSSELL, P.F., SHAPER, A.G., POCOCK, S.J., and COOK, D.G. (1982). Water quality and cardiovascular disease in British towns. Water Research Centre Technical Report; TR 178.

SCHROEDER, H.A. (1966). Municipal drinking water and cardiovascular death rates. JAMA 195:81–5.

SCHWARZ, K., PUNSAR, S., RICCI, B.A., and KARVONEN, M.J. (1977). Inverse relation of Si in drinking water an atherosclerosis in Finland. Lancet I:538–9.

SHAPER, A.G., PACKHAM, R.F., and POCOCK, S.J. (1980). The British Regional Heart Study: cardiovascular mortality and water quality. J. Env. Path. and Toxic 4:89–111.

SHAPER, A.G., POCOCK, S.J., WALKER, M., COHEN, N.M., WALE, C.J., and Thomson, A.G. (1981). British Regional Heart Study: cardiovascular risk factors in middle-aged men in 24 towns. Br Med. J 283:179–86.

SHAPER, A.G. (1984). Geographic variations in cardiovascular mortality in Great Britain. Br Med Bulletin 40:366–373.

SHAPER, A.G., COOK, D.G., WALKER, M. and MACFARLANE, P.W. (1984). The prevalence of ischaemic heart disease in middle-aged British men. Br Heart J 51:595–605.

THELLE, D.S., SHAPER, A.G., WHITEHEAD, T.P., BULLOCK, D.G., ASHBY, D., and PATEL, I. (1983). Blood lipids in middle-aged British men. Br Heart J 49:205–13.

CHAPTER XIII

W.H.O. STUDIES ON WATER HARDNESS AND CARDIOVASCULAR DISEASES

R. Masironi
World Health Organization, Geneva, Switzerland

ABSTRACT

Evidence from many epidemiological studies shows that hardness of drinking water is inversely associated with cardiovascular mortality. Although it has not yet been possible to establish a cause to effect relationship, the existence of an association with mortality cannot be dismissed. The mechanism of action is not understood. The significance of the association is critically reviewed. Further research on this topic may not be justified.

INTRODUCTION

Perhaps the first evidence of an association between human health and water composition was presented by Kobayashi (1957) who found that, in Japan, death rates from cerebrovascular haemorrhage were positively correlated with the SO_4/CO_3 content, which is an indicator of the acidity of the river waters in the various districts of that country. After Kobayashi, a number of investigators (Anderson et al., 1975; Crawford et al., 1971; Masironi et al., 1979; Schroeder, 1966; Stitt et al., 1973) in several other countries have reported negative relationships between the hardness of drinking water and mortality, particularly from cardiovascular diseases. Areas served by relatively hard waters were characterized by a lower death rate from arteriosclerotic and coronary heart disease (CHD), from hypertensive heart disease or sudden coronary deaths.

The negative associations were best evident in studies that covered very wide geographical areas and involved large numbers of people. Smaller studies which compared, for instance, different districts within the same town, or counties within the same state or province, or which compared a few cities among themselves, often produced inconsistent results (Bierenbaum et al., 1975; Keil, 1979; Meyers and Williams, 1977). Some of these small-scale studies, which initially failed to show any clear association, were later expanded by the same or other authors and the usual negative relationship between water hardness and cardiovascular mortality appeared. (Keil, 1979; Mulcahy, 1966; Winton and McCabe, 1970).

Of course, studies in such relatively small geographic areas are likely to be influenced by the small population size, by population mobility and by factors such as the use of water softeners in homes.

Many investigators dealt with treated municipal water supplies, but others (Kobayashi, 1957; Masironi, 1970; Masironi et al., 1976) analyzed raw river waters and showed associations between geochemical factors and human health.

Within the framework of its Cardiovascular Diseases Programme, WHO has also investigated the relationship between water hardness and cardiovascular diseases in various countries. These investigations will be summarized here.

A W.H.O. study of 15 European cities (Masironi et al., 1979) revealed a negative association between hardness of municipal water supplies and incidence of heart attacks, both in males and females. Another study (Masironi, 1970) examined the cardiovascular mortality rates in populations living along four rivers in the U.S. having different levels of water hardness, namely the Ohio, Missouri, Colorado and Columbia rivers. Mortality rates from hypertensive heart disease and, less markedly, from arteriosclerotic heart disease were significantly lower in the populations living along the hard-water Colorado and Missouri rivers than in the populations living along the soft-water Columbia and Ohio rivers. The non-cardiovascular mortality rates did not differ in the four areas.

Neither in Japan (Kobayashi, 1957) nor in the U.S. do people drink raw water as it is, but primitive communities which live in relatively isolated areas with very little exposure to industrialization are more likely to be in a close relationship with the geochemical environment. One such community was studied in New Guinea by a WHO team and blood pressure was measured in the inhabitants of eleven villages located along the Wogupmeri river. The villagers subsist on a non-cash economy and drink the river water as it is. The main calcium concentration of the water decreases downstream from about 8 to about 3 ppm as the river flows away from the limestone mountains where it originates. Contrary to this trend of decreasing calcium content in water, the mean of the blood pressure measurements was found to increase from 97 to 110 mm/Hg. (Masironi et al., 1976).

The WHO studies are in line with many other reports on the negative association between water hardness and cardiovascular diseases. However, no single water component has ever been found to be clearly associated with water hardness on the one hand, and disease or health on the other. Calcium, magnesium, chromium, fluorine, lithium and other elements present in hard water have been alternatively hypothesized as exerting a beneficial effect on cardiovascular health. Cadmium and lead dissolved from the pipes by soft water have been, instead, considered harmful.

The mechanism of action has not been ascertained. The specificity of the reported association between water hardness and cardiovascular diseases is not very high, either. Numerous other diseases and causes of death have been found to be occasionally associated with water hardness, some of them as strongly and negatively correlated as cardiovascular disease. This was the situation for cancer, liver cirrhosis, peptic ulcer, urinary stone formation, bronchitis and even infant mortality (Churchill et al., 1980; Crawford et al., 1972; Roberts, 1976). However, these associations did not have the degree of repeatability and the geographic consistency with water hardness that the large scale cardiovascular epidemiology studies have shown.

Water hardness is a geographical variable and it varies according to broad geographical patterns. However, other factors also vary in a similar manner and this prevents an understanding of the association.

For instance, it has been suggested that the regional variation in cardiovascular mortality rates may be accounted for in terms of climatic conditions. In the British studies (Crawford et al., 1972), water hardness is related to both temperature and rainfall, and both temperatures and rainfall are related to cardiovascular death rates, but not as strongly as water calcium is. This suggests that the rainfall and temperature really add little, if anything, to the prediction of cardiovascular mortality rates.

In the W.H.O. survey of fifteen European cities mentioned above, a strong relationship between the frequency of myocardial infarction and latitude has been reported (Masironi et al., 1979). The incidence rates of myocardial infarction were higher and water was softer at more northerly latitudes. The relationship was consistent with the myocardial infarction rates, doubling for each 15° of latitude.

The relationship between water hardness and latitude arises from the geological trends across the continents. In Europe, northern countries with a higher cardiovascular death rate are underlain by very old geological substrata (Masironi, 1979). These are poor sources of minerals essential to life, and the waters are soft. In Europe, this pattern occurs in a north to south direction, but a similar association of higher cardiovascular mortality with lower levels of trace elements in soils and water is present in the U.S. in an east to west direction (Masironi, 1979; Shacklette et al., 1972). Latitude, therefore, does not seem to play the same role in cardiovascular mortality in northern Europe and in North America, whereas water hardness shows a more consistent type of inverse relationship with cardiovascular mortality in both continents.

Many of the inconsistent epidemiological findings could be attributed to inadequate experimental design, e.g., the population groups under study were too small, the range of water hardness was too narrow, adequate control populations were lacking, etc. Another source of potential mis-classification is the insufficient knowledge about the proportion of daily water intake that comes from the tap. Bottled water is drunk quite extensively in many areas. Additional problems arise if a considerable proportion of the residences are equipped with water softening devices. It is also possible that the negative association between water hardness and cardiovascular diseases is not a linear one, or it may be present only within a certain hardness range. This fact alone could account for many discordant results.

At this point, the question arises as to whether these studies on the relationship between water hardness and cardiovascular diseases should be continued. In 1971, a group of experts met at W.H.O. and their recommendation was that "water quality studies in relation to cardiovascular diseases should be particularly encouraged." Another group of experts met again in Geneva in 1973 and recommended that "W.H.O. should consider suggesting to appropriate national authorities that they pay increased attention to the problem of cardiovascular mortality in relation to the softness of drinking water, and should ask its Member States to supply information on any proposed changes to be made in the quality of water supplied to a large city or area." Evidently, at that time, the outlook was promising and investigators were optimistic.

The recommendations of a European Symposium on Hardness of Drinking Water and Public Health, which was held in Luxembourg in 1975 under the auspices of the Commission of the European Communities, as well as another W.H.O. meeting, again emphasized the need for further research on the relationship between water hardness and human health (Commission of European Communities, 1976; World Health Organization, 1979).

Many years have passed now and many studies have been carried out. Some of them, like the British Regional Heart Study (Pocock et al., 1980) are very comprehensive. These studies, however, have failed to provide a better knowledge of the association between water hardness and cardiovascular diseases, with respect to the knowledge which had alredy been acquired with the pioneer work of Kobayashi, Crawford, Schroeder and other investigators in the sixties and early seventies.

Even the last Conference that was held in Amherst, and other Conferences (Water Research Center, 1976) have failed to provide insight into the controversial association between water hardness and cardiovascular diseases. It seems that research in this field has now reached a point of diminishing returns. With research money badly needed in other important areas, it is doubtful that massive financial support and manpower would still be justified for research on the association between hard water and cardiovascular diseases. At W.H.O. this type of research has been abandoned.

REFERENCES

ANDERSON, T.W., NERI, L.C., SCHREIBER, G.B., TALBOT, F.D.F. and ZDRO-JEWSKI, A. (1975). Ischemic heart disease, water hardness and myocardial magnesium. Can. Med. Assoc. J. 113:199–203.

BIERENBAUM, M.L., FLEISCHMAN, A.I., DUNN, J.P. and ARNOLD, J. (1975). Possible toxic water factor in coronary heart disease. Lancet 1:1008–10.

CHURCHILL, D.N., MALONEY, C.M., BEAR, J., BRYANT, D.G., FODOR, G., GAULT, M.H. (1980). Urolithiasis—A study of drinking water hardness and genetic factors. J. Chron. Dis. 33:727–31.

COMMISSION OF THE EUROPEAN COMMUNITIES. (1976). Hardness of drinking water and public health. Report of a symposium, Luxembourg, 1975, 553 pp, (R. Amavis, W.J. Hunter, J.G.P.M. Smeets, eds). Oxford, Pergamon Press.

CRAWFORD, M.D. (1972). Hardness of drinking water and cardiovascular disease. Proc. Nutr. Soc. 31:347–53.

CRAWFORD, M.D., GARDNER, M.J., SEDGWICK, P.A. (1972). Infant mortality and hardness of local water supplies. Lancet 1:988–92.

KEIL, U. (1979). Geomedizine in Forschung und Lehre. In *Geographische Zeitschrift*. Beitrage zur Geoökologie des Menschen. Weisbaden: F. Steiner Verlag, 76 pp.

KOBAYASHI, J. (1957). On geographical relationship between the chemical nature of river and death-rate from apoplexy. Ber. Ohara Inst. Landwirtsch. Biol. **11**:12–21.

MASIRONI, R. (1970). Cardiovascular mortality in relation to radioactivity and hardness of local water supplies in the U.S.A. Bull. World Health Org. **43**:687–97.

MASIRONI, R. (1979). Geochemistry and cardiovascular diseases. Phil. Trans. Royal Soc. London Sec. B **288**:193–203.

MASIRONI, R., KOIRTYOHANN, S.R., PIERCE, J.O. and SCHAMSCHULA, R.G. (1976). Calcium content of river water, trace element concentrations in toenails, and blood pressure in village populations in New Guinea. Sci. Total Envir. **6**:41–53.

MASIRONI, R., PISA, Z. and CLAYTON, D. (1979). Myocardial infarction and water hardness in the WHO myocardial infarction registry network. Bull. World Health Org. **57**:291–99.

MEYERS, D.H. and WILLIAMS, G. (1977). Mortality from all causes and from ischemic heart disease in Australian capital cities. Med. J. Aust. **2**:504–06.

MULCAHY, R. (1966). The influence of water hardness and rainfall on cardiovascular and cerebrovascular mortality. J. Ir. Med. Assoc. **59**:14–15.

POCOCK, S.J., SHAPER, A.G., COOK, D.G., PACKHAM, R.F., LACEY, R.F., POWELL, P. and RUSSELL, P.F. (1980). British regional heart study: geographic variation in cardiovascular mortality, and the role of water quality. Br. Med. Jr. **280**:1243–49.

ROBERTS, C.J. (1976). Commission of the European Communities, 1976. *Hardness of drinking water and public health*. Report of a Symposium, Luxembourg, 1975, 553 pp.

SCHROEDER, H.A. (1966). Hardness of local water supplies and mortality from cardiovascular disease. Lancet **1**:1171.

SHACKLETTE, H.T., HAMILTON, J.C., BOERNGEN, J.C. and BOWLES, J.W. (1971). Elemental composition of surficial materials in the coterminous United States. U.S. Geol. Surv. Prof. Pap. No. 574-D. Washington, D.C., U.S. Govt. Printing Office.

STITT, F.W., CLAYTON, D.G., CRAWFORD, M.D. and MORRIS, J.N. (1973). Clinical and biochemical indicators of cardiovascular diseases among men living in hard and soft water areas. Lancet **1**:122–26.

WATER RESEARCH CENTRE. (1976). Drinking water quality and public health. Medmenham Laboratory, Medmenham, Marlow, Bucks., U.K.

WINTON, E.F. and MC CABE, L.J. (1970). Studies relating to water mineralization and health. J. Am. Water Works Assoc. **63**:26–30.

WORLD HEALTH ORGANIZATION. (1979). Health effects of the removal of substances occurring naturally in drinking water with special reference to demineralized and desalinated water. Rep. Working Group, Brussels, 20-23 Mar. 1978, EUR Rep. Studies, 16, Copenhagen, 24 pp.

CHAPTER XIV

DRINKING WATER INORGANICS AND CARDIOVASCULAR DISEASE: A CASE-CONTROL STUDY AMONG WISCONSIN FARMERS

E.A. Zeighami,* M.D. Morris,† E.E. Calle,*
P.S. McSweeny,‡ and B.A. Schuknecht‡
*Health and Safety Research Division
†Engineering Physics and Mathematics Division
Oak Ridge National Laboratory
Oak Ridge, Tennessee 37831

‡Wisconsin State Laboratory of Hygiene
State of Wisconsin
University of Wisconsin
Madison, Wisconsin 53706

ABSTRACT

A case-control study of Wisconsin farmers has examined the relationship of coronary artery disease death or cerebrovascular disease death to levels of 19 inorganic parameters in drinking water. The study included 505 cases and 854 controls, all of whom obtained their drinking water from an individual non-chlorinated well on the farm. Drinking water of cases was significantly softer than that of controls. Differences between the two groups were limited to the range of total hardness below 200 mg/L. The relationships were as strong or stronger when respondents reporting artificial softening were removed. A variety of potential confounders of the relationship were examined, and none were found to explain the difference in hardness in the two groups. Drinking water of cases also had significantly lower carbonate hardness (alkalinity). Of the metals, cadmium, lead, and zinc levels were significantly higher for cases. Levels of iron, copper, manganese, nitrate, sodium, and fluoride were not different in the two groups. The levels of cadmium and lead in the water were extremely low, and the significant difference between the groups was limited to the percentage of samples with values above analytic detection limits.

INTRODUCTION

The possibility that intake of trace and bulk elements in food and water may contribute to cardiovascular system change has been examined in a variety of ways for some time. The elements present in food and water which had received the most attention are calcium, magnesium, cadmium, lead, and sodium. Other trace elements (e.g., selenium, lithium, copper, zinc, chromium, manganese) have been suggested as having either a beneficial or deleterious effect to the cardiovascular system.

There is substantial evidence that both cadmium and lead ingestion can produce hypertension in experimental animals (Sharrett, 1979; Saltman, 1983; Ohanian et al., 1980). Cadmium intake can produce hypertension in rats at levels which are approaching environmental exposure levels for humans (Kopp et al., 1982). Calcium deficiency and magnesium deficiency enhance the effect of either cadmium or lead on the hypertensionogenic animal (Sandstead, 1979; Revis et al., 1979).

Elements present in drinking water are also present in food, often in considerably larger quantities. Bioavailability of some of the elements from food and water may not be comparable. In addition, food cooked in water acquires some of the elemental content of the water (Haring, 1981).

Studies in humans of intake of inorganic elements and cardiovascular diseases have generally concentrated on drinking water intake for several reasons. An estimate of intake over a period of time can often be made more meaningfully for drinking water than for food. The existence of public regulatory standards for inorganics in drinking water have also created a focus on that route.

Historically, evidence for a relationship between inorganics in water has arisen from geographic correlation studies of regional averages of water constituents and death rates for various cardiovascular disease categories. Overall, soft water areas have higher cardiovascular disease death rates than hard water areas. Hardness of water is defined by total calcium and magnesium content. Several authors have reviewed the evidence regarding the various aspects of the "water story" (Comstock, 1979; Sharrett, 1979; Neri et al., 1974). Evidence from individual studies is scarce. Comstock et al. (1980) conducted a prospective study of residents of Washington County, Maryland, using death with arteriosclerotic heart disease as an endpoint and water hardness estimates based on water samples from private taps. There was no clear evidence of an association between water hardness and arteriosclerotic heart disease death rates.

The existence of a statistical association between water hardness and cardiovascular disease death rates is established. Whether a causal relationship exists between some set of water constituents and some form of cardiovascular disease is much more debatable. If such a relationship exists, the true causal factors may not be hardness (or a constituent of hardness) but other water element(s) present in greater quantities in soft water. The present report presents results from a case-control study of Wisconsin male farmers in which the drinking water content of persons dying with coronary artery disease (ICD8 410-414) or cerebrovascular disease (ICD8 430-438) was compared to the content of drinking water drawn from control farms.

METHODS

Cases were ascertained by monitoring of death certificates in the state of Wisconsin for certificates which met the criteria that at least one cause of death was coronary artery disease or arteriosclerotic cardiovascular disease, and that the occupation listed on the death certificate was farmer. The next of kin was contacted by mail during the period of time 2-3 months after the date of death. The mailing included two 250-ml polyethylene sampling bottles, one pH vial, and a respondent questionnaire. For each non-coroner certified death identified through death certificate screening, the certifying physician was asked by mail to provide more detailed information on cardiovascular disease history and causes of death. Persons for whom the physician did not verify a cardiovascular disease cause of death were excluded. However, persons for whom a physician questionnaire was not received were retained in the study and causes of death were assumed to be those on the death certificate. A total of 259 of the 396 non-coroner certified cases (65 percent) had physician verification of causes of death and a cardiovascular disease history.

Respondent questionnaires were completed by telephone interview with the spouse (wife) for both case and control series. In instances for which a telephone interview could not be arranged, the respondent mailed in a completed questionnaire. The questionnaire included questions verifying occupation, place and length of residence, time spent working off the farm, smoking, diet (principally intake of fatty foods), liquid intake, some medical history, water sources, use of water-softening equipment, and type of farm.

Controls were selected from the Brucellosis Testing List maintained by the state of Wisconsin and updated yearly. All farms which sell Grade A milk are given by address and county on the list. Controls were selected by stratified random sampling, stratified by county to represent the distribution by county of all farms in the state of Wisconsin with sales of $2500 or more in 1974. Controls were contacted in the same fashion as cases. Only farms in which a white male ≥ 35 years of age resided were included in the study. The procedure for contacting and obtaining information was the same for cases and controls.

Differences in sources for identification of cases and controls introduce the possibility of fundamental differences between cases and controls. In particular, it is likely that control farms contained a higher percentage of dairy farms than did the case series. However, 63 percent of farms in the state of Wisconsin are classified as principally dairy, while 77 percent are either dairy or other livestock (U.S. Census Bureau, 1976). It is likely, therefore, that both series contained principally individuals who were or had been dairy or livestock farmers. Only persons who had resided on the farm for at least the previous 2 years and had not been employed off the farm more than 40 percent of that time were included in the study.

For purposes of examining geographic variations, Wisconsin counties were divided into six geographic regions shown in Fig. 1. The map indicates the proportion of all Wisconsin farms in each region, percent of controls, and percent of cases.

Water samples were first-draw morning water samples from the kitchen cold water tap. Respondents used a standard set of instructions to fill two 250-ml polyethylene bottles and one gas-tight glass vial for pH determination. Samples were mailed to the Wisconsin State Hygiene Laboratory in Madison, where all water analyses were carried out. One 250-ml bottle was acidified upon receipt and was used for metals analyses. Parameters analyzed, method of analysis, and analytic detection limits are shown in Table 1.

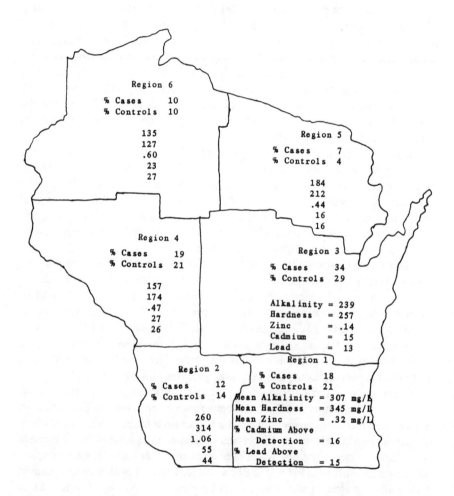

FIGURE 1. Location of cases and controls within the state of Wisconsin and mean water constituent values for controls.

TABLE 1
List of Parameters, Methods of Preservation, and Detection Limits

Parameter	Method	Preservation	Detection Limit
Calcium	AAS-flame[a]	HNO_3	1.0 mg/L
Magnesium	AAS-flame	HNO_3	1.0 mg/L
Iron	AAS-flame	HNO_3	0.1 mg/L
Zinc	AAS-flame	HNO_3	0.02 mg/L
Copper	AAS-flame	HNO_3	0.05 mg/L
Barium	AAS-flame	HNO_3	0.4 mg/L
Lead	AAS-HGA[b]	HNO_3	0.003 mg/L
Manganese	AAS-flame	HNO_3	0.04 mg/L
Tin	AAS-flame	HNO_3	1.0 mg/L
Sodium	AAS-flame	HNO_3	1.0 mg/L
Potassium	AAS-flame	HNO_3	1.0 mg/L
Chromium	AAS-HGA	HNO_3	0.003 mg/L
Cadmium	AAS-HGA	HNO_3	0.0002 mg/L
Nickel	AAS-HGA	HNO_3	0.01 mg/L
Fluoride	AAS-HGA	HNO_3	0.1 mg/L
Alkalinity	H_2SO_4 titration	none	1.0 mg/L $CaCO_3$
Hardness	Calculation	n/a	1.0 mg/1 $CaCO_3$
Nitrate	Automated Cd reduction	none	0.02 mg/L-N
pH	Potentiometric	none	n/a

[a] Atomic absorption spectrophotometry, flame atomizer.

[b] Atomic absorption spectrophotometry, heated graphite furnace atomizer.

RESULTS

Table 2 shows the criteria used for inclusion of cases in the study. Of the 505 total cases, 217 had specific physician verification of either myocardial infarction (MK) or cerebrovascular accident (CVA). The remainder of cases were included on the basis of death certificate information.

The age distribution of cases and controls is shown in Table 3. Cases are considerably older than controls, since no attempt was made to match or stratify for age during control selection. All analyses of water parameters

TABLE 2

Distribution of Cases by Criteria for Inclusion

Physician-Verified Diagnoses	Number
Myocardial Infarction	148
Cerebrovascular Accident	69

Death Certificate Information Only[a]	Number
Coronor-certified sudden death, listed as myocardial infarction or heart attack	109
Myocardial Infarction (ICD 410), listed on death certificate only (non-coroner)	69
Other coronary artery disease on death certificate (ICD 411-414)	203
Cerebrovascular Disease (ICD 430-438) on death certificate	45

[a] Some persons are counted in more than one category because of multiple listings on death certificate. Does not include persons with physician-verified causes of death.

include an adjustment for age by including age as an independent variable in the logistic regression. Table 4 shows the rank correlation coefficients for selected variables for both the case and control series. Total hardness and alkalinity (carbonate hardness) are highly correlated, and calcium and magnesium levels are closely correlated. Age is not related to hardness variables, but is generally related to metal content. One possible explanation is that older individuals have older homes and pipes, from which greater leaching of metals occurs.

Table 5 shows the results of logistic regressions for which age and a single constituent are the independent variables. The results are presented for the entire group, and separately for persons with vary hard water (> 200 mg/L) versus persons with soft to moderately hard water (≤ 200 mg/L). Elements or parameters for which some evidence of a difference between cases and controls exist are alkalinity (carbonate hardness) and total hardness, and the metals

TABLE 3

Age Distribution of Cases and Controls
Number of Persons (Percent)[a]

Age	Cases	Controls
35-54	21(5)	472(56)
55-64	86(17)	287(33)
65+	399(78)	95(11)

TABLE 4
Rank Correlations Among Water Constituents and Age

Cases	Alkalinity	Hardness	Calcium	Magnesium	pH	Cadmium	Zinc	Lead	Age
Alkalinity	–	0.83[a]	0.80[a]	0.84[a]	0.15[a]	-0.04	0.00	-0.10[b]	0.04
Hardness	0.83[a]	–	0.97[a]	0.97[a]	0.05	0.00	0.09	-0.06	0.06
Calcium	0.80[a]	0.97[a]	–	0.92[a]	0.00	0.03	0.11[b]	-0.03	0.05
Magnesium	0.84[a]	0.97[a]	0.92[a]	–	0.09[b]	0.00	0.07	-0.05	0.04
pH	0.15[a]	0.05	0.00	0.09[b]	–	-0.18[a]	-0.17[a]	-0.22[a]	0.00
Cadmium	-0.04	0.00	0.03	0.00	-0.18[a]	–	0.67[a]	0.40	0.07
Zinc	0.00	0.09	0.11[b]	0.07	-0.17[a]	0.67[a]	–	0.48[a]	0.09[b]
Lead	-0.10[b]	-0.06	-0.03	-0.05	-0.22[a]	0.40[a]	0.48[a]	–	0.10[b]
Age	0.04	0.06	0.05	0.04	0.00	0.07	0.09[b]	0.10[b]	–

Controls	Alkalinity	Hardness	Calcium	Magnesium	pH	Cadmium	Zinc	Lead	Age
Alkalinity	–	0.77[a]	0.72[a]	0.77[a]	0.13[a]	-0.05	-0.06	-0.12[a]	0.00
Hardness	0.77[a]	–	0.97[a]	0.98[a]	0.02	0.00	0.08[b]	-0.05	0.00
Calcium	0.72[a]	0.98[a]	–	0.91[a]	-0.03	0.01	0.09[a]	-0.04	0.00
Magnesium	0.77[a]	0.98[a]	0.91[a]	–	0.06	-0.01	0.07[b]	-0.06	0.00
pH	0.13[b]	0.02	-0.03	0.06	–	-0.13	-0.11[a]	-0.18[a]	0.04
Cadmium	-0.05	0.00	0.01	-0.01	-0.13	–	0.58[a]	0.32[a]	0.07[b]
Zinc	-0.06	0.08[b]	0.09[a]	0.07[b]	-0.11[a]	0.58[a]	–	0.35[a]	0.15[a]
Lead	-0.12[a]	-0.05	-0.04	-0.06	-0.18[a]	0.32[a]	0.35[a]	–	0.03
Age	0.00	0.00	0.00	0.00	0.04	0.07[b]	0.15[a]	0.03	–

[a] $p < 0.01$
[b] $p < 0.05$

TABLE 5
Significance of Single Constituents by Categories of Hardness[a]

Constituent	p-values		
	All Persons	Hardness < 200	Hardness ≥ 200
Alkalinity[b]	0.06(Neg)	0.19	0.72
Total Hardness[b]	0.17(Neg)	0.10	0.52
Calcium	0.37	0.35	0.27
Magnesium	0.21	0.84	0.91
Cadmium (Indicator)[c]	0.03(Pos)	0.22	0.07(Pos)
Lead (Indicator)[c]	0.03(Pos)	0.15	0.12
Zinc	0.08(Pos)	0.36	0.13
Fluoride	0.85	0.77	0.83
Nitrate	0.84	0.12	0.41
pH	0.45	0.31	0.60
Copper	0.69	0.84	0.21
Potassium	0.44	0.35	0.52
Sodium	0.48	0.42	0.54
Iron	0.76	0.60	0.81

[a]In each instance the result presented is that for the logistic regression for which the independent variables are age and the single constituent only. Each comparison represents an estimate of effect after accounting for the effect of age. The word in parentheses indicates the sign of the regression coefficient.

[b]Alkalinity is defined as capacity of the water to neutralize acid at a fixed pH, and in natural water is determined by carbonate and bicarbonate ions.

[c]Cadmium and lead are treated as binary variables (present or absent) because of the very limited range of values above analytic detection limits.

cadmium, lead, and zinc. Alkalinity and total hardness were both lower in cases than in controls, while levels of cadmium, lead, and zinc were higher. These parameters were, therefore, selected for further analysis.

Alkalinity, Hardness, and pH. Table 6 shows the results of analyses for several combinations of elements. Although pH itself was not different in cases and controls, the inclusion of pH in the regression equations strengthens the relationship of both alkalinity and total hardness to case-control status.

The results in Table 6 illustrate clearly that the differences in alkalinity and hardness levels between cases and controls are restricted almost entirely to differences at the lower levels of both parameters. Neither alkalinity nor hardness levels are at all different in the two groups when the analysis is confined to levels above 200 mg/L (CACO$_3$) of either parameter. When analysis is confined to units below that value, both alkalinity and hardness are significantly lower in

TABLE 6

Relationships of Water Parameters to Case-Control Studies

Independent Variables[a]	Group All	Alkalinity $\leq$ 200 Significance of Individual Variables p-Value	Alkalinity $\geq$ 200 p-Value
Alkalinity	0.02 (Neg)	0.05 (Neg)	0.54
pH	0.13 (Pos)	0.03 (Pos)	0.97
Significance of Regression[b]	$p < 0.05$	$p < 0.05$	NS
Hardness	0.13	0.03 (Neg)	0.62
pH	0.33	0.05 (Pos)	0.56
Significance of Regression[b]	NS	$p < 0.05$	NS
Hardness	0.12	0.03 (Neg)	
Cadmium	0.19	0.15	
Lead	0.13	0.43	
Zinc	0.64	0.98	
pH	0.10	0.02 (Pos)	
Significance of Regression[b]	$p < 0.05$	$p < 0.10$	NS

[a]Logistic regression include combinations of variables given and age—as independent variables. Cadmium and lead are treated as binary variables (above or below detection).

[b]Significance of regression containing all variables given, plus age, compared to that containing only age as an independent variable. Test was likelihood ratio test.

TABLE 7
Mean pH Values by Level of Alkalinity

Alkalinity	Controls	Cases	(% Cases) ÷ (% Controls)
	Mean pH (No.)	Mean pH (No.)	
0-49	6.4(58)	6.5(46)	1.34
50-100	7.1(75)	7.3(60)	1.35
100-149	7.5(82)	7.7(48)	1.00
150-199	7.7(106)	7.8(64)	1.02
200-249	7.7(128)	7.7(70)	0.93
250+	7.5(405)	7.6(217)	0.91

cases than in controls. The slope of the regression line for pH is positive, indicating that at a given age and level of either hardness or alkalinity, water samples from cases have higher pH values. The differences in both alkalinity and pH levels among cases and controls are apparent in Table 7.

Table 8 shows results separately for cases in the coronary artery disease category (CAD) and cases with cerebrovascular disease (CVD). The coronary artery disease category includes persons with physician-documented myocardial infarction, all persons with ICD 410-414 listed as a cause of death, and all persons with coroner-certified sudden death presumed to be myocardial infarction. The CVD category includes all persons with ICD 430-438 on the death certificate and all persons with physician-documented cerebrovascular accident. A total of 40 persons satisfied the conditions for both groups.

The slope of the regression equation for the combination of alkalinity and pH is approximately the same in the two groups, although smaller sample sizes in the CVD group reduce the significance of the regression. Relationships with metals will be discussed in the next section.

Age is not a confounder of the relationship of alkalinity or hardness to the disease endpoint, since the regression of either alkalinity or hardness including age as an independent variable is nearly the same as that when age is not included. This corresponds to the lack of evidence of a relationship between those two exposure variables and age in either the case group or the control group, as illustrated by the correlations shown in Table 4.

Total hardness is calculated as a function of the calcium and magnesium content of the water. Considerable speculation has arisen concerning the potential physiological impacts of these two components of hardness, and which of the two might account for the observed negative correlations between cardiovascular disease death rates and average total hardness in the United States. In the data set presented here, calcium and magnesium levels are highly correlated (see Table 4). It is difficult for that reason to separate the relationships of the two variables as to status. For the subgroup with alkalinity ≤ 200, the logistic regression including calcium and magnesium indicates that calcium levels are

TABLE 8
Relationships of Water Constituents to Case-Control Status Within Diagnostic Categories

Independent Variables[a]	Coronary Artery Disease (N = 424)	Cerebrovascular Disease (N = 121)
Alkalinity[b]		
Slope	−0.0017	−0.0016
Standard Error	0.0008	0.0013
Significance	p < 0.03	NS
Cadmium		
Slope	0.29	0.88
Standard Error	0.19	0.29
Significance	NS	p < 0.01
Zinc		
Slope	0.16	0.13
Standard Error	0.08	0.14
Significance	p < 0.06	NS
Lead		
Slope	0.47	0.29
Standard Error	0.20	0.30
Significance	p < 0.01	NS

[a]All regressions include age as an independent variable. Cadmium and lead are included as binary variables (above or below detection), so that significance of those variables indicates only that the case group has a significantly higher percentage above detection.

[b]Regression also includes pH. Although pH itself was not significant in either group, the inclusion of pH improves the fit for the Coronary Artery Disease group.

significantly lower in cases than in controls, while magnesium levels are not different.

Table 9 gives the case-control ratio by categories of each variable. The rows of the table represent the ratio of cases to controls (in percentage) for each variable within a fixed level of the other. Although neither pattern is totally consistent, the pattern of decreasing ratios across each row appears to be somewhat more consistent for changing calcium levels (top table) than it is for changing magnesium levels (bottom table).

The ratio of calcium to magnesium is distributed virtually identically in the case and control groups, and is therefore not helpful in separating effects.

Calcium, Lead, and Zinc. As Table 5 showed, the metals which are significantly different in cases and controls are cadmium, lead, and zinc. Cadmium and zinc are highly correlated, as Table 4 illustrates. Lead levels are also

TABLE 9
Relationship of Calcium and Magnesium Levels to Case-Control Status, for Persons with Alkalinity Below 200

Case-Control Ratios by Levels of Calcium and Magnesium

Ratio: % Cases at Magnesium Level ÷ % Controls at Magnesium Level

Magnesium (mg/L)	Calcium (mg/L)				N_1^a	N_2^a
	<10	10-24	25-39	40+		
<5	68/55	32/41	0/4	_b	41	34
5-9	_b	83/84	15/14	2/2	48	64
10-19	_b	19/13	60/64	20/23	75	155
20+	0/2	7/2	27/23	65/73	55	68
	$N_1 = 28$	$N_1 = 71$	$N_1 = 67$	$N_1 = 53$		
	$N_2 = 20$	$N_2 = 90$	$N_2 = 126$	$N_2 = 85$		

Ratio: % Cases at Calcium Level ÷ % Controls at Calcium Level

Calcium (mg/L)	Magnesium (mg/L)				N_1^a	N_2^a
	0-5	5-10	10-19	20+		
0-9	100/95	_b	_b	0/5	28	20
10-24	18/16	56/60	20/23	6/1	71	90
25-39	0/1	10/7	67/79	22/13	67	126
40+	3/1	22/37	56/46	19/16	53	85

[a] N_1 = number of cases; N_2 = number of controls.
[b] No observations in cell.

TABLE 10

TABLE 10
Levels of Cadmium, Zinc, and Lead by Age and Status

	Percent in Category					
	Cadmium Level (µg/L)					
	Below Detection[a]		0.2-0.5		≥0.6	
	Cases	Controls	Cases	Controls	Cases	Controls
35-54	86	81	9	11	5	8
55-64	66	81	16	10	18	9
65+	64	70	14	14	22	17

	Lead (µg/L)					
	Below Detection[a]		3-6		≥7	
	Cases	Controls	Cases	Controls	Cases	Controls
35-54	90	80	10	10	0	10
55-64	69	80	16	8	15	12
65+	65	76	13	14	22	11

	Zinc (mg/L)							
	Below Detection[a]		0.02-0.15		0.15-0.84		≥0.85	
	Cases	Controls	Cases	Controls	Cases	Controls	Cases	Controls
35-54	5	8	53	45	28	39	14	8
55-64	1	8	33	39	46	41	20	12
65+	4	2	27	34	43	45	26	19

[a]Detection limits are 0.2 µg/L for cadmium, 3 µg/L for lead, and 0.02 mg/L for zinc.

significantly correlated with both cadmium and zinc levels. Lead is negatively correlated with alkalinity, although not strongly, while cadmium and zinc levels are not related to alkalinity. All three metals have higher levels in more acid waters as indicated by the negative correlations with pH. All the above results are typical relationships for drinking water supplies (National Research Council, 1977; Greathouse, 1979). Actual levels of the three metals found are shown in Table 10. Levels of cadmium and lead are quite low, as the table clearly shows. Levels of zinc are somewhat higher. Nevertheless, the actual measured levels of the metals in the drinking water would result in a direct drinking water intake far below the intake levels ordinarily found in food, for example. The question of possible different bioavailability of the forms in food and water remains. Buhler et al. (1981) found no differences in uptake of cadmium in rats ingesting the metal through food or water.

Table 8 presented the results by cause category for the three metals. The relationships for metal are not clearly limited to either of the groups.

Although the metals are clearly related to pH (Table 4), the inclusion of pH in the regression equation does not change the predictive value of any of the three,

TABLE 11
Values of Metals by Five-Year Age Groups

Age	Cadmium (% Above Detection)				
	Cases		Controls	
	Percent	N	Percent	N
50-54	20	15	21	141
55-59	27	30	19	161
60-64	38	55	18	126
65-69	31	94	29	56
70+	37	289	32	37

Age	Lead (% Above Detection)			
	Cases		Controls	
	Percent	N	Percent	N
50-54	13	13	20	113
55-59	27	30	20	161
60-64	34	56	21	126
65-69	35	94	23	56
70+	35	305	26	39

Age	Zinc (Mean Values, mg/L)[a]			
	Cases		Controls	
	Percent	N	Percent	N
50-54	0.38	15	0.49	141
55-59	0.50	30	0.46	160
60-64	0.61	56	0.36	126
65-69	0.80	94	0.71	56
70+	0.86	305	0.54	39

[a]Values below detection are included as zeroes.

nor does the inclusion of alkalinity or hardness have any effect. For all of the three metals, the relationship to case-control status is relatively independent of either total hardness or alkalinity (see Table 5).

Because cadmium, zinc, and lead are clearly age-related, a comparison of differences by narrow age groups is worthwhile. Table 11 shows the percentages of persons having cadmium and lead levels above detection, and mean zinc values. Below age 50, the number of cases is too small for analysis. Above age 50, the differences between the two groups are spread across all ages and are relatively consistent.

Confounders and Effect-Modifiers. Possible explanatory variables for the observed relationships between the water parameters and disease status include:

(A) Small differences do exist between cases and controls in region of

TABLE 12
Logistic Regressions by Regions[a]

Region	Cadmium(ind) β	p	Lead(ind) β	p	Zinc β	p	Alkalinity β	p	pH β	p	N Cases	Controls
1	0.63	0.16	0.21	0.65	0.45	0.09	-0.0010	0.67	-0.16	0.84	89	184
2	0.99	0.05	0.83	0.11	0.58	0.01	0.0009	0.81	0.51	0.60	63	121
3	0.03	0.93	0.47	0.18	-0.03	0.82	-0.0010	0.50	0.56	0.10	171	249
4	0.21	0.58	0.04	0.92	0.11	0.54	-0.0049	0.09	0.38	0.39	94	177
6	0.24	0.63	0.48	0.32	0.07	0.67	-0.0093	0.03	0.95	0.07	52	86

[a]Regions are shown by number in Figure 1. Region 5 was omitted because of inadequate sample size.

149

TABLE 13
Relationships of Water Parameters and Disease Status, Including Only Dairy Farms[a]

Independent Variables	Significance of Individual Variable
Alkalinity	< 0.03
pH	0.30
Hardness	$p < 0.02$
pH	0.58
Cadmium (indicator)	0.79
Zinc	0.23
Lead (indicator)	0.77

[a] Regressions for hardness and alkalinity include only respondents with alkalinity ≤ 200. Others include all alkalinity levels. All logistic regressions include age as an independent variable.

residence, and there are substantial differences by region in hardness and alkalinity, as well as in the levels of metals. It would have been inappropriate to eliminate differences in geographic location, since that would have substantially reduced the opportunity for differences between the groups. It it appropriate, however, to examine differences within regions. Table 12 shows the coefficients of regressions and the significance of the coefficients for the logistic regressions carried out within region. Although the smaller sample sizes do introduce considerable variation, the values make it clear that the pattern of relationship occurs within regions as well. Notably, the evidence of effect for alkalinity and hardness is greatest in Regions 4 and 6, which have the softest water. Regions 1 and 2, with very hard water, show little evidence of differences between cases and controls. Although some differences in geographic origin of cases and controls could exist within the regions, such differences do not seem to be a likely explanation for the lower hardness and alkalinity levels in cases. Because Regions 4 and 6 have the stronger relationships for hardness and alkalinity, mean values of those two parameters were analyzed by county for these regions. A total of 11 counties in the two regions had at least five cases and five controls after deleting persons reporting water softener use. Of these, in eight counties mean hardness and alkalinity were lower in cases than in controls.

(B) A substantially higher proportion of controls than cases report on the questionnaire that the major product of the farm is dairy products. This is expected since the source of the case series admits all farmers, while the source of the control series admits only farms with herd registered for brucellosis testing. The previous paragraph discussed the geographic similarities of the two groups. Lifestyle factors such as exercise level, dietary fat intake, or smoking

150

TABLE 14
Number of Years Lived at Present Residence, by Class and Age

Age	N	Percent in Category		
		<10 Years	10-19 Years	20+ Years
35-54				
Cases	21	14	9	77
Controls	468	18	27	55
55-64				
Cases	85	21	9	70
Controls	283	7	11	82
65+				
Cases	390	13	14	73
Controls	93	8	7	85

habits may differ between the two groups. The question of interest for the present study is whether these risk factors for disease are related to the water parameters, since to be confounders they must be related to both outcome and exposure (Miettinen, 1970, 1974).

Exercise level is a variable which could not be measured, so its relationship to water content is not possible to determine. The likelihood of a relationship seems small, however. Questions on dietary fat intake, particularly consumption of dairy products, were included in the respondent questionnaire. There was no evidence of any relationship between respondent-estimated intake of any dietary element and any water parameter.

There were clear differences between cases and controls in reported dietary habits. Within age groups, controls reported clearly higher average consumption of milk, butter, and cheese than did cases, and reported a somewhat higher consumption of red meat. Although dietary questions were phrased to request an average over the last 5 years, these differences may reflect recent habits and a reduction in consumption of high cholesterol foods by cases.

The major products of the farm were an item reported in the respondent questionnaire. Respondents were divided according to whether dairy products were listed as a major product of the farm. Logistic regressions were repeated, using that subset of respondents. Table 13 shows the results of the regressions, using only farms with alkalinity below 200. The relationships with metals are not significant in this subgroup, however.

Persons reporting dairy products as a major farm product were not significantly different in either region of origin or age distribution from persons not reporting such products, in either the case group or the control group.

TABLE 15
Relationship of Hardness and Alkalinity to Disease Status, Deleting Persons Reporting Use of a Softener

| | Significance of Coefficients | | | |
| | Alkalinity $\leq$ 200 | | Hardness $\leq$ 200 | |
	All Persons	Softened[a] Deleted	All Persons	Softened Deleted
Alkalinity	0.05	0.03	0.03	0.13
pH	0.03	0.02	0.04	0.06
Hardness	0.03	0.06	0.04	0.001
pH	0.05	0.06	0.11	0.009

[a]All persons reporting softener use excluded from the analysis.

Cigarette smoking clearly emerges as a risk factor for case status. Results of the logistic regression including estimated number of cigarettes smoked per day and age as independent variables gives an odds ratio for smoking one pack per day (previous 5 years) of 2.3. However, within both the case series and the control series, smoking and water constituents were unrelated, so that smoking is not a confounder of the exposure-disease relationships. This is borne out by the fact that the inclusion of the smoking variable in the regression analyses does not alter the observed water-disease relationships.

(C) Another factor which could be different in the two groups is the number of years spent on the farm. This is a variable which could be related to water constituents and would also be related to length of exposure at that location.

Above age 55, the proportion of cases having spent 20 or more years on the farm is clearly lower for cases than for controls. Table 14 shows the distribution of reported years lived at the present residence. The proportions probably reflect a higher number of recent moves by cases precipitated by either ill health or retirement. However, all persons had resided a minimum of 2 years at the current residence.

There was no evidence that length of time spent at the present residence was related to levels of alkalinity, hardness, or pH. There was some evidence of a relationship to levels of metals, however, although the relationship was not very consistent and appeared to be principally accounted for by adjusting for age. The water-disease regressions were repeated adding number of years spent on the farm as an independent variable. There was little or no effect on the logistic regressions for metals, or for hardness and alkalinity. Amount of time spent working off the farm was not significantly different for cases and controls, once

152

TABLE 16
Odds Ratios Associated with a Specified Increase or Decrease in Constituent

Contituent	Odds Ratio[a]	Change	95% Confidence Limits[a]
Alkalinity	1.15	100 mg/L decrease	1.00, 1.32
Alkalinity (with pH included)	1.18	100 mg/L decrease	1.02, 1.38
Alkalinity (entries with alkalinity ≤200 only, pH included)	1.73	100mg/L decrease	1.00, 2.74
Hardness	1.07	100 mg/L decrease	0.97, 1.19
Hardness (with pH included)	1.08	100 mg/L decrease	0.98, 1.20
Hardness (entries with alkalinity ≤200 only, pH included)	1.47	100 mg/L decrease	1.03, 2.08
Hardness (entries with hardness ≤200, persons reporting softeners deleted, pH included)	2.64	100 mg/L decrease	1.45, 4.81
Cadmium	1.47	above detection versus below detection	1.03, 2.11
Lead	1.48	above detection versus below detection	1.03, 2.12
Zinc	1.15	1 mg/L increase	0.98, 1.37

[a]All regressions include age as an independent variable, so that the odds ratio and the 95% confidence limits both are calculated with adjustment for age.

age was taken into account. Ninety-four percent of controls and 90 percent of cases reported no work off the farm.

(D) Use of water softeners is a variable which could affect the results for hardness considerably. The respondent questionnaire included questions regarding use of water softeners. Also, since the water analysis included both sodium and total hardness (calcium and magnesium), it was generally possible to ascertain whether a fully-recharged softener was being used when the water sample was taken by determining whether the water had a high sodium content and low total hardness.

A total of 14 percent of cases and 24 percent of controls reported having water softeners attached to either the cold water line or both hot and cold water lines. An examination of sodium and hardness values for respondents reporting such softeners indicated that either many were not fully operational or respondents were incorrectly reporting the use of the softener.

Analyses of the data taking water softening into account were made in two ways. First, exposure-disease relationships were reexamined after eliminating all persons reporting use of a cold-water softener. Second, the relationships were reexamined using the algorithm of elimination of a respondent if sodium level was at least 25 mg/L and total hardness was less than 50 mg/L. That algorithm eliminated a total of 23 cases and 54 controls.

Table 15 shows the results of regressions for hardness and alkalinity, including pH, deleting persons reporting use of softeners. Results are reported both for the subgroup with alkalinity ≤ 200 and for the group with total hardness ≤ 200. The one major change produced by deleting persons with softeners is for the relationship with hardness among the subgroup having total hardness below 200. The deletion of persons reporting softeners strengthened that relationship considerably. The change occurs because among the group reporting artificially softened water, the proportion of controls with very soft water was higher than the proportion of cases with soft water. All of the relationships reported were in the same direction as previously reported—either hardness or alkalinity negatively related to disease status (cases having softer water or less total carbonate), while the relationship with pH has a positive sign.

The logistic regressions involving hardness were repeated omitting persons who reported having water softeners attached to the cold water line, and limiting the analysis to persons having hardness below 200 mg/L. Cases in this group still have higher lead levels, but the relationship with cadmium and zinc disappears. Alkalinity loses significances, even when pH is included in the equation.

Odds Ratios. Table 16 presents the estimated odds ratios for the specified changes in water constituents. These values are presented for perspective only. The fact that the odds ratio is above one does not necessarily imply a causal relationship, only a significant association.

The estimate of the odds ratio for a given water parameter was usually heavily dependent on what other factors were taken into account (i.e., what other independent variables were included in the logistic regression). Also, the estimated odds ratios for various subgroups varied considerably. For alkalinity and hardness, for example, the odds ratio estimates for the subgroup with alkalinity ≤ 200 were considerably higher than for the total group.

It should also be remembered that the estimate of exposure is based on a single sample. The presumption that this provides some quantitative estimate of actual exposure is better for some constituents than others. A single sample probably provides a fairly good relative ranking for metals, but actual levels may vary considerably dependent on conditions under which the sample was taken. For alkalinity and hardness, on the other hand, the fact that the water source is local ground water probably means that those two parameters are fairly stable. In addition, the esposure estimate does not take into account the length of exposure—only the quantity present at one point in time.

DISCUSSION

Hardness Variables. The negative relationship of total hardness and alkalinity (carbonate hardness) to disease status is consistent, and there is no evidence in the data set to indicate that confounding variables can explain the differences.

The effect is clearly limited to the lower part of the range of either alkalinity or hardness. In this analysis, that point was taken to be below 200, although there was no analytical reason for that cutoff value. The better predictive power of alkalinity compared to total hardness in the entire group is probably totally explained by the lack of relationship of alkalinity to artificial softening, which proved to be more prevalent in the control group. When those persons are eliminated, hardness is a better predictor of disease status. The fact that a higher proportion of controls than cases have artificially softened water seems to indicate that the higher risk associated with soft water applies only to naturally soft water. The sample size of individuals having softeners is too small for definitive conclusions, however.

Separation of the calcium and magnesium components of hardness is very difficult in this data set. As Table 9 showed, there is some indication that the relationship of cases' status to calcium level is a little more consistent than the relationship with magnesium level. For the logistic regressions in which calcium and magnesium are both included, neither is significant. Calcium is invariably more predictive of case status, however, although not individually reaching significance.

It is not entirely possible to rule out the existence of some set of unmeasured or unknown confounders which explain the softer water among cases. The most likely confounders of the relationship seem to be age and/or some set of variables which vary with geography or type of farm. However, age was not related at all to either hardness or alkalinity. Cases and controls did not differ greatly in region of origin (see Figure 1). The analysis of Regions 4 and 6 indicates that the lower water hardness in cases holds true at the county level.

It is possible that some basic difference for cases and controls produces a fundamental difference in the two groups related to softer water. However, all water sources were individual drilled or dug wells, and there was no evidence that the type of farm was systematically related to the exposure variables. The relationships of hardness and alkalinity to disease status appear when the analysis is confined only to self-reported dairy farmers.

The contribution of pH is consistent, and the water of cases clearly had was higher pH than that of controls, once alkalinity is taken into account. Alkalinity and pH are positively correlated, so that higher pH is to some extent associated with higher alkalinity. Hardness and pH are not significantly correlated. However, higher pH is also associated with lower metal content, and less leaching ability of the water. Thus, if metal content were a contributor to risk, one would expect lower pH levels among cases than controls. The difference in pH level in the two groups remains unexplained at this point.

Cadmium, Lead, and Zinc. The levels of metals in both cases and controls in this series are lower than the levels found in most drinking water series (Greathouse, 1979; National Research Council, 1977), most of which are drawn from public water supplies. The specificity of the association of these three metals is intriguing, since cadmium and lead are the two metals known to be toxic, both to humans and to the cardiovascular system of animals. Zinc is not toxic at the levels found in this series, and is an essential nutrient. No other metal, including iron, copper, and manganese, was at all different in cases and controls. Some metals (nickel, chromium, and tin) were present only rarely at detectable levels.

The higher levels of cadmium and zinc in cases would be expected if cases had greater leaching from galvanizing material of pipes. Cadmium occurs as a contaminant of the zinc coating material. Very few of the respondents reported having lead pipes, and it is likely that the primary source of lead in the drinking water was from lead solder.

The relationship of the three metals to case-control status was essentially independent of the relationships of hardness, alkalinity, and pH to disease status. The addition of any of these three variables to the equations relating a metal to disease status generally does not change the metal-disease relationship substantially.

Differences between cases and controls in cadmium and lead levels are not significant when only respondents with values above detection are included. The major difference between the two groups is apparently in the proportion having amounts above detection. This argues against a causal relationship, since the amount just above detection is very low for both metals. It is possible that true levels of the two metals are higher than the analysis indicates. The most likely reason for that would be adsorption onto container walls during the 24 to 72 hour period in transit. Some adsorption could have occurred. However, a number of spiked samples were tested before and after 24 to 72 hours, and the tests showed little or no adsorption onto walls in that time.

Other Elements. Sodium is an element for which evidence exists of a relationship between drinking water intake and blood pressure (Tuthill, 1979; Saltman, 1983; Tobian, 1975; Folsom, 1982). For that reason, it has been speculated that sodium intake may also be related to the cardiovascular diseases. No evidence of such a relationship was found in the current study. Two recent reports have provided evidence in rats that the sodium-blood pressure relationship may in fact be a relationship with chloride (Whitescarver et al., 1984; Kurtz et al., 1984). Unfortunately, chloride levels were not measured in the present series. However, none of the water was chlorinated, so that chloride levels would probably not be high in this series.

It is also noteworthy that no differences were found in either fluoride content or nitrate content of the drinking water. Nitrate intake through water is a known cause of methemoglobinemia, and one study found a relationship between blood pressure levels in army recruits in Colorado and nitrate levels in their geographic home region (Morton, 1971).

SUMMARY

There is convincing evidence in the present study of an association between hardness of drinking water and coronary artery disease and cerebrovascular disease. Because 424 of the 505 cases had evidence of coronary artery disease, the evidence is strongest for that endpoint.

One of the difficulties in interpreting the observed statistical associations of water hardness and cardiovascular disease has been the fact that the relationship was considerably stronger when the geographic unit was large (e.g., states), than when the unit was small (e.g., cities or counties within a state). Since the measurement of average hardness is more meaningful in small areas than in large ones, this tended to argue against a causal relationship. The British Regional Heart Study (Pocock et al., 1980) has examined regional variations in cardiovascular disease in Great Britain in relation to drinking water, climate, rainfall, socioeconomic status and other variables. The geographic units were 253 towns in England, Wales, and Scotland. They found a significant negative association between water hardness and cardiovascular mortality rates, not explained by other geographic variables. Interestingly, all or nearly all the effect occurred in the range of 0 to 150-200 mg/L total hardness. They also found a significant independent effect of alkalinity (carbonate hardness). The results of that study and the work reported here thus appear to corroborate each other strongly. The contribution of calcium and magnesium nutrition to cardiovascular disease risk needs to be investigated thoroughly.

ACKNOWLEDGEMENTS

This research was sponsored by the Environmental Protection Agency under Interagency Agreement 40-1063-80 under Martin Marietta Energy Systems, Inc., contract DE-AC05-840R21400 with the U.S. Department of Energy.

Although the research described in this paper has been funded wholly or in part by the United States Environmental Protection Agency (EPA) through Interagency Agreement 40-1063-80 to Oak Ridge National Laboratory, it has not been subjected to EPA review and therefore does not necessarily reflect the views of EPA and no official endorsement should be inferred.

The authors would like to acknowledge Dr. Frank Dickson of the Chemistry Division and Dr. Annetta Watson of the Health and Safety Research Division for their advice during this study.

REFERENCES

BUHLER, D.R., WRIGHT, D.C., SMITH, K.L. and TINSLEY, I.J. (1981). Cadmium absorption and tissue distribution in rats provided low concentrations of cadmium in food or drinking water. J. Toxicol. Envir. Health 8:185–197.

COMSTOCK, G.W. (1979). Water hardness and cardiovascular diseases. Am. J. Epidemiol. 110:375–400.

COMSTOCK, G.W., CAUTHEN, G.M. and HELSING, K.J. (1980). Water hardness at home and deaths from arteriosclerotic heart disease in Washington County, Maryland. Am. J. Epidemiol. 112:209–216.

FOLSOM, A.R. and PRINEAS, R.J. (1982). Drinking water composition and blood pressure: A review of the epidemiology. Am. J. Epidemiol. 115:818–832.

GREATHOUSE, D.G. (1979). A preliminary report on a nationwide study of drinking water and cardiovascular diseases, in Drinking Water and Cardiovascular Diseases. Pathotox Publishers, Park Forest South, Illinois, pp. 65–76.

HARING, B.S.A. and VAN DELFT, W. (1981). Changes in the mineral composition of food as a result of cooking in "hard" and "soft" waters. Arch. Evn. Health 36(1):35–38.

KOPP, S.J., GLONEK, T., PERRY, H.M., ERLANGER, M. and PERRY, E.F. (1982). Cardiovascular actions of cadmium at environmental exposure levels. Science 217:837–839.

KURTZ, T.W. and MORRIS, R.C. (1983). Dietary chloride as a determinant of "sodium-dependent" hypertension. Science 222:1139–1141.

MIETTINEN, O.S. (1970). Matching and design efficiency in retrospective studies. Am. J. Epidemiol. 91:111–118.

MIETTINEN, O.S. (1974). Confounding and effect-modification. Am. J. Epidemiol. 100:350–353.

MORTON, W.E. (1971). Hypertension and drinking water constituents in Colorado. Am. J. Public Health 61:1371–1378.

NATIONAL RESEARCH COUNCIL (1977). Drinking Water and Health. National Academy of Sciences, Washington, D.C.

NERI, L.C., HEWITT, D. and SCHREIBER, G.B. (1974). Can epidemiology elucidate the water story? Am. J. Epidemiol. 99:75–99.

OHANIAN, E.V., and IWAI, J. (1980). Etiological role of cadmium in hypertension in an animal model. J. Environ. Pathol. Toxicol. 4-2-3:229–241.

POCOCK, S.J., SHAPER, A.G., COOK, D.G., PACKHAM, R.F., LACEY, R.F., POWELL, P. and RUSSELL, P.F. (1980). British Regional Heart Study: Geographic variations in cardiovascular mortality, and the role of water quality. Brit. Med. J. 280:1243–1248.

REVIS, N.W., MAJOR, T.C. and HORTON, C.Y. (1979). The effects of calcium, magnesium, lead, or cadmium on lipoprotein metabolism and arteriosclerosis in the pigeon, in Drinking Water and Cardiovascular Disease. Pathotox Publishers, Park Forest South, Illinois, pp. 293–303.

SALTMAN, P. (1983). Trace elements and blood pressure. Ann. Int. Med. 98:823–827.

SANDSTEAD, H.H. (1979). Some interaction among elements and binding ligands that may relate to cardiovascular disease, in Geochemistry of Water in Relation to Cardiovascular Disease. National Academy of Sciences, Washington, D.C., pp. 39–43.

SHARRETT, A.R. (1979). The role of chemical constituents of drinking water in cardiovascular diseases. Am. J. Epidemiol. 110:401–419.

TOBIAN, L. (1975). Current status of salt in hypertension, in Epidemiology and Control of Hypertension. Stratton Intercontinental Book Corporation, New York, pp. 131–146.

TUTHILL, R.W., SONICH, C., OKUN, A. and GREATHOUSE, D. (1979). The influence of naturally and artificially elevated levels of sodium in drinking water on blood pressure in school children, in Drinking Water and Cardiovascular Disease. Pathotox Publishers, Park Forest South, Illinois, pp. 173–182.

WHITSCARVER, S.A., OTT, C.E., JACKSON, B.A., GUTHRIE, G.P., and KOTCHEN, T.E. (1984). Salt-sensitive hypertension: contribution of chloride. Science 223:1430–1432.

CHAPTER XV

OVERVIEW OF EPIDEMIOLOGIC STUDIES ON THE ASSOCIATION OF HARD AND SOFT WATER WITH CARDIOVASCULAR DISEASE

Gunther F. Craun
U.S. Environmental Protection Agency
Cincinnati, Ohio

ABSTRACT

Since Kobayashi (1957) first reported a statistical correlation between cerebrovascular disease mortality and the acidity of water supplies in Japan some 27 years ago, more than 40 publications have described an association between drinking water quality and cardiovascular disease. Several excellent reviews on this subject have recently been published (Folsom and Prineas, 1982; Masironi and Shaper, 1981; Comstock, 1980; NRC, 1980; Comstock, 1979; Sharrett, 1979; NRC, 1979). In general, studies have shown a negative association between cardiovascular disease mortality and water hardness, that is, lower cardiovascular mortality is found in areas where the hardness of drinking water is high. However, the association is presently considered to be statistical rather than causal. Although biologically plausible in some respects, the epidemiologic evidence for an association between water quality and cardiovascular disease is not specific.

INTRODUCTION

The association of drinking water quality and cardiovascular disease has been obtained primarily from descriptive epidemiologic and statistical-correlational studies of mortality rates in areas having different water characteristics. Individual exposures and possible confounding by individual risk indicators have generally not been considered in the studies, the results are inconsistent, and the observed associations are relatively weak. Water hardness and total dissolved solids in water have also been shown to be negatively associated with numerous other causes of death, including total mortality, cancer mortality, sudden death from other than arteriosclerotic heart disease, cirrhosis, and peptic ulcer and positively associated with fatal accidents, congenital malformations, and chronic obstructive pulmonary disease.

A negative association of water hardness and cardiovascular mortality has been reported in most, but not all, studies involving large geographic areas. However, numerous studies have failed to find similar negative associations within small geographic areas and among communities. It is possible that the observed association of water quality with cardiovascular mortality is due to the correlation of some other geographically related factors, such as demographic, socio-economic, and cultural characteristics, with water quality. Altitude, climate, latitude, humidity, air temperature, and socio-economic status have been found in some studies to influence the correlation of water quality with cardiovascular mortality.

I have not been active in this research area as long as Lee McCabe and have not become as discouraged with our inability at this time to draw definitive conclusions on the resolution of the so-called "water factor" and cardiovascular disease. Rather, I have become encouraged of late, not because I think we'll necessarily be able to provide individuals such as Joe Cotruvo and Peter Toft with all the information they might need for developing drinking water regulations in this area in the near future but because I see a logical progression of epidemiologic studies from the descriptive and statistical-correlational studies to the more recent studies where investigators have attempted to quantify the possible effects, estimate individual exposures to specific water constituents, and assess or control some of the likely confounding and modifying factors.

Few studies have provided an estimate of the possible effect of influence of a water factor on cardiovascular disease. In areas of the United Kingdom where drinking water supplies are extremely soft, cardiovascular mortality is about 40% higher than in areas where drinking water supplies are extremely hard. In the United States a difference of about 15% in cardiovascular mortality is found between areas with soft and hard water supplies. It has been suggested that this might be the "maximum effect or influence" of a water factor in these countries. More recently Neri et al. (1974, 1975) estimated that the "maximum effect or influence" of a water factor in Canada might be 20%. Comstock (1971; NRC, 1979) calculated the relative risks for total cardiovascular mortality for white males aged 45–64 due to soft water −1.25 in the United States and 1.19 in England and Wales. Using multiple regression techniques to assess the association of water hardness and standardized mortality ratios while controlling for climate and socio-economic factors, Shaper, Packham, and Pocock (1980) reported preliminary results of the British Regional Heart Study indicating a 3 to 4% increase in cardiovascular mortality for every 100 mg/L decrease in total hardness. Perhaps Dr. Pocock will comment further on this during his presentation. At the American Medical Association's Symposium on Drinking Water and Health in 1983, Sharrett et al. (1984) discussed a similar analysis of 484 cities in the United States; when soft water cities were compared with hard water cities in the same region and the results adjusted for demographic variables, the mortality rates were found to be approximately 5% higher in soft water cities. I hope Dr. Sharrett will discuss this further during his presentation.

Lee McCabe noted two recent epidemiologic studies reporting no association between water quality and cardiovascular disease. I reviewed two additional articles published in 1983, which I feel provide inconclusive results (Lanzola et al., 1983; Luoma et al., 1983). I do not intend to provide a critical review of these studies, as the studies included only a small number of individuals, but I do offer these brief comments. In Italy Lanzola et al. (1983) studied the diets of thirty-three families in which one family member had experienced a death due to coronary heart disease and 66 population control families matched on age, family size, and occupation. No difference was found between case and control families in total mineral intake for calcium, magnesium, zinc, lead, and cadmium from samples of drinking water collected in spring and winter and food from a 1-week market basket survey. In Finland, Luoma et al. (1983) assessed the association between calcium, magnesium, and fluoride in drinking water and acute myocardial infarction. Cases were males (30–64 years of age) who had been discharged with a first acute myocardial infarction from Kotka Central Hospital. A population control and a hospital control (surgical patients) matched for age and type of community were selected for comparison. Analysis of 50 case-hospital control pairs and 50 case-population control pairs indicated no association with calcium, but a positive association between low fluoride water (≤ 0.1 ppm) and low magnesium water (≤ 1.2 ppm) and acute myocardial infarction was reported. The relative risk for acute myocardial infarction in cases compared to population controls was 4.67 (95% confidence interval 1.30, 25.32) for low magnesium water and 4.40 (95% confidence interval 1.62, 14.87) for low fluoride water. However, the wide confidence intervals suggest unstable risk estimates from this study.

My final comment concerns the evaluation of drinking water exposures in epidemiologic studies of drinking water quality and cardiovascular disease. Gillies and Paulin (1983) showed more than a ten-fold variation in the amount of water people drink daily and noted that the only reliable way to determine mineral intakes from water is to analyze representative samples of water actually consumed. The lack of a precise estimate of exposure to various minerals in water has likely affected the results of epidemiologic studies conducted in this area, and the use of total hardness as the exposure variable rather than specific water constituents may be inappropriate. It is important to accurately assess exposure not only to increase the sensitivity of epidemiologic analyses but also to assist in the possible development of drinking water regulations.

It has been suggested that trace metals leached from water piping by soft or corrosive water may be responsible for increased cardiovascular mortality. If this is the case, we have the option, at least in the United States, of revising the drinking water standard for each metal or adjusting various water parameters to make drinking water less corrosive to plumbing materials. Calcium and magnesium are likely possibilities as beneficial constituents in hard water. High calcium concentrations in hard water may reduce or prevent the absorption of low levels of metals such as lead or cadmium. Another possibility is that hard water is a source of an essential element, such as calcium or magnesium, that is deficient in the diet. If it is shown that the magnesium content of hard water is sufficient to prevent a deficiency where dietary magnesium is marginal and is important in reducing cardiovascular mortality, water utilities could consider a modification in the lime softening process which would precipitate calcium but not precipate magnesium. This is theoretically possible because excess lime is required to precipate $Mg(OH)_2$, and maximum precipitation of $Mg(OH)_2$ occurs at pH 10.5 while the maximum precipitation of $CaCO_3$ occurs at pH 9.5.

In conclusion, the epidemiologic studies conducted to date, while suggestive of an association between hard water and decreased cardiovascular mortality or between soft water and increased cardiovascular mortality, have provided insufficient evidence to support recommendations that municipal waters not be artificially softened by lime-soda ash treatment or ion exchange. Artificial softening of water by ion exchange at the municipal water plant or individual home can increase the sodium concentration of drinking water, and the increased sodium concentrations could adversely affect those on low sodium diets. Additional research is needed, however, before recommendations can be made regarding the advisability of removing calcium or magnesium from drinking water by either ion exchange or lime-soda ash softening. There are benefits associated with reducing the corrosiveness of drinking water and preventing the leaching of metals from plumbing materials, but it is not clear at this time whether this will also result in decreased cardiovascular mortality.

ACKNOWLEDGEMENTS

The research described in this paper has been subject to the Agency's review and it has been approved for publication as an EPA document. Mention of trade names or commercial products does not constitute endorsement or recommendation for use.

REFERENCES

COMSTOCK, G.W. (1971). Fatal arteriosclerotic heart disease, water at home, and socio-economic characteristics. Am. J. Epidemiol. **94**:1–10.

COMSTOCK, G.W. (1979). Water hardness and cardiovascular diseases. Am. J. Epidemiol. **110**:375–400.

COMSTOCK, G.W. (1980). The epidemiologic perspective: water hardness and cardio-vascular disease. J. Environ. Path. Toxicol. **4**:9–25.

FOLSOM, A.R. and PRINEAS, R.J. (1982). Drinking water composition and blood pressure: a review of the epidemiology. Am. J. Epidemiol. **115**:818–832.

GILLIES, M.E. and PAULIN, H.V. (1983). Variability of mineral intakes from drink-ing water: a possible explanation for the controversy over the relationship of water quality to cardiovascular disease. Inter. J. Epidemiol. **12**:45–50.

KOBAYASHI, J. (1957). On geographic relationship between the chemical nature of river water and death rate from apoplexy. Berichte des Ohara Institut fur Landwirt-schaftliche Biologie **11**:12–21.

LANZOLA, E., TURCONI, G., ALLEGRINI, M., deMARCO, R., MARINONI, A., and MIRACCA, P. (1983). Relation between coronary heart disease and certain elements in water and diet. Prog. Biochem. Pharmacol. **19**:80–88.

LUOMA, H., AROMAA, A., HELMINEN, S., MARTOMAA, H., KIVILAOTO, L., PUNSAR, S. and KNEKT, P. (1983). Risk of myocardial infarction in Finnish men in relation to fluoride, magnesium, and calcium concentration in water. Acta. Med. Scand. **213**:171–176.

MASIRONI, R. and SHAPER, A.G. (1981). Epidemiologic studies of health effects of water from different sources. Ann. Rev. Nutr. **1**:375–400.

NATIONAL RESEARCH COUNCIL. (1979). *Geochemistry of Water in Relation to Cardiovascular Disease*. National Academy of Sciences, Washington, D.C.

NATIONAL RESEARCH COUNCIL. (1980). *Drinking Water and Health, Vol. 3* National Academy Press, Washington, D.C., pp. 21–24.

NERI, C.C., NEWITT, D. and SCHREIBER, G.B. (1974). Can epidemiology elucidate the water story? Am. J. Epidemiol. **99**:75–88.

NERI, C.C., HEWITT, D., SCHREIBER, G.B., ANDERSON, T.W., MANDEL, J.S. and ZDROJEWSKY, A. (1975). Health aspects of hard and soft waters. J. Am. Water Works Assoc. **67**:403–08.

SHAPER, A.G., PACKHAM, R.F. and POCOCK, S.J. (1980). The British regional heart study: cardiovascular mortality and water quality. J. Environ. Path. Toxicol. **4**:89–111.

SHARRETT, A.R. (1979). The role of chemical constituents of drinking water in cardiovascular diseases. Am. J. Epidemiol. **110**:401–419.

SHARETT, A.R., MORIN, M.M., FABSITZ, R.R. and BAILEY, K.R. (1984). Water hardness and cardiovascular mortality. *Drinking Water and Human Health*, In Bell, J.A. and Doege, T.C., eds., American Medical Assoc., Chicago, IL., pp. 57–68.

CHAPTER XVI

EFFECT OF MULTIPLE ELEMENT VARIATION ON BLOOD PRESSURE

Ben H. Douglas,* P.T. McCauley† and R.J. Bull†
**University of Mississippi Medical Center
Jackson Mississippi*

*†Health Effects Research Laboratory
Cincinnati, Ohio*

ABSTRACT

The present study was designed to determine the effect of varying the dietary intake of Na, K, Cd and Pb on the blood pressure of 16 groups of rats (10 each group). The animals received 80% of the minimum daily requirement (MDR) of Ca and 120% MDR Mg. Control levels were established for weight and blood pressure. The animals were then given diets containing high or low levels of the minerals for 16 weeks. High levels were 0.07% Na, 0.24% K, and 0.048% Mg (percent by weight of the total diet) plus 30 Mg $PbCl_2$/1 in the drinking water and 5 mg Cd/1 in the drinking water. Low levels were 0.48% Na, 0.16% K, and 0.448% Ca, no Pb and no Cd. The values for Na, K, Ca and Mg represent intakes of 20% above or 20% below the normal dietary intake. The blood pressure of the animals which received Cd rose and became labile. This effect was modified by the presence or absence of the other minerals.

INTRODUCTION

A reasonable physiological basis by which water hardness can protect against cardiovascular mortality has hampered studies of this relationship. Hypertension is a major cardiovascular risk factor. If the elements in hard water could protect against hypertension or soft water could enhance the development of hypertension, this would offer a partial explanation for the observation.

Ca intake is perhaps important. It has been shown that the blood pressure of rural high school children in Hinds County, Mississippi is higher than that of urban school children and that in the city the higher the socio-economic status of the family, the lower the blood pressure (Langford et al., 1968). The findings were present in individual race/sex groups. Some factor, presumably diet, is likely responsible for the differences in blood pressure. Dietary histories of these children showed an inverse correlation of Ca intake with blood pressure. Other investigators (McCarron et al., 1984) have reported that Ca intake is higher in normotensive individuals than in hypertensive individuals.

Excess Na has been shown to raise blood pressure (Langston et al., 1963), especially when there is concomitant reduction of functional renal tissue (Douglas et al., 1964) or a decrease in glomerular filtration coefficient (Norman et al., 1978). Na and K have been implicated in the control of aldosterone secretion (Nicholls et al., 1978).

The detrimental effects of Pb (Cramer et al., 1974; Goyer, 1968) and Cd (Kanisawa and Schroeder, 1969) have received considerable attention in recent years. Pb produces renal damage and encephalopathy. Some investigators have reported that hypertension can be induced by chronic ingestion of Cd or by acute administration of the element (Perry et al., 1977). Others have been unable to produce hypertension in experimental animals by exposing them to Cd (Porter et al., 1974).

The contribution of hard drinking water to the nutritional requirement for Ca is small (Hankin et al., 1970). The contribution may be important though, since it has been suggested (Seelig and Heggtveit, 1974) that the intake is marginal in the diet of substantial segments of the population. A marginal amount of Ca should unmask, or at least not blunt, the pressure-raising effects of other minerals. In the present studies, adequate Mg was given since it has been shown that Mg deficiency is associated with cardiovascular pathology (Seelig and Heggtveit, 1974).

Pb can induce chronic nephrotoxicity in humans (Cramer et al., 1974) and in experimental animals (Goyer, 1968). Any agent which damages renal glomeruli can affect the level to which blood pressure rises. Pb could enhance the toxic effect of Cd or other agents. Pb has been demonstrated to be leached from water distribution systems (Craum and McCabe, 1975).

The level to which blood pressure rises cannot be predicted on the basis of one mineral alone. Adequate Ca is necessary for normal cardiac function such as excitation-contraction coupling (Fleckstein, 1977). High levels of dietary Ca decrease serum lipids (Yacowitz et al., 1965). As noted above, Mg deficiency has been associated with cardiovascular pathology. K is necessary for proper cardiovascular function. Excess Na, at least in sensitive animals, will raise the blood pressure. Pb, Cd and other agents which may be toxic to the kidney could raise the blood pressure by altering the arterial pressure-urinary output relationship for blood pressure control. The long-term hypertensive effect of minerals on blood pressure is likely a result of their effect on the kidney to raise the set-point for blood pressure control to a higher level. The present studies were designed to provide additional information regarding the effects of these minerals on blood pressure.

METHODS

Sixteen groups of male Sprague Dawley rats (10 rats each group) were used in the study. The rats weighed approximately 200 g initially. They were housed in a temperature controlled (22 ± 2° C) room. The relative humidity was 50% and the light-dark cycle was 12 hours. Blood pressures were measured weekly both during the two week control period and the sixteen week experimental period using the tail cuff method (Friedman and Freed, 1949). The sixteen groups of animals were run simultaneously, they were housed in the same location and they were handled by the same personnel. After control levels were established for weight and blood pressure the animals received high or low density levels of Na, K, Ca, Mg, Pb and Cd. The groups and the dietary mineral variations are shown in Table 1.

High dietary levels of the elements varied were 0.07% Na, 0.24% K, 0.672% Ca, 0.048% Mg plus 300 Mg $PbCl_2$/l in the drinking water and 5 mg Cd/l in the drinking water. The percentages given are percent by weight of the total diet. Low dietary levels were 0.048% Na, 0.16% K, 0.448% Ca, 0.03% Mg, no Pb and no Cd. The values for Na, K, Ca and Mg represent values which would be 20% above or 20% below the normal intake. The animals were on the diets for 16 weeks.

TABLE I
Dietary Mineral Variation

Group	Ca	Mg	Pb	Cd	Na	K
1	L	H	H	H	H	H
2	L	H	H	H	H	L
3	L	H	H	H	L	H
4	L	H	H	H	L	L
5	L	H	L	H	H	H
6	L	H	L	H	H	L
7	L	H	L	H	L	H
8	L	H	L	H	L	L
9	L	H	H	L	H	H
10	L	H	H	L	H	L
11	L	H	H	L	L	H
12	L	H	H	L	L	L
13	L	H	L	L	H	H
14	L	H	L	L	H	L
15	L	H	L	L	L	H
16	L	H	L	L	L	L

Groups studied are shown. Groups receiving high (H) or low (L) dietary levels of Ca, Mg, Cd, Pb, Na and K are indicated. See text for description of composition of diet.

The diets were prepared by Teklad Test Diets (Wisconsin) and included 18.2% protein, 71.6% carbohydrate, 5% fat, 2.65% moisture, 0.40% phosphorous, 0.05% chloride, 103 ppm Fe, 0.35 ppm I, 10 ppm Cu, 55 ppm Mn, 20 ppm Zn and an adequate vitamin content. The diets were mixed to provide adequate nutritional requirements (National Academy of Sciences, 1972).

At the end of the study kidneys were collected from each animal and placed in 10% formalin solution. The tissue was sectioned, paraffin embedded, stained with hematoxylin and eosin and mounted for examination by light microscopy. Electron microscopic examination was done.

RESULTS

Table II shows the blood pressure changes (mmHg systolic) of the animals in groups 1 through 8. All blood pressures are reported as Mean ± Standard Error of Mean. All of the animals in groups 1 through 8 received diets low in Ca, high in Mg and high in Cd. The Na, K and Pb was varied. Within two weeks after starting the experimental regimen the blood pressure of group 1 had increased ($p < 0.05$) by 15 mmHg (from 122 ± 2 mmHg to 137 ± 2 mmHg). Thereafter, the blood pressure became variable but remained predominantly 10–20 mmHg above control levels. The blood pressure of group 2 increased during treatment but was not as variable nor as high as that of group 1. The diet was similar to that of group 1 except for the low K.

The blood pressure response of group 3 was similar to that of group 1. It rose initially. Thereafter, there was considerable variation in the blood pressure; sometimes near normal (week 5), at other times elevated (week 9). The blood pressure of the animals in group 4 rose following the initiation of treatment and became variable. During the experimental period the blood pressure ranged from a low of 123 ± 3 mmHg to a high of 149 ± 4 mmHg. The blood pressure of group 5 rose during the experimental period. It was variable and remained above control levels throughout the study. The blood pressure of the animals in group 6 rose within 2 weeks. It was variable throughout the experimental period ranging from 124 ± 1 mmHg to 142 ± 2 mmHg. The blood pressure response of the animals in group 7 was typical of that of the other groups of animals which received Cd. The blood pressure was variable during the experimental period and remained above control levels. The variability of the blood pressure of group 8 was just as evident as that of the other groups which received Cd. During the experimental period it ranged from 121 ± 1 mmHg to 140 ± 3 mmHg.

Table III shows the blood pressure changes in groups 9 through 16. All of the animals in groups 9 through 16 received diets low in Ca and high in Mg. None of the animals received Cd. As in the previous 8 groups the Na, K and Pb was varied.

The diet of group 9 was low in Ca and high in Mg, Ma and K. The diet contained Pb but no Cd. As shown in Table III the blood pressure during eight of the last ten weeks of the experimental period was below 130 mmHg. (Com-

TABLE II
Blood Pressures (mmHg)

Week	Group 1	2	3	4	5	6	7	8
1	122 ± 2	124 ± 3	123 ± 3	114 ± 2	113 ± 3	115 ± 3	126 ± 3	122 ± 3
2	117 ± 2	117 ± 2	125 ± 2	124 ± 3	121 ± 1	123 ± 2	121 ± 3	122 ± 3
3	129 ± 2	123 ± 3	132 ± 4	138 ± 3	135 ± 2	130 ± 4	131 ± 3	135 ± 3
4	137 ± 2	136 ± 3	135 ± 2	123 ± 3	140 ± 3	133 ± 3	130 ± 3	131 ± 2
5	134 ± 3	120 ± 1	120 ± 2	135 ± 3	120 ± 3	124 ± 1	134 ± 3	123 ± 3
6	130 ± 3	125 ± 2	134 ± 2	123 ± 3	133 ± 3	129 ± 2	123 ± 1	128 ± 2
7	128 ± 2	120 ± 3	128 ± 6	124 ± 2	132 ± 3	129 ± 2	132 ± 2	124 ± 2
8	135 ± 2	128 ± 2	128 ± 2	128 ± 2	132 ± 2	136 ± 1	140 ± 4	136 ± 2
9	143 ± 4	135 ± 2	143 ± 4	149 ± 4	137 ± 4	142 ± 2	144 ± 4	140 ± 3
10	141 ± 2	129 ± 2	140 ± 2	124 ± 3	134 ± 3	139 ± 2	130 ± 3	130 ± 1
11	133 ± 2	132 ± 2	133 ± 3	127 ± 3	127 ± 3	138 ± 3	129 ± 3	136 ± 3
12	137 ± 1	133 ± 3	126 ± 3	132 ± 2	131 ± 1	125 ± 2	141 ± 5	121 ± 1
13	137 ± 1	131 ± 3	126 ± 2	136 ± 3	136 ± 3	130 ± 2	140 ± 3	126 ± 2
14	137 ± 1	131 ± 2	128 ± 4	133 ± 2	137 ± 2	136 ± 2	138 ± 3	135 ± 2
15	124 ± 2	130 ± 1	131 ± 3	131 ± 2	131 ± 1	127 ± 3	138 ± 2	134 ± 3
16	122 ± 2	123 ± 2	131 ± 2	130 ± 1	136 ± 3	135 ± 2	140 ± 1	133 ± 2
17	139 ± 2	130 ± 3	133 ± 3	134 ± 2	129 ± 3	128 ± 4	129 ± 1	129 ± 2

Systolic pressures (MEAN ± SEM) of animals in Groups 1–8 are shown. The first 2 pressures (weeks 1–2) are control pressures.

pare to the blood pressures of group 1. Group 1 had the same diet plus Cd.) The diet of group 10 was similar to that of group 9 except for the low K. No consistent pattern of sustained elevation of blood pressure was apparent. The blood pressure of the animals in group 11 exhibited some variability but the blood pressures during the last half of the experimental period were not higher than during the first half. The animals were not hypertensive. A similar pattern was observed in group 12. The diet of group 13 contained neither Cd nor Pb. The animals demonstrated no tendency toward developing a sustained hypertension and the blood pressure changes were generally unremarkable. Group 14, which also received neither Pb nor Cd, responded in a similar fashion. The blood pressure response of group 15 was almost identical to that of group 14. The blood pressure remained near or below control levels throughout the study. Group 16 did not demonstrate a consistent pattern of sustained elevation of blood pressure.

Renal morphological changes in the Cd-ingesting animals included areas of non-specific foot process fusion in the epithelial cells, inclusion bodies and a thickening of the glomerular membrane. Chronic nephrotoxicity as a result of Pb ingestion was not observed.

TABLE III
Blood Pressures (mmHg)

Week	Group 9	10	11	12	13	14	15	16
1	137 ± 4	128 ± 2	138 ± 2	132 ± 3	131 ± 5	134 ± 3	133 ± 3	135 ± 3
2	129 ± 3	134 ± 3	129 ± 3	120 ± 3	135 ± 3	134 ± 3	134 ± 4	134 ± 3
3	130 ± 3	136 ± 2	135 ± 3	139 ± 3	137 ± 2	131 ± 7	139 ± 3	133 ± 2
4	135 ± 2	133 ± 2	134 ± 2	130 ± 1	126 ± 2	134 ± 2	133 ± 3	130 ± 2
5	138 ± 2	142 ± 3	128 ± 4	131 ± 4	138 ± 2	134 ± 1	131 ± 3	131 ± 2
6	136 ± 3	138 ± 2	141 ± 2	127 ± 2	127 ± 5	140 ± 3	132 ± 2	136 ± 2
7	134 ± 5	133 ± 3	132 ± 1	128 ± 2	132 ± 4	136 ± 3	133 ± 2	143 ± 3
8	136 ± 2	127 ± 3	135 ± 3	124 ± 3	129 ± 2	133 ± 2	145 ± 3	131 ± 2
9	128 ± 3	130 ± 3	134 ± 3	124 ± 1	139 ± 3	135 ± 4	127 ± 2	135 ± 4
10	129 ± 3	129 ± 2	125 ± 3	131 ± 3	125 ± 3	128 ± 3	133 ± 3	128 ± 3
11	129 ± 2	131 ± 2	132 ± 2	131 ± 3	128 ± 3	127 ± 3	128 ± 1	119 ± 3
12	125 ± 2	132 ± 2	120 ± 3	124 ± 3	131 ± 3	132 ± 3	134 ± 2	132 ± 3
13	131 ± 3	152 ± 3	131 ± 2	121 ± 2	137 ± 2	135 ± 2	131 ± 2	129 ± 4
14	125 ± 2	130 ± 3	138 ± 3	129 ± 3	125 ± 2	136 ± 2	130 ± 2	124 ± 4
15	128 ± 3	131 ± 7	127 ± 2	116 ± 3	124 ± 3	135 ± 2	133 ± 2	122 ± 3
16	123 ± 3	141 ± 3	128 ± 3	125 ± 2	139 ± 2	133 ± 3	126 ± 2	122 ± 1
17	126 ± 3	133 ± 3	134 ± 2	121 ± 2	133 ± 4	134 ± 1	133 ± 3	118 ± 5
18	136 ± 2	134 ± 2	122 ± 3	124 ± 3	135 ± 4	127 ± 2	123 ± 2	120 ± 2

Systolic pressures (MEAN ± SEM) of animals in Groups 9–16 are shown. The first 2 pressures (weeks 1–2) are control pressures.

DISCUSSION

The mineral content of the diet of the animals in the present study affected the blood pressure. The eight groups of animals which received Cd had two common features. First, the blood pressure tended to increase within a few weeks. Secondly, the blood pressure tended to exhibit an unusual degree of variability. The blood pressure of the eight groups of animals which did not receive Cd generally showed a contrasting response. No consistent pattern of sustained elevation of blood pressure was apparent.

The presence or absence of the other minerals modified the Cd effect on blood pressure. For example, the blood pressure response of the animals in group 7 (reduced Na intake) was typical of that of the other groups of animals which received Cd except that they were on the experimental regimen approximately six weeks before the blood pressure rose. This delay in blood pressure elevation was not observed in group 5. Group 5 was on a high Na intake. All other components of the diet were the same as that of group 7.

Pb can induce chronic nephrotoxicity (Cramer et al., 1974; Goyer, 1968) but it was not observed in the animals in this study which received Pb. An increased intake or a longer duration of ingestion of Pb might be necessary to produce nephrotoxicity.

The reduced Ca intake probably unmasked, or at least did not blunt, the pressure-raising effects of the other minerals. We have shown that less Na is required to raise the blood pressure of animals on a Ca-deficient diet (Langford et al., 1968). Conversely, a high Ca intake (120% MDR) blunts the hypertensive effect of an increased Na intake (Douglas and Bull, 1980).

The increase in blood pressure observed in this study was likely due to damage sustained to the kidney glomeruli, thus reducing the functional renal mass. This would alter the arterial pressure-urinary output relationship for blood pressure control. A higher blood pressure would then be necessary in order to maintain fluid balance. The level to which blood pressure rises as a result of mineral ingestion cannot be predicted on the basis of one mineral alone.

ACKNOWLEDGEMENTS

The research described in this paper has been subject to the Agency's review and it has been approved for publication as an EPA document. Mention of trade names or commercial products does not constitute endorsement or recommendation for use.

REFERENCES

CRAMER, K., GOYER, R.A., JAGENBURG, R. and WILSON, M.H. (1974). Renal ultrastructure, renal function and parameters of lead toxicity in workers with different periods of lead exposure. Brit. J. Ind. Med. 31:113–127.

CRAUM, G.F. and McCABE, L.J. (1975). Problems associated with metals in drinking water. J. Am Water Assn. pp. 593–599.

DOUGLAS, B.H. and BULL, R.J. (1980). The influence of multiple trace elements on blood pressure in the rat. J. Environ. Path. Toxi. 4–2,3:243–249.

DOUGLAS, B.H., GUYTON, A.C., LANGSTON, J.B. and BISHOP, V.S. (1964). Hypertension caused by salt loading. II. Fluid volume and tissue pressure changes. Am. J. Physiol. 207:669–671.

DOUGLAS, B.H. and LANGFORD, H.G. (1965). Effect of DCA and post DCA hypertension upon the course of pregnancy in the rat. Proc. Soc. Exper. Biol. Med. 120:238.

FLECKSTEIN, A. (1977). Specific pharmacology of calcium in myocardium, cardiac pacemakers and vascular smooth muscle. Ann. Rev. Pharmacol. Toxicol. 17:149–166.

FRIEDMAN, M. and FREED, S. (1949). Microphonic manometer for indirect determination of systolic blood pressure in the rat. Proc. Soc. Exper. Biol. Med. 70:670–672.

GOYER, R.A. (1968). Mitochondrial swelling and aminoaciduria. Lab. Invest. 19:71–77.

HANKIN, J.H., MERGEN, S. and GOLDSMITH, N.F. (1970). Contribution of hard water to calcium and magnesium intakes of adults. J. Am. Dietet. Assn. 56:212–224.

KANISAWA, M. and SCHROEDER, H.A. (1969). Renal arteriolar changes in hypertensive rats given cadmium in drinking water. Exper. & Molec. Pathol. 10:81–98.

LANGFORD, H.G., WATSON, R.L. and DOUGLAS, B.H. (1968). Factors affecting blood pressure in population groups. Transactions Assoc. Amer. Physicians **LXIII**:135–146.

LANGSTON, J.B., GUYTON, A.C., DOUGLAS, B.H. and DORSETT, P.E. (1963). Effect of changes in salt intake on arterial pressure and renal function in partially nephrectomized dogs. Cir. Res. **12**:508.

McCARRON, D.A., MORRIS, C.D., HENRY, H.J. and STANTON, J.L. (1964). Blood pressure and nutrient intake in the United States. Science **224**:1292–1398.

NICHOLLS, M.G., TREE, M., BROWN, J.J., DOUGLAS, B.H., FRASER, R., HAY, G.D., LEVER, A.F., MORTON, J.J. and ROBERTSON, J.I.S. (1978). Angiotensin II/aldosterone dose-response curves in the dog: Effect of changes in sodium balance. Endocrinol. **102**:485:493.

NORMAN, R.A., JR., ENOBAKHARE, J.A., DECLUE, J.W., DOUGLAS, B.H. and GUYTON, A.C. (1979). Arterial pressure-urinary output relationship in hypertensive rats. Am. J. Physiol. **234**(3):98.

PERRY, H.M., JR., ERLANGER, M. and PERRY, E.F. (1977). Elevated systolic pressure following chronic low-level cadmium feeding. Am. J. Physiol. **232**: H114–H121.

PORTER, M.C., MIYA, T.S. and BOUSQUET, W.F. (1974). Cadmium's inability to induce hypertension in the rat. Toxicol. Appl. Pharmacol. **27**:692–695.

SEELIG, M.S. and HEGGTVEIT, H.A. (1974). Magnesium interrelationships in ischemic heart disease: A review. Am. J. Clin. Nutrition **27**:59–79.

YACOWITZ, H., FLEISCHMAN, A.I. and BIERENBAUM, M.L. (1965). Effects of oral calcium upon serum lipids in man. Brit. Med. J. **1**:1352–1354.

CHAPTER XVII

EFFECTS OF LOW LEVEL CADMIUM EXPOSURE ON BLOOD PRESSURE AND MYOCARDIAL FUNCTION AND METABOLISM

Stephen J. Kopp,* Robert C. Prentice, * H. Mitchell Perry, Jr.,†
Janice M. Feliksik,* June P. Tow* and Margaret Erlanger†
*Department of Physiology and Nuclear Magnetic
Resonance Laboratory
Chicago College of Osteopathic
Medicine, Chicago, Illinois

†Medical Service, Veterans Administration Medical Center
Hypertension Division, Department of Internal Medicine
Washington University School of Medicine,
St. Louis, Missouri

ABSTRACT

Cadmium-hypertension has been reported following chronic oral exposure by approximately 55-60% of the laboratories that have studied this phenomenon. In addition 85-90% of the research groups that have examined the pressor effect of cadmium following chronic intraperitoneal injection have reported a significant pressure response. A defined-dose-response relationship exists with an optimal dose range between 9×10^{-6} to 5×10^{-5} mol/kg body wt producing maximal pressor effects. Generally, the duration of the exposure period in the chronic feeding studies that have failed to induce a significant hypertensive effect has been comparatively short, often less than six months. Moreover, studies of this nature that have involved male rats have been distinguished from each other by the fact that the control groups appear different. When nonsignificant blood pressure effects have been reported following chronic oral exposure, systolic blood pressures have averaged 15 to 20 mmHg above the values reported for control groups in studies that have described the hypertensive effect of oral cadmium doses. This difference generally represents the magnitude of the pressor response that commonly occurs in response to chronic cadmium treatment. Overall, cadmium-hypertension has been reported in a variety of animal models including different strains of rats, in rats of both sexes, and in studies that have utilized different dietary conditions. Hypertension has not been reported in response to cadmium either in studies which have used purified diets, or in the few studies in which cadmium has been administered in the food. Thus, the ability of cadmium to induce hypertension is not strain-, sex-, or diet-specific, and the cross-species findings add credence to the possibility that similar effects may occur in humans. Accompanying the hypertensive effect of cadmium are significant changes in the functional and metabolic properties of cardiovascular tissues. The results obtained from chronic studies have demonstrated that oral cadmium exposure leads to significant changes in *in vivo* myocardial contractility, responsiveness of the cardiovascular system to exogenously administered norepinephrine, calcium sensitivity of the myocardium, and myocardial phosphoglyceride metabolism. These observations support the hypothesis that cadmium acts to disrupt cellular processes mediated by calcium, leading to altered phospholipid structure and molecular dynamics of the cell membrane. The resultant pathophysiologic responses to cadmium in part reflect these actions of cadmium on the cell membrane and the calcium-dependent processes of the cell.

INTRODUCTION

Historically, cadmium-hypertension has been viewed as an esoteric finding that manifests itself under only certain rigorous experimental conditions, in only relatively few laboratories and in only highly selected animal populations (Fleischer et al., 1974; Friberg et al., 1974; Templeton and Cherian, 1983; Whanger, 1979). Comprehensive, rather than perfunctory evaluation of the literature pertaining to this subject, however, does not support this traditional viewpoint (Kopp, 1985). Overall, cadmium-hypertension has been induced in a variety of animal models (rats, rabbits, dogs) including different strains of rats (Long-Evans, Sprague-Dawley, Fischer 344, but not Wistar and Oregon State University Brown), in rats of both sexes, and in studies that have utilized diverse dietary conditions—e.g., rye-based and commercial chow diets, mineral fortified water and deionized water (Boscolo et al., 1980, 1981; Eakin et al., 1980; Hadley et al., 1979; Kopp et al., 1980a-d; Kopp, 1985; Ohanian et al., 1978; Perry and Erlanger, 1974, 1982; Perry et al., 1976, 1979; Revis, 1978; Revis et al., 1981, 1983; Schroeder and Vinton, 1962; Schroeder and Buckman, 1967; Tomera and Harakal, 1980). Hypertension has not been reported, however, in response to cadmium either in studies which have used purified diets (Doyle et al., 1974), or in the few studies in which cadmium has been administered in the food (Frickenhaus et al., 1976; Loeser and Lorke, 1977a). Thus, based on existing literature evidence, the ability of cadmium to induce hypertension is not necessarily animal-, species-, sex-, diet- or laboratory-specific.

Nine (Boscolo et al., 1980, 1981; Hadley et al., 1979; Kopp et al., 1980a-d, 1983; Ohanian et al., 1978; Perry and Erlanger, 1974; Perry et al., 1979; Schroeder and Vinton, 1962; Tomera and Harakal, 1980; Walker and Moses, 1979) of sixteen (Doyle et al., 1974; Eakin et al., 1980; Fingerle et al., 1982;

Frickenhaus et al., 1976; Kotsonis and Klaassen, 1978; Loeser and Lorke, 1977a,b; Petering et al., 1979) laboratories that have studied the pressor effect of cadmium have reported a significant increase in blood pressure in experimental animals in response to chronic, orally administered cadmium doses. In certain of the studies where cadmium exposure was not associated with a significant pressor effect, the duration of the exposure period was relatively short, often six months or less (Doyle et al., 1974; Fingerle et al., 1982; Frickenhaus et al., 1976; Kopp and Hawley, 1978; Kotsonis and Klaassen, 1978; Loeser and Lorke, 1977a). Closer inspection of the blood pressures reported for male control populations has yielded an interesting observation. When cadmium has had a nonsignificant effect on the blood pressure of treated male rats, the corresponding control populations have had systolic blood pressures that have averaged 15 to 20 mmHg above the control values reported in studies in which a hypertensive response to cadmium was described (Figure 1). This difference between male control populations is somewhat disconcerting, considering that the mag-

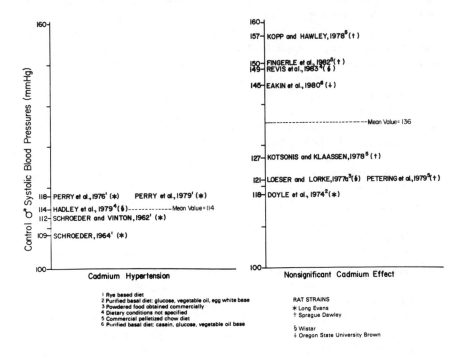

FIGURE 1. Comparison of reported control (male) systolic pressure values from representative studies in which cadmium added to the drinking water had either a significant (hypertension) or non-significant pressor effect. The respective dietary considerations are indicated with a numerical superscript and the rat strains used in each study are indicated with a symbol superscript. Since other differences exist among these studies, such as the duration of the individual exposure periods, the mean values (average of the values shown) shown adjacent to the dotted lines are presented for illustrative purposes, rather than to indicate a rigorous statistical treatment of these results.

nitude of this difference generally represents the magnitude of the pressor response induced by cadmium. As a result, this phenomenon may be a contributing factor to the absence of a statistically significant response to cadmium in these studies.

Further assessment of reported literature findings has revealed that six of seven additional research groups have demonstrated a significant pressor response to cadmium following chronic or acute intraperitoneal injection (Fadloun and Leach, 1981; Hall and Nasseth, 1980; Hall and Hungerford, 1982; Porter et al., 1974; Roach and Damude, 1980; Thind et al., 1970; Watkins, 1980). Similarly, acute intravascular administration of cadmium has been shown to induce a sustained pressor response in four of five studies that have examined cadmium's effect on systemic blood pressure using this method (Dalhamn and Friberg, 1954; Fadloun and Leach, 1981; Hall and Nasseth, 1980; Perry and Yunice, 1965; Perry et al., 1970). Generally, results from the cited studies indicate that oral and intraperitoneal routes of cadmium exposure are characterized by parabolic dose-pressor response curves that have defined maxima, corresponding to the optimal effective dose of cadmium for each route of exposure. A chronic, oral intake level of approximately 10 μ g/day has been shown to induce near maximal increases in systolic pressure in rats receiving cadmium via the drinking water (Kopp et al., 1982). Alternatively, cadmium administered chronically by intraperitoneal injection has a maximal effective dose, ranging between 10^{-6} to 10^{-5} mol cadmium per kilogram body weight, as illustrated in Figure 2. This figure was compiled from existing literature findings. By comparison, the dose-response relationship for cadmium administered intravascularly and the resultant pressor effect on the cardiovascular system appear less well-defined, as illustrated in Figure 3. Collectively, the cited literature findings are consistent with the overall interpretation that cadmium causes a significant pressor effect within the cardiovascular system, irrespective of the exposure method, and that the dose-response relationship is essentially parabolic with a defined maximum well below the concentration of cadmium that elicits overt, toxic manifestations.

Although the aforementioned analysis of the pressor response to cadmium suggests that hypertension is a more reproducible and generalized finding than is commonly recognized, other cardiovascular manifestations have been reported in conjunction with cadmium exposure which indicate that cadmium also causes significant functional and metabolic disturbances within cardiovascular tissues (Kopp, 1985). At present the relationship between these effects and the pressor effect of cadmium is unresolved. To a certain extent the preoccupation with the hypertension controversy has hindered the evaluation of these other cardiovascular actions of cadmium and obscured the significance of recent findings. Ex vivo analysis of hearts obtained from chronically treated rats has revealed significant biochemical and functional disturbances within hearts from cadmium-exposed animals. Cadmium-induced changes identified by this technique include reduced myocardial high-energy phosphate levels, decreased cardiac myofibrillar protein phosphorylation activity involving phosphoproteins linked to the regulation of myocardial contractility, diminished myocar-

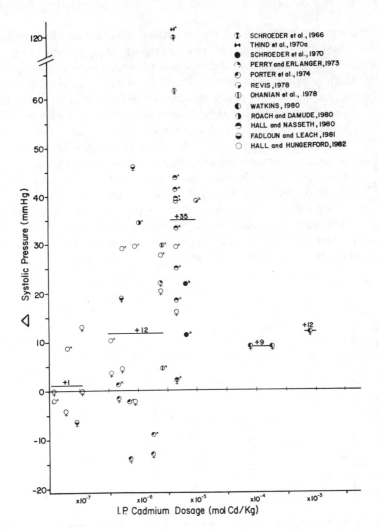

FIGURE 2. Graphic depiction of reported cadmium-induced changes in systolic blood pressure when administered chronically by intraperitoneal (i.p.) injection. The numerical value shown above each solid horizontal line represents the average of the reported values included within the cadmium dose range indicated by the width of the horizontal line. These mean values are presented to illustrate the qualitative aspects of the relationship between the dose of cadmium administered by intraperitoneal injection and the resultant pressor response.

dial contractile activity and reduced excitability of the cardiac conduction system (Kopp et al., 1980a-d; Kopp et al., 1983). By performing these biochemical and physiologic analyses under *ex vivo* conditions it was assumed that the findings obtained by this method would reflect intrinsic *in vivo* changes associated with chronic cadmium exposure, rather than changes complicated by combined effects of cadmium and the *ex vivo* procedures. As will be demonstrated in the studies reported herein, this assumption may not be entirely valid.

The present study was performed to extend these earlier observations to include *in vivo* analyses of the functional and metabolic properties of cardiovascular tissues following chronic oral exposure to cadmium (Kopp, 1983). These *in vivo* findings permit comparison with previous results obtained by *ex vivo* analytical procedures, thus enabling more definitive evaluation of the direct actions of cadmium. Implicit within this overall approach has been the goal to identify putative cellular sites and mechanisms of cadmium's action on the cardiovascular system. The findings described herein give credence to the hypothesis that cadmium acts to disrupt functional and cellular processes of the heart mediated by calcium, possibly leading to altered phospholipid structure and molecular dynamics of the sarcolemma. Comparison of these *in vivo* findings with previous *ex vivo* observations appears to indicate that chronic cadmium exposure interferes with the post-ischemic functional and metabolic recovery processes of the myocardium giving rise to quantitatively exaggerated, but qualitatively similar responses under *ex vivo* analytical conditions.

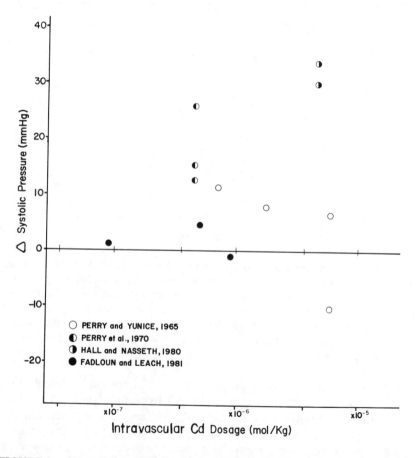

FIGURE 3. Graphic representation of reported cadmium-induced changes in systolic blood pressure when administered acutely by intravascular injection.

METHODS

Chronic Feeding Studies

General animal care and diet. Female, Long-Evans rats were used exclusively in the chronic exposure studies. Rats obtained as weanlings from Blue Spruce Farms, Altamont, New York were individually earmarked for identification and maintained according to routine practices in specially designed, low contamination quarters for the duration of each study (Perry et al., 1979). Room temperature and relative humidity were maintained at 21°C and 45% respectively. All rats were weighed periodically as a measure of group well-being. The animals were followed for either 12 or 18 mos.

The only water provided for drinking was the fortified water described by Schroeder (Schroeder and Vinton, 1962), which is deionized water supplemented with the essential trace elements cobalt, molybdenum, copper, manganese and zinc. Depending upon the group to which the rats were assigned, the drinking water was supplemented as follows: no added cadmium (control); or 1.0 ppm cadmium (1 μg Cd per ml, or 8.9×10^{-6} M Cd). The drinking water was provided *ad libitum* in glass bottles with rubber stoppers and stainless steel drinking tubes. Each rat group had its own supply of bottles, stoppers and tubes for the duration of each experiment. The volume of water consumed by each group was approximated for 1 week each month.

All animals received a standard rye-based diet (Kopp et al., 1983; Perry et al., 1979; Schroeder and Vinton, 1962), low in heavy metal content. Random batches of this diet were assayed for metal content as a quality control check. Food intake was approximated for each group for 1 week each month.

Conscious blood pressure determinations. At defined intervals (not exceeding 3 months) during the course of each study indirect systolic blood pressures were measured in the conscious state from each rat, using tail cuff plethysmographic procedures described previously (Perry and Erlanger, 1982).

Ex vivo myocardial contractility. Control (n = 14) and 1 ppm Cd (n = 13)-fed rats from the 18 month exposure groups were used in these studies. Hearts from treated rats were analyzed according to standard *ex vivo* perfusion techniques developed for this purpose (Kopp et al., 1978; 1980d). Briefly, rats [control (n = 9); cadmium-treated (n = 8)] were selected in random order from the respective groups, heparinized and sacrificed by cervical dislocation. The chest cavity was immediately opened, the heart excised, and placed in precooled perfusion fluid (5°C) to induce diastolic arrest. While in this cold buffer, the aorta was cannulated and tied to the catheter for retrograde perfusion, superfluous connective and adipose tissues were removed, and a single open silk (4-0) loop was sutured to the apical region of the heart and attached to a Grass FT0.03C force displacement transducer through a submersed string-pulley arrangement for recording isotonic contractile tension. Hearts were then perfused for a 30 min equilibration period during which time the physiologic activity was monitored as a basis for assessing the stability of the preparation. Following this 30 min stabilization period the cardiac contractile activity [peak active tension, rate of tension development (dT/dt) and pulse rate] was recorded and analyzed. After permanent tracings of myocardial contractile activity had been recorded, each heart continued to perfuse briefly during which time it was rapidly frozen by compression in a liquid N_2-chilled Wollenberger clamp (Kopp et al., 1983). The frozen heart tissue was stored briefly in liquid N_2 prior to preparation of the tissue perchloric acid extract.

Alternatively, the remaining rats [control (n = 5) and cadmium-fed (n = 5)] were heparinized by intraperitoneal injection and anesthetized with sodium pentobarbital (45 mg/kg body wt, i.p.). A tracheal intubation was performed and each rat was ventilated with intermittant positive pressure using a Phipps and Bird small animal respirator. The chest cavity was opened, and the heart was exposed from the pericardial sac and arrested with a bolus injection of a potassium-based, chilled (5°C) cardioplegic solution [30mM KCl, and 10mM Tris-HCl (pH 7.4) in isotonic saline]. The heart was then immediately frozen by compression in a liquid N_2-chilled Wollenberger clamp and the tissue perchloric acid extract was prepared for subsequent biochemical analysis.

In vivo myocardial contractility. A detailed methodologic presentation of this surgical procedure has been reported elsewhere; therefore, only an abbreviated description is provided herein (Kopp, 1983). Rats from 12 month exposure groups [control-fed (n = 7) or 1 ppm Cd-fed (n = 7)] were individually weighed and anesthetized with sodium pentobarbital (45 mg/kg, i.p.). Subcutaneous needle electrodes were inserted into each limb for monitoring heart electrical activity during surgery. A superficial, medial incision was made in the ventral surface of the neck, the right common carotid artery was isolated by blunt dissection and ligated superior to the heart. A Millar Instruments catheter-tip pressure transducer was then inserted into the right common carotid artery and advanced into the left ventricle for recording myocardial contractility indices [e.g., left intraventricular pressure, rate of pressure development (dP/dt)]. Following completion of all surgical and catheter-placement procedures, a 20 min stabilization period was allowed to permit accommodation to the catheters prior to recording mechanical events with an Electronics for Medicine VR-12 recording system for analysis. Included among the various functional characteristics derived from this *in vivo* cardiologic assessment procedure are peak left intraventricular pressure, peak dP/dt, the peak left intraventricular isovolumic pressure, and the contractile element shortening velocity of cardiac muscle fibers (V_{CE}). The contractile element shortening velocity was calculated to provide a more definitive assessment of the ventricular contractile state (Parmley and Sonnenblick, 1967). Although dP/dt is generally considered to be a valid measure of the ventricular inotropic state, changes in ventricular preload (end-diastolic pressure) and afterload (arterial diastolic pressure) can significantly affect contractility interpretations based solely on a single contractile parameter.

Following completion of the physiologic recordings the intracardiac catheter was removed and the carotid artery was ligated. A tracheal intubation was performed and each rat was ventilated with intermittent positive pressure using a small animal respirator. After a bilateral thorachotomy was performed, a cold

(5°C) 1 to 2 ml bolus of isotonic saline containing 30mM KCl and 10mM Tris-HCl (pH 7.4) was injected into the left ventricle, resulting in essentially instantaneous myocardial arrest. The heart was then immediately frozen by compression in a cryogenically cooled Wollenberger clamp. The frozen heart tissue was stored briefly in liquid N_2 until the tissue perchloric acid (PCA) extract was prepared for subsequent biochemical analysis.

Analysis of Myocardial Metabolite Concentrations. Lyophilized polyvalent cation purged heart PCA extracts were prepared from both perfused and non-perfused hearts according to procedures detailed elsewhere (Kopp, 1983; Kopp et al., 1983). Immediately prior to phosphorus-31 nuclear magnetic resonance (P-31 NMR) analysis, the extracts were dissolved in 0.8 ml of 20% D_2O, a 0.2 ml volume of potassium Chelex-100 (BioRad) was added to the sample, the pH adjusted to 10.0, and the suspension was filtered through glass wool into a precision 12 mm tube microcell assembly for subsequent spectroscopic determination of phosphatic metabolite levels. The chemical conditions employed: pH 10.0, K^+ countercation, 20% D_2O, saturated $KClO_4$, Chelex-100 pretreatment were adopted to optimize spectral resolution of the P-31 resonance signals.

The NMR spectrometer, the analytical and signal averaging conditions, the acquisition parameters, and the resonance peak chemical identification and quantification procedures used in this study were identical to those described elsewhere (Kopp, 1983). Briefly, the NMR spectrometer was a Nicolet NT-200 system operating at 80.987663 MHz for ^{31}P, interfaced to a wide-bore (89 mm) Oxford superconducting magnet (4.7 Tesla). The heart extracts were analyzed at 24°C, with proton-decoupling, while spinning to enhance signal resolution. The acquisition parameters were the same as those cited previously (Kopp, 1983): pulse sequence, 1 pulse; pulse width, 8 μ sec (45° flip angle); acquisition delay, 200 μ sec; cycling delay, 250 μ sec; number of data points per free induction decay; 16,384; number of acquisition scans, 4000; acquisition time, 1.64 sec; sweep width $\pm$ 2500 Hz; and free induction decay exponential multiplication factor, 0.6 Hz.

Spectral data reduction, resonance peak chemical shift determination and identification, and quantification of spectral resonance peak distributions based on peak area integration were achieved by standardized spectral computer analysis detailed elsewhere (Kopp, 1983). Relative resonance signal areas were corrected for small differential spectroscopic saturation and nuclear Overhauser enhancement through a calibration procedure based on the quantitative addition of reference compounds to the tissue extracts (Bárány and Glonek, 1983). Absolute tissue metabolite concentrations (as μ mol/g tissue wet wt) were computed as the product of the mole percentage of the metabolite detected in the ^{31}P NMR spectrum times the extract total tissue phosphate content per gram tissue wet weight (Kopp et al., 1983; Kopp, 1983). The latter determination was performed for each extract after completion of the ^{31}NMR analysis and was based on a modified Fiske-SubbaRow molybdate colorimetric analysis of Kjeldahl digested samples, aminonaphtholsulfonic acid reduction, and absorbance measurement at 660 nm.

181

In vivo assessments of cardiovascular norepinephrine sensitivity and reactivity. A second group of rats chronically exposed to either no cadmium (control, n = 12), or 1 ppm Cd (1 μ g Cd/ml of fortified drinking water, n = 8) for 12 mos were studied using the same *in vivo* method, as has been described for analysis of myocardial contractility characteristics. Rats were anesthetized with 80 mg ketamine hydrochloride per kg body weight and 8 mg xylazine hydrochloride per kg body weight to minimize anesthetic induced changes in the measured responses. As before, a Millar Instruments catheter-tip pressure transducer was inserted into the right common carotid artery and advanced into the left ventricle. In addition a hollow intravenous catheter was inserted in the right jugular vein for intravenous administration of the norepinephrine (Levophed® bitartrate, Breon Laboratories) doses. Basal recordings of myocardial contractility parameters (left intraventricular pressure and dP/dt) were made prior to injection of the lowest norepinephrine (NE) dose (6×10^{-11} mol NE per kg body weight). Each dose trial was performed in triplicate, and the concentration range examined (6×10^{-11} to 6×10^{-8} mol NE per kg body weight) elicited minimal and near maximal positive inotropic responses. Only peak contractile (dP/dt) responses involving a sinus rhythm were considered to represent valid appraisals of the NE response. The duration of the NE response was measured, as well, from the onset of the positive inotropic response to the restoration of pre-injection-peak left intraventricular pressure levels to within 5mmHg.

Ex Vivo Heart Studies Involving Acute Cadmium Exposure

Myocardial phospholipid derivatives: Interactive effects of calcium and cadmium. Isolated intact heart perfusions were performed according to a modified Langendorff technique detailed elsewhere (Kopp et al., 1978). Male Sprague-Dawley rats (250-300g) were used in this acute phase of these studies. Following the standard 30 min equilibration period, hearts (n = 6 per group) were perfused for an additional 60 min with either the control buffer (1.8 mM Ca) or the identical buffer containing either an increased or decreased final calcium concentration: 0.9, 3.5 or 5.0 mM $CaCl_2$ with and without added cadmium, 3×10^{-6} M $CdCl_2$. All experiments were performed at 37°C and the physiologic perfusate used in these experiments was the same as that used throughout the *ex vivo* perfusion studies, except for the stated changes in perfusate calcium levels or the addition of cadmium: 152 mM NaCl, 5.4 mM KCl, 1.05 mM $MgCl_2$, 1.8 mM $CaCl_2$, 5.6 mM glucose, and 10 mM Tris (Sigma) buffer (pH 7.4 at 37°C). Time-dependent, calcium- and cadmium induced changes in myocardial contractile activity were determined based on active contractile tension and dT/dt analysis. These results have been reported elsewhere (Prentice et al., 1984) and will not be specifically presented because these physiologic findings are peripheral to the points to be emphasized.

Following completion of the 60 min experimental perfusion period, hearts briefly continued to perfuse whereupon they were frozen instantaneously by compression in a liquid N_2-chilled Wollenberger clamp. Heart PCA extracts were prepared and analyzed by P-31 NMR spectroscopy as described herein. In addition to the metabolic findings that have already been reported to occur in conjunction with this experimental approach (Prentice et al., 1984), emphasis is given here to the effects of calcium and cadmium on the concentration of the phosphoglyceride derivatives, glycerol 3-phosphate (G3-P) and glycerol 3-phosphorylcholine (GPC). The effects of these cations on these metabolites were determined and evaluated in the context of a molar ratio (GPC/G3-P) as a basis for identifying possible effects on phosphatidylcholine formation and breakdown. This approach enabled comparison of findings obtained from both *in vivo* and *ex vivo* studies and provided a mechanism for interpreting the effects of cadmium on these metabolites.

Statistical Methods. Quantitative evaluation of the contractility characteristics of individual hearts entailed analysis and averaging of ten separate cardiac contraction events to compute representative values for each heart or animal preparation. This procedure was used for both *ex vivo* analytical procedures to determine peak active contractile tension, dT/dt and contraction rate and *in vivo* assessments of peak left intraventricular pressure, peak left intraventricular isovolumic pressure, peak dP/dt, contractile element shortening velocity and pulse rate. These individual values were used to calculate respective group means for each of the various contractile parameters reported. All data obtained by *in vivo, ex vivo* physiologic and metabolic analytical procedures were evaluated for statistical significance by the one-way analysis of variance method and the Scheffé comparison procedure. In all cases a probability value <0.05 was accepted as indicating a significant difference relative to control.

RESULTS

In all instances control and cadmium-treated rats survived the 12- and 18-month experimental periods without incident. There were no differences in growth rates and the average final body weights for experimental and control groups were essentially the same, within experimental error. The dose of cadmium given in the drinking water (1 μ g/ml) did not alter water or food consumption relative to control at any time during the experiments. Moreover, by visual examination the rats receiving cadmium in their drinking water were physically indistinguishable from their control counterparts.

Blood Pressure Response To Chronic Cadmium Exposure

Rats receiving cadmium (1 μ g/ml) in their drinking water were characterized by significant pressor responses, which appeared as early as 2 mos after exposure to cadmium commenced (Table 1). The values presented represent the average differences in conscious blood pressures between cadmium-exposed and control animals. This response was observed in all groups of rats receiving cadmium and was persistent throughout the duration of the exposure period. A tendency towards a time-dependent, progressive increase in systolic pressure was evident.

TABLE 1

Pressor Effects of Cadmium Following Chronic Exposure Via The Drinking Water For 12 or 18 Mos

A. __18 mos Exposure__

<u>Change in Conscious Systolic Pressure (mmHg)[a]</u>

	2 mos	4 mos	6 mos	8 mos	10 mos	12 mos	15 mos	18 mos
1 ppm Cd	+19[**]	+13[*]	+11[*]	+15[*]	+28[**]	+25[**]	+24[**]	+31[**]

B. __12 mos Exposure__

<u>Change in Conscious Systolic Pressure (mmHg)</u>

	3 mos	6 mos	9 mos	12 mos
1 ppm Cd	+12[**]	+14[**]	+18[**]	+20[**]

[a]Values represent the change relative to control

Significance relative to respective control populations: [*]P < 0.05   [**]P < 0.01

Myocardial Contractility Following Chronic Cadmium Exposure

Ex vivo analysis at 18 mos. The contractile activity of *ex vivo* hearts obtained from rats chronically exposed to cadmium was altered significantly relative to control (Table 2). Peak active tension and maximal rate of tension development were diminished significantly in hearts from cadmium-treated rats. The contraction rate was comparable among the two groups, suggesting that contraction frequency was not a factor contributing to the observed effect.

In vivo analysis at 12 mos. The most notable change detected in the myocardial contractility characteristics of cadmium treated animals was the reduced contractile element shortening velocity of cardiac muscle fibers (Table 2). The maximal rate of pressure development (dP/dt) in hearts of cadmium-treated animals was diminished (85% of control value); however, this difference was not statistically significant. These findings indicated that despite an ability to generate normal to supranormal pressures, the velocity mechanisms of cardiac muscle contraction are diminished as a consequence of chronic cadmium exposure.

In vivo cardiovascular reactivity to norepinephrine. The reactivity of the cardiovascular system to norepinephrine (6×10^{-11} to 6×10^{-8} mol/kg body wt) was significantly attenuated in rats following 12 mos oral exposure to cadmium (1 μg/ml of drinking water). This relationship is illustrated in Figure 4, which depicts the dose-dependent effects of norepinephrine on the maximal dP/dt generated by the myocardium. Moreover, although the contractile responsiveness of the myocardium to norepinephrine was diminished in rats exposed chronically to cadmium, the duration of the positive inotropic response was

TABLE 2
Myocardial Contractility Following Exposure To 1 ppm Cadmium
$(8.9 \times 10^{-6}$ M Cd) Via The Drinking Water

A. *Ex Vivo* Analysis at 18 mos

	Active Tension (g)	dT/dt (g/sec)	Contraction Rate (bts/min)
Control	16.4 ± 1.0^a	1983.6 ± 75.2	149 ± 9
Cd-Treated	$10.4 \pm 1.3^{**}$	$1259.2 \pm 160^{**}$	139 ± 8

B. *In Vivo* Analysis at 12 mos

	Peak Left Intraventricular Pressure (mmHg)	dP/dt (mmHg/sec)	V_{CE} at Peak dP/dt (muscle lengths/sec)	Pulse Rate (bts/min)
Control	113 ± 6	7644 ± 1171	2.5 ± 0.1	298 ± 15
Cd-Treated	120 ± 7	6481 ± 1191	$1.8 \pm 0.1^{**}$	294 ± 16

[a] Values represent Mean $\pm$ SE

[**] Significantly different relative to control, $P < 0.01$

prolonged significantly relative to the control group in these animals at each of the two highest norepinephrine concentrations. Following intravenous bolus infusion of 6×10^{-9} mol NE/kg body wt, the increased contractile response persisted for 3.9 min in the control group versus 5.3 min in the cadmium-treated rats. Similarly, intravenous injection of 6×10^{-8} mol NE/kg body wt resulted in a positive inotropic response that lasted 5.6 min in the controls, as opposed to 9.8 min in the cadmium group. These findings indicate that the sensitivity of the cardiovascular system to norepinephrine is shifted to the right, indicating a diminished responsiveness, but that the pressor response persists longer, reflecting an increased norepinephrine half-life.

Effect of Chronic Cadmium Exposure on Myocardial Metabolite Concentrations

Ex Vivo analysis at 18 mos. Post-perfused hearts from cadmium-fed (1 μ g/ml) rats were characterized by significantly reduced adenosine triphosphate (ATP) and phosphocreatine (PCr) concentrations and increased tissue adenosine diphosphate (ADP), and inorganic phosphate (Pi) levels (Table 3). The cardiac tissue phosphorylation potential which characterizes the relative ability of myocardial cells to sustain cellular energy-dependent processes, was markedly reduced in hearts from cadmium-fed rats (46% of control). In addi-

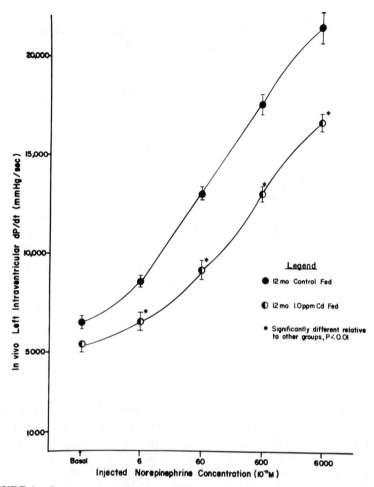

FIGURE 4. *In vivo* myocardial contractility as a function of intravenous norepinephrine dose in rats that received control and cadmium-containing (1μ g/ml) drinking water for 12 mos. Graph illustrates the shift in myocardial sensitivity to adrenergic stimulation that occurred following chronic cadmium exposure.

tion the glycerol 3-phosphorylcholine content of these hearts was also significantly reduced relative to control suggesting an effect on phosphatidylcholine metabolism. In contrast the total perchloric acid extractable phosphate concentration of hearts from cadmium-treated animals was comparable to control, suggesting that the metabolic changes reflect an effect on overall cellular metabolism, rather than a consequence of cellular degeneration.

Non-perfused heart analysis at 18 mos. As shown in Table 3, the magnitude of the metabolic changes associated with chronic cadmium exposure were less pronounced, when the hearts were not subjected to *ex vivo* perfusion, as compared to the effects measured in post-perfused hearts. As before, myocardial ATP and GPC levels were reduced and Pi levels were elevated significantly relative to identically treated control hearts. The tissue phosphorylation poten-

TABLE 3

Specific Myocardial Phosphatic Metabolite Concentrations Following 18 mos Exposure to 1 ppm Cadmium (8.9×10^{-6} M Cd) Via The Drinking Water

A. Perfused Hearts

	Concentrations (μ mol/g tissue wet wt)					$\dfrac{[ATP]}{[ADP][Pi]}$
	ATP	ADP	PCr	Pi	GPC	
Control	6.3 ± 0.1	1.3 ± 0.04	6.7 ± 0.2	2.8 ± 0.2	0.4 ± 0.04	1.93 ± 0.23
Cd-Treated	$4.9 \pm 0.2^{**}$	$1.9 \pm 0.15^{*}$	$5.6 \pm 0.2^{**}$	$3.8 \pm 0.3^{**}$	$0.2 \pm 0.04^{*}$	$0.88 \pm 0.12^{**}$

B. Non Perfused Hearts

Control	6.5 ± 0.2	1.4 ± 0.1	7.8 ± 0.3	2.3 ± 0.1	0.2 ± 0.02	2.00 ± 0.1
Cd-Treated	$6.1 \pm 0.1^{*}$	1.6 ± 0.1	7.3 ± 0.2	$2.9 \pm 0.2^{*}$	$0.1 \pm 0.02^{**}$	$1.34 \pm 0.1^{**}$

Values represent Mean $\pm$ SE

Significantly different relative to control: $^{*}P < 0.05$
$^{**}P < 0.01$

GPC: Glycerol 3-phosphorylcholine

tial was also diminished significantly in hearts from cadmium-fed rats. The decrease in the magnitude of the apparent cadmium-induced effect on myocardial metabolism indicates a differential response of the cadmium hearts to the *ex vivo* perfusion conditions, rather than a generalized response of hearts from both groups. This observation may reflect an inability of hearts from cadmium-fed rats to compensate and recover from the isolation and perfusion procedure.

Influence of Calcium and Cadmium on Myocardial Phosphoglyceride Derivatives

As shown in Figure 5, the ratio of glycerol 3-phosphorylcholine (GPC) to glycerol 3-phosphate (G 3-P) is markedly influenced by the perfusate calcium concentration, approaching a maximum at 3.5 mM. This relationship was evident, as well, in hearts from rats maintained on the control dietary regimen for 18 mos (Figure 6). This apparent calcium-activated lypolytic and phosphoglyceride activity was disrupted significantly in hearts exposed acutely to 3×10^{-6} M cadmium added to the perfusate (Figure 5), and in hearts from rats exposed chronically to cadmium via their drinking water [1 μ g/ml (8.9×10^{-6} M $CdCl_2$)] for 18 mos (Figure 6). In hearts perfused with a similar cadmium concentration the calcium-activated increase in the GPC/G3-P ratio was completely abolished. Conversely, chronic cadmium-exposure attenuated, rather than inhibited the absolute increase in this ratio that occurred in control hearts in response to the *ex vivo* perfusion conditions. Qualitatively, these effects were

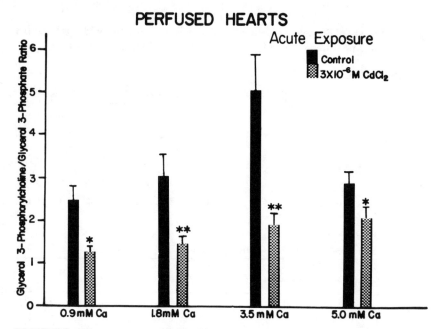

FIGURE 5. Dose-response relationship between the extracellular (perfusate) calcium concentration and the ratio of glycerol 3-phosphorylcholine to glycerol 3-phosphate in the isolated perfused rat heart. Note that acute exposure of the hearts to cadmium by addition of 3×10^{-6} M $CdCl_2$ to the perfusion medium completely inhibited the calcium-activated increase in phosphoglyceride activity as reflected by an increase in this ratio. Asterisks denote significantly different changes relative to the respective controls (*$P < 0.05$; **$P < 0.01$).

remarkably similar and suggest that this response may provide a useful predictive index for estimating the effective myocardial calcium concentration.

DISCUSSION

The present studies have demonstrated that chronic exposure to cadmium at relatively low intake levels results in systemic hypertension, and significant, potentially detrimental physiologic and metabolic changes in the rat myocardium. Perusal of reported findings concerned with the pressor effects of cadmium appear to support the contention that chronic cadmium exposure will induce hypertension (Boscolo et al., 1981; Hadley et al., 1979; Iannaccone et al., 1981; Kopp et al., 1980a-d; 1982; 1983; Perry et al., 1977; 1979; Perry and Erlanger, 1982; Revis, 1978; Revis et al.; 1983; Schroeder and Vinton; Schroeder et al., 1970; Walker and Moses, 1979), and that the dose-response relationship for this effect is a parabolic function (Kopp et al., 1982). However, until the mechanistic basis for the pressor response is elucidated, the issue of cadmium hypertension will remain controversial. Various mechanisms have been postulated to explain the cadmium-induced hypertension in experimental

IN VIVO VERSUS EX VIVO ANALYSIS

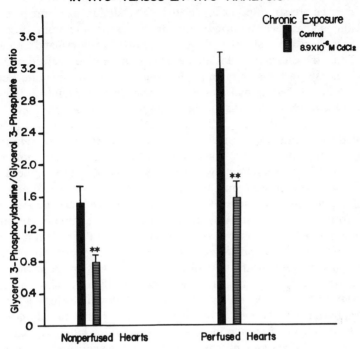

FIGURE 6. Molar relationship between phosphatidylcholine degradation-product (glycerol 3-phosphorylcholine) and precursor (glycerol 3-phosphate) in hearts (perchloric acid extracted) non-perfused or artificially perfused (1.8 mM calcium, glucose as exogenous substrate) following 18 mos chronic exposure to 1 ppm cadmium via the drinking water (8.9 × 10^{-6} M $CdCl_2$). Note the increase in this ratio resulting from *ex vivo* perfusion of control hearts and the attenuated response by the hearts from cadmium-treated rats. Asterisks denote significantly different changes relative to the respective controls (**P < 0.01).

animals (for review see Kopp, 1985). One, which has received attention recently has suggested that altered norepinephrine metabolism may be involved as a causative factor in this response (Revis; 1978; Revis et al., 1983). This hypothetical mechanism is based on experimental findings demonstrating an increased plasma norepinephrine concentration and an increased plasma norepinephrine half-life following chronic cadmium exposure (Revis, 1978; Revis et al., 1983). The findings reported herein, which were concerned with the responsiveness of the myocardium to norepinephrine, only partially support this hypothesis. The prolonged response to norepinephrine that occurred at higher norepinephrine doses was consistent with the interpretation of an increased norepinephrine half-life in cadmium-exposed animals. However, the diminished norepinephrine sensitivity of the myocardium suggests the possibility that the elevated levels of circulating norepinephrine detected in cadmium-exposed animals may represent a compensatory response of the cardiovascular system to a decreased sensitivity to norepinephrine, rather than a mechanistic basis for the hypertension. As shown recently in several human studies, various putative mediators involved in the pressor response associated with cadmium exposure in experimental animals have been reported in humans exposed to cadmium (Boscolo et al., 1978; Iannaccone et al., 1979; Revis et al., 1981; Vorobreva and Eremeeva, 1980). Thus, these experimental animal studies appear to provide pertinent findings relevant to at-risk human populations exposed to cadmium. Further work with established animal models may provide new insights in this area regarding the mechanistic basis for the cadmium hypertension.

As shown herein, the myocardial metabolic and functional disturbances associated with chronic cadmium exposure were exacerbated by *ex vivo* heart perfusion. Although the actual cause for this differential response is uncertain, comparison of *in vivo* and *ex vivo* findings suggests that the compensatory functional reserve of hearts from cadmium-treated animals may be diminished. A change of this nature would render these hearts less able to accommodate and recover from physiologic stress conditions, such as those imposed during the preparation of the heart for *ex vivo* perfusion. The effect of cadmium became apparent after analyzing and comparing the metabolite concentrations of perfused and non-perfused hearts obtained from rats of the same population that had received cadmium in the drinking water for 18 mos. This concept is supported further by the relative differences that were detected between myocardial contractility results obtained in control and cadmium-treated groups by *ex vivo* and *in vivo* methods. Although this latter comparison is somewhat biased due to the different duration of the exposure periods of the compared studies, these findings suggest that the myocardium is responsive to the actions of cadmium and that these effects are qualitatively similar, but quantitatively exaggerated when the response is measured in conjunction with physiologic stress conditions.

Experimental evidence reported herein and elsewhere has consistently implicated disturbances in cellular calcium metabolism as the basis for the deleterious effects of cadmium on the heart (Bers and Langer, 1979; Kopp et al., 1980a; Kopp, 1985; Langer et al., 1974; Lee and Tsien, 1983; Prentice et al., 1984). The apparently compromised functional reserve capacity of the myocardium following chronic *in vivo* exposure to cadmium is consistent with this hypothesis. Cadmium has been shown to interact with membrane phospholipid binding sites, thereby displacing Ca^{2+} from rapidly exchangeable calcium binding sites (Bers and Langer, 1979; Langer et al., 1974). In addition cadmium (Cd^{2+}) exhibits the properties of a slow calcium channel inhibitor, interfering with membrane calcium conductance (Lee and Tsien, 1983). Cadmium has also been shown to antagonize calcium-mediated cellular processes through a competition with calcium for functional binding sites (for review see Kopp, 1985; Prentice et al., 1984). As a consequence, the responsiveness of the myocardium to changes in ionized calcium levels is attenuated, as evidenced by the truncation of the normal calcium-activated lypolysis and phosphoglyceride activity that was manifested in conjunction with *ex vivo* perfusion conditions (Kopp et al., 1980a; Hron et al., 1977; Prentice et al., 1984). Although these changes were more dramatic following *ex vivo* analysis of hearts from animals exposed chronically to cadmium, this effect was evident regardless of the analytical conditions employed. The acute, *ex vivo* calcium perfusion studies, which have demonstrated the calcium-dependent lypolytic activity of the myocardium, have suggested that the action of cadmium may be linked to a partial inhibition of the calcium activation of this response. This interpretation is supported by the observation that the most pronounced changes were those that involved metabolites sensitive to changes in cellular calcium levels. Presumably, the differences detected in control hearts not artificially perfused relative to those that were perfused reflect the difference between the ionized calcium levels of the perfusate and blood. The disturbances in myocardial phosphoglyceride metabolism that were manifested in conjunction with chronic and acute cadmium exposure appeared to affect primarily phosphatidylcholine derivatives (accumulation of glycerol 3-phosphate and reduced levels of glycerol 3-phosphorylcholine). The phosphocholine content of the hearts was not affected significantly in conjunction with the effects on GPC and G3-P. Therefore, these changes in phosphoglyceride derivatives cannot be attributed to an increased catabolism of GPC. Instead, these findings appear to represent a partial inhibition of phosphatidylcholine biosynthesis by cadmium through an effect on the calcium-regulated enzyme, choline phosphotransferase (for review see Kopp, 1985). Since phosphatidylcholine and its derivatives are major constituents of the sarcolemma membrane, changes in the biosynthesis or turnover of this membrane constituent may provide a mechanistic basis for the biochemical and functional changes that occur in response to cadmium. Presumably, an inhibition in the formation of this phospholipid and its derivatives by cadmium would alter the structural and functional characteristics of cardiac cell membranes, possibly leading to (a) unbalanced calcium influx and extrusion rates; (b) altered bioelectrical and biophysical properties of the membranes, which would influence cardiac excitability and contractility; and (c) modified receptor-site sensitivity, which would lead to modified responsiveness of the myocardium to adrenergic stimulation. Evidence compiled to date, which has been admittedly indirect, is wholly consistent with this proposed mechanism. Moreover, the ability of cadmium to induce significant changes in membrane phospholipids and lipid metabolism is certainly not unprecedented and has been shown in other systems (Datson, 1982; Henderson et al., 1979).

In vivo analysis of myocardial contractility following chronic cadmium exposure has demonstrated that cadmium primarily affects the velocity components of cardiac muscle contraction. The contractile element shortening velocity (V_{CE}) of hearts from rats receiving cadmium in the drinking water for 12 mos was 72% of the control value. This attenuated V_{CE} appears to reflect impaired ATP coupling to mechanical work, which may be related to a partial inhibition; either direct or indirect, of the myosin ATPase activity (Kopp et al., 1980 a,c). It should be noted that the activity of this enzyme is calcium-dependent; therefore, cadmium-induced disturbances in cellular calcium activity would be expected to affect the activity of this enzyme. Paralleling these physiologic findings are those reported by Vorobieva and Eremeeva (1980), which have described altered myocardial contractility and dystrophic changes in cardiac muscle of workers chronically exposed occupationally to cadmium oxide fumes. The occurrence of similar clinical manifestations corroborates the potential significance of the present experimental findings to humans.

Overall, the experimental findings and the biologic inferences derived from these studies are consonant with the hypothesis that chronic daily intake of cadmium at levels approaching those encountered from environmental sources can adversely affect the metabolic and functional integrity of the myocardium. Thus, the purported effects of cadmium on the cardiovascular system are not limited to hypertension, but include the heart, as well. In addition chronic cadmium exposure appears to impair the functional reserve capacity of the myocardium. As a consequence, these hearts intrinsically have a limited compensatory capacity, which limits their ability to respond to increased functional and metabolic demands imposed by additional physiologic (inotropic) stressors (Kopp et al., 1980 a,c). These results indicate that cadmium is cardiotoxic at very low levels and that further studies are needed to assess the impact of chronic cadmium exposure from environmental and industrial sources on human health.

ACKNOWLEDGEMENTS

The authors thank Kay Keenan and Rose Sage for expert typing and proofing of this manuscript. The expert assistance of Ruth Zelkha in the preparation of the illustrations is gratefully acknowledged. This research was supported by Grant ES02397 from the National Institute of Environmental Health Sciences (SJK), an award from the Chicago Community Trust Fund (SJK), the Chicago College of Osteopathic Medicine and the Veterans Administration (HMP).

REFERENCES

BÁRÁNY, M. and GLONEK, T. (1983). Identification of diseased states by P-31 NMR. In: *Phosphorus-31 NMR Principles and Applications* (D. Gorenstein, Ed.). Academic Press, New York, in press.

BERS, D.M. and LANGER, G.A. (1979). Uncoupling cation effects on cardiac contractility and sarcolemmal Ca^{2+} binding. Am. J. Physiol. 237:H332–341.

BOSCOLO, P., CECCHETTI, G., IANNACCONE, A., PORCELLI, G. and SALIMEI, E. (1978). La callicreina urinaria nell'esposizione professionale al cadmio. Ann. Ist Super. Sanita. 14:597–600.

BOSCOLO, P., PORCELLI, G., CARMIGNANI, M. and FINELLI, V.N. (1981). Urinary kallikrein and hypertension in cadmium exposed rats. Toxicol. Lett. 7:189–194.

DALHAMN, T. and FRIBERG L. (1954). The effect of cadmium on blood pressure and respiration and the use of dimercaprol (BAL) as antidote. Acta. Pharmacol. Toxicol. 10:199–203.

DATSON, G.P. (1982). Toxic effects of cadmium on the developing rat lung. II. Glycogen and phospholipid metabolism. J. Toxicol. Environ. Hlth. 9:51–61.

DOYLE, J.J., BERNHOFT, R.A. and SANDSTEAD, H.H. (1974). The effects of a low level of dietary cadmium on some biochemical and physiological parameters in rats. In: *Trace Substances in Environmental Health Vol. VIII.* (D.D. Hemphill, Ed.). University of Missouri Press, Columbia, pp. 403–409.

EAKIN, D.J., SCHROEDER, L.A., WHANGER, P.D. and WESWIG, P.H. (1980). Cadmium and nickel influence on blood pressure, plasma renin, and tissue mineral concentrations. Am. J. Physiol. **238**:E53–E61.

FADLOUN, Z. and LEACH, G.D.H. (1981). The effects of cadmium ions on blood pressure, dopamine-β-hydroxylase activity and on the responsiveness of *in vivo* preparations to sympathetic nerve stimulation, noradrenaline and tyramine. J. Pharm. Pharmacol. **33**:660–664.

FINGERLE, H., FISCHER, G. and CLASSEN, H.G. (1982). Failure to produce hypertension in rats by chronic exposure to cadmium. Fd. Chem. Toxic. **20**:301–306.

FLEISCHER, M., SAROFIM, A.F., FASSETT, D.W., HAMMOND, P., SHACK-LETTE, H.T., NISBET, I.C.T. and EPSTEIN, S. (1974). Environmental impact of cadmium: a review by the panel on hazardous trace substances. Environ. Hlth. Perspect. **7**:253–323.

FRIBERG, L., PISCATOR, M., NORDBERG, G.F. and KJELLSTRÖM. (1974). Cadmium In The Environment. CRC Press, Boca Raton, pp. 23–135.

FRICKENHAUS, B., LIPPAL, J., GORDON, T. and EINBRODT, H.J. (1976). Blutdruck und pulsfrequenz bei oraler belastung mit cadmiumsulfid im tier versuch. Zentbl. Bakt. Hyg. I. Abt. Orig. B **161**:371–376.

HADLEY, J.G., CONKLIN, A.W. and SANDERS, C.L. (1979). Systemic toxicity of inhaled cadmium oxide. Toxicol. Lett. **4**:107–111.

HALL, C.E. and NASSETH, D. (1980). Factors affecting the acute pressor response to bolus cadmium injections. Physiol. Behavior **24**:373–380.

HALL, C.E. and HUNGERFORD, S. (1982). Influence of dosage, consciousness, and nifedipine on the acute pressor response to intraperitoneally administered cadmium. J. Toxicol. Environ. Hlth. **9**:953–962.

HENDERSON, R.F., REBAR, A.H., PICKRELL, J.N. and NEWTON, G.J. (1979). Early damage indicators in the lung. III. Biochemical and cytological response of the lung to inhaled metal salts. Toxicol. Appl. Pharmacol. **50**:123–136.

HRON, W.T., JERMOK, G.J., LOMBARDO, Y.B., MENAHAN, L.A. and LECH, J.J. (1977). Calcium dependency of hormone stimulated lipolysis in the perfused rat heart. J. Mol. Cell. Cardiol. **9**:733–748.

IANNACCONE, A., PORCELLI, G. and BOSCOLO, P. (1979). The urinary kallikrein activity in cadmium exposure. Adv. Exp. Med. Biol. **120B**:683–684.

IANNACCONE, A., CARMIGNANI, M. and BOSCOLO, P. (1981). Reattivita cardiovascolare nel ratto dopo cronica esposizione a cadmio o piombo. Ann. Ist. Super. Sanita. **17**:655–660.

KOPP, S.J. and HAWLEY, P.L. (1978). Cadmium feeding: apparent depression of atrioventricular - His Purkinje conduction system. Acta Pharmacol. et Toxicol. **42**:110–116.

KOPP, S.J., BAKER, J.C., D'AGROSA, L.S. and HAWLEY, P.L. (1978). Simultaneous recording of His bundle electrogram, electrocardiogram, and systolic tension from intact modified Langendorff rat heart preparations: Effects of perfusion time, cadmium, and lead. Toxicol. Appl. Pharmacol. **46**:475–487.

KOPP, S.J., BARANY, M., ERLANGER, M., PERRY, E.F. and PERRY, H.M., Jr. (1980a). The influence of chronic low-level cadmium and/or lead feeding on myocardial contractility related to phosphorylation of cardiac myofibrillar proteins. Toxicol. Appl. Pharmacol. **54**:48–56.

KOPP, S.J., GLONEK, T., ERLANGER, M., PERRY, E.F., BARANY, M. and

PERRY, H.M., JR. (1980b). Altered metabolism and function of rat heart following chronic low level cadmiu /lead feeding. J. Mol. Cell. Cardiol. 12:1407–1425.

KOPP, S.J., GLONEK, T., ERLANGER, M., PERRY, E.F., PERRY, H.M., Jr. and BARANY, M. (1980c). Cadmium and lead effects on myocardial function and metabolism. J. Environ. Path. Toxicol. 4:205–227.

KOPP, S.J., PERRY, H.M., Jr., GLONEK, T., ERLANGER, M., PERRY, E.F., BARANY, E.F. and D'AGROSA, L.S. (1980d). Cardiac physiologic-metabolic changes after chronic low-level heavy metal feeding. Am. J. Physiol. 239:H22–H30.

KOPP, S.J., GLONEK, T., PERRY, H.M., Jr., ERLANGER, M. and PERRY, E.F. (1982). Cardiovascular actions of cadmium at environmental exposure levels. Science 217:837–839.

KOPP, S.J. (1985). Cd and the cardiovascular system. In: *Handbook of Experimental Pharmacology: Cadmium.* (Ed. E.C. Foulkes) Springer-Verlag, Berlin. In press.

KOPP, S.J., PERRY, H.M., Jr., PERRY, E.F. and ERLANGER, M. (1983). Cardiac physiologic and tissue metabolic changes following chronic low-level cadmium and cadmium plus lead ingestion in the rat. Toxicol. Appl. Pharmacol. 69:149–160.

KOPP, S.J. (1983). Vascular intracardiac catheterization technique for multiphasic evaluation of rat heart *in vivo*. Toxicol. Appl. Pharmacol. 70:273–282.

KOTSONIS, F.N. and KLAASSEN, C.D. (1978). The relationship of metallothionein to the toxicity of cadmium after prolonged oral administration to rats. Toxicol. Appl. Pharmacol. 46:39–54.

LANGER, G.A., SERENA, S.D. and NUDD, L.M. (1974). Cation exchange in heart cell culture: correlation with effects on contractile force. J. Mol. Cell. Cardiol. 6:149–161.

LEE, K.S. and TSIEN, R.W. (1983). Mechanism of calcium channel blockade by verapamil, D600, diltiazem and nitrendipine in single dialyzed heart cells. Nature 302:790–794.

LOESER, E. and LORKE, D. (1977a). Semichronic oral toxicity of cadmium. 1. Studies on rats. Toxicology 7:215–224.

LOESER, E., and LORKE, D. (1977b). Semichronic oral toxicity of cadmium. 2. Studies in dogs. Toxicology 7:225–232.

OHANIAN, E.V., IWAI, J., LEITL, G. and TUTHILL, R. (1978). Genetic influence on cadmium-induced hypertension. Am. J. Physiol. 235:H385–H391.

PARMLEY, W.W. and SONNENBLICK, E.H. (1967). Series elasticity in heart muscle. Its relation to contractile element velocity and proposed muscle models. Circ. Res. 20:112–123.

PERRY, H.M., Jr. and YUNICE, A. (1965). Acute pressor effects of intra-arterial cadmium and mercuric ions in anesthetized rats. Proc. Soc. Exp. Biol. Med. 120:805–808.

PERRY, H.M., Jr. ERLANGER, M., YUNICE, A., SCHOEPFLE, E. and PERRY, E.F. (1970). Hypertension and tissue metal levels following intravenous cadmium, mercury, and zinc. Am. J. Physiol. 219:755–761.

PERRY, H.M., Jr., and ERLANGER, M. (1974). Metal induced hypertension following chronic feeding of low doses of cadmium and mercury. J. Lab. Clin. Med. 83:541–547.

PERRY, H.M., Jr., ERLANGER, M. and PERRY, E.F. (1977). Elevated systolic blood pressure following chronic low-level cadmium feeding. Am. J. Physiol. 232:H114–H121.

PERRY, H.M., Jr., ERLANGER, M. and PERRY, E.F. (1979). Increase in the systolic pressure of rats chronically fed cadmium. Environ. Hlth. Perspect. 28:251–260.

PERRY, H.M., Jr., and ERLANGER, M. (1982). Effect of diet on increases in systolic pressure induced in rats by chronic cadmium feeding. J. Nutr. 112:1983–1989.

PETERING, H.G., MURTHY, L., SORENSON, J.R.J., LEVIN, L. and STEMMER, K.L. (1979). Effect of sex on oral cadmium dose responses in rats: blood pressure and pharmacodynamics. Environ. Res. 20:289–299.

PORTER, M.C., MIYA, T.S. and BOUSQUET, W.F. (1974). Cadmium: inability to induce hypertension in the rat. Toxicol. Appl. Pharmacol. 27:692–695.

PRENTICE, R.C., HAWLEY, P.L., GLONEK, T. and KOPP, S.J. (1984). Calcium-dependent effects of cadmium on energy metabolism and function of perfused rat heart. Toxicol. Appl. Pharmacol. 75:198–210.

REVIS, N. (1978). A possible mechanism for cadmium-induced hypertension in rats. Life Sci. 22:479–488.

REVIS, N.W., and ZINSMEISTER, A.R. (1981). The relationship of blood cadmium level to hypertension and plasma norepinephrine level: a Romanian study. Proc. Soc. Exp. Biol. Med. 167:254–260.

REVIS, N.W., MAJOR, T.C. and HORTON, C.Y. (1983). The response of the adrenergic system in the cadmium-induced hypertensive rat. J. Am. Coll. Toxicol. 2:165–174.

ROACH, M.R. and DAMUDE, L.R. (1980). The effect of daily injections of cadmium on the systolic pressure of conscious rats. J. Environ. Path. Toxicol. 4:443–449.

SCHROEDER, H.A. and VINTON, W.H., Jr. (1962). Hypertension induced in rats by small doses of cadmium. Am. J. Physiol. 202:515–518.

SCHROEDER, H.A., KROLL, S.S., LITTLE, J.W., LIVINGSTON, P.O. and MYERS, M.A.G. (1966). Hypertension in rats from injection of cadmium. Arch. Environ. Hlth. 13:788–789.

SCHROEDER, H.A. and BUCKMAN, J. (1967). Cadmium hypertension. Its reversal in rats by a zinc chelate. Arch. Environ. Hlth. 14:693–697.

SCHROEDER, H.A., BAKER, J.T., HANSEN, N.M. Jr., SIZE, J.G. and WISE, R.A. (1970). Vascular reactivity of rats altered by cadmium and a zinc chelate. Arch. Environ. Hlth. 21:609–614.

TEMPLETON, D.M., and CHERIAN, M.G. (1983). Cadmium and hypertension. Trends Pharmacol. Sci. 4:501–503.

THIND, G.S., KARREMAN, G., STEPHAN, K.F. and BLAKEMORE, W.S. (1970). Vascular reactivity and mechanical properties of normal and cadmium–hypertensive rabbits. J. Lab. Clin. Med. 76:560–568.

TOMERA, J.F. and HARAKAL, C. (1980). Cyclic nucleoside changes in aortic segments derived from hypertensive rabbits. Eur. J. Pharmacol. 68:505–508.

VOROBIEVA, R.S. and EREMEEVA, E.P. (1980). Cardiovascular function in workers exposed to cadmium. Gig. Sanit. 10:22–25.

WALKER, H.L., and MOSES, H.A. (1979). Cadmium: hypertension induction and lead mobilization. J. Natl. Med. Assn. 71:1187–1189.

WATKINS, B.E. (1980). Effects of cadmium injections on arterial pressure regulation in the rat. Clin. Exp. Hypertension 2:153–162.

WHANGER, P.D. (1979). Cadmium effects in rats on tissue iron, selenium, and blood pressure; blood and hair cadmium in some Oregon residents. Environ. Hlth. Perspect. 28:115–121.

CHAPTER XVIII

INVESTIGATIONS INTO THE EFFECT OF DRINKING WATER BARIUM ON RATS

P.T. McCauley,* B.H. Douglas,†
R.D. Laurie,* and R.J. Bull*
*Health Effects Research Laboratory
26 West St. Clair Street
Cincinnati, Ohio

† University of Mississippi Medical Center
Jackson, Mississippi

ABSTRACT

Barium in excess of drinking water standards has been measured in isolated ground water aquifers. Studies were initiated to investigate the histologic and cardiovascular effects on rats of barium (Ba) in drinking water. Histologic examination of 34 tissues stained with hematoxylin and eosin demonstrated no significant changes from control after up to 68 weeks of exposure to up to 1, 10, 100, or 250 ppm Ba. Rats exposed to 250 ppm Ba for 5 months were challenged with an arrhythmagenic dose of L-norepinephrine (N.E.) (5 μg/kg I.V.). These rats demonstrated no significant ECG changes when compared to controls. However, at 4 minutes post I.V. N.E., the heart rate of the exposed group was significantly lower than that of the control group. In another experiment Sprague Dawley (SD) rats were exposed for 20 weeks to drinking water containing from 0 to 100 ppm Ba as barium chloride (BaCl$_2$). Similarly, Dahl salt sensitive and uninephrectomized rats exhibited no Ba related changes in blood pressure when exposed for 16 weeks to 1000 ppm Ba in either distilled water or 0.9 % saline. Animals which received highest dose of Ba (1000 ppm) exhibited ultrastructural changes in the glomeruli, which included basement membrane thickening, epithelial foot process fusion, and the presence of myelin figures.

INTRODUCTION

Acute Ba toxicity from oral exposure to BaCl$_2$ is reported to occur in humans at doses of 80 mg/kg (NIOSH, 1976). The primary actions of Ba in an acute

197

toxic episode are primarily stimulatory manifestations on all forms of muscle tissue in nearly every body organ (Chernick, 1971). Symptoms include nausea, vomiting, diarrhea, and abdominal pain. Cardiovascular effects involve a substantial rise in blood pressure due primarily to generalized vasoconstriction and Ba induced cardiac arrhythmia. This hypertension is acetylcholine resistant and thus baroreceptor reflex resistant. Additional hypertensive activity results from Ba induced catecholamine release from the adrenal medulla (Shanbaky, 1978). In extreme cases cardiac extrasystoles, convulsions, and extremity paralysis may be observed. Gastrointestinal and renal hemorrhages often occur. Death results from cardiac arrest (Chernick, 1971).

Oral doses of barium sulfate ($BaSO_4$) are used clinically as a radiopaque aid to X-ray diagnosis. When $BaSO_4$ is administered in large doses, very small fractions are absorbed. Conversely similar, accidental doses of $BaCl_2$ have been lethal since large amounts of Ba are absorbed from oral $BaCl_2$ (Hammond and Beliles, 1980). However, when $BaCl_2$ or $BaSO_4$ is administered in 10 mg/kg doses their absorption rates are nearly equivalent. Ba from $BaSO_4$ or $BaCl_2$ is distributed to soft tissues such as the kidney and liver and even concentrated in the heart, skeletal muscle, and eye (McCauley and Washington, 1983).

Little is known about the low-dose chronic effects of Ba. Miller et al. (1984) have reported that children from a town with high Ba drinking water concentrations (10 mg/l) demonstrated 5 times higher Ba/Ca ratio in teeth than children from a town with lower Ba concentrations (0.2 mg/l) in drinking water. Since the Miller paper demonstrates the possibility of low-dose chronic Ba exposure to humans the need to study the health effects of chronic Ba exposure is self evident.

The current paper addresses three areas of investigation into chronic drinking water Ba exposure. They are (1) light microscopic histology of 35 tissues, (2) electrocardiographic result during L-norepinephrine challenge, and (3) blood pressure effects in normal and hypertension susceptible rate species with electron micrographic examinations of renal morphology. All studies were conducted in rats chronically exposed to Ba.

METHODS

Histology Studies. Chronic Ba exposure studies were conducted using three different exposure regimes. (1) Male SD rats given free access to Purina Rat Chow (12/group) were exposed to 0, 1, 10, 100, or 250 ppm Ba in drinking water for 36 weeks. (2) Male SD rats (10/group) were exposed to 0, 1, 10, or 100 ppm Ba in drinking water for 68 weeks. (3) Female SD rats (12/group) were exposed to 0 or 250 ppm Ba for 46 weeks. Food and water consumption as well as body weight gain records were kept.

On the last day of the exposure period all rats were sacrificed. During dissection, an examination for gross pathology was conducted and hematocrit values taken. Tissues were formalin fixed, dehydrated, embedded, sectioned, and hematoxylin and eosin stained for light microscopic analysis of pathology.

The following tissues were examined microscopically from all rats: mesenteric lymph node, salivary glands, sternebrae including marrow, thyroids, parathyroids, small intestine, colon, liver, ovaries and uterus (or testis and prostate), lungs with mainstem bronchi, nasal cavity and nasal turbinates, heart, esophagus, stomach, brain (frontal cortex and basal ganglia, parietal tissue cortex and thalamus, cerebellum and pons), thymus, trachea, pancreas, spleen, kidneys, adrenals, urinary bladder, pituitary, eyes, mammary gland, larynx, aorta, femur, gross lesions, and tissue masses with regional lymph nodes, if possible.

Electrocardiogram Studies (ECG). SD rats were given free access to Purina Rat Chow and drinking water containing either 0 or 250 ppm Ba as $BaCl_2$ for 5 months. Control and Ba exposed group sizes were 11 and 10 rats, respectively. Animals were anesthetized with 50 mg/kg Nembutal. Recordings were made from a standard 3 lead placement with a Nicolet 1170 Digital Signal Averaging System using only a single sweep. After a baseline ECG was established rats were given I.V. injections of 0.5 μg/kg L-norepinephrine (Levophed). Data were obtained at 0, 4, and 60 minutes after the N.E. injection. Data was analyzed by a two-way analysis of variance for repeated measures (BMDP2V).

Blood Pressure Studies. Twenty-six groups of animals (6/group) were given free access to Tekland Rat Chow (< 1 ppm Ba) and drinking water for 16 weeks. Five groups of SD rats received 0, 3, 10, 30, or 100 ppm Ba in their drinking water, while 5 additional SD groups received equivalent amounts of Ba in 0.9% NaCl. These animals were not nephrectomized. Four groups of uninephrectomized, SD animals received higher levels of Ba—1, 10, 100, or 1000 ppm—in either drinking water, or in 0.9% NaCl. In the next set of experiments, two specially bred rat strains were used: the Dahl salt sensitive and Dahl salt resistant. Their names adeptly describe their degree of susceptibility to hypertension in the presence of NaCl. Four groups each of Dahl sodium sensitive and Dahl sodium resistant rats received 1, 10, 100, or 1000 ppm Ba in 0.9% NaCl.

Blood pressures for each animal in each group were taken weekly by the conventional tail cuff method for unanesthetized rats. At the termination of the study, the animals were perfused with 2% glutaraldehyde fixative and the kidneys were removed. Routine electron microscopic technique was employed to prepare the kidney samples for ultrastructural analysis. (Of particular interest were the effects of Ba ingestion on the glomeruli of the renal cortex.)

RESULTS

Barium Histology Studies. Food and water consumption data as well as body weights were recorded for all animals in all groups. Analysis of variance for repeated measures demonstrated no significant differences in any category between dosage groups.

A total of 21 neoplasms were observed in all groups. They were all benign and uniformly distributed among control treatment groups (data not shown). All but 6 neoplasm were adenomas of the pituitary gland, which is a common tumor in older SD rats.

A variety of non-neoplastic observations were also detected in control and treated rats. The incidence and severity of these microscopic observations were

TABLE 1
Ba Histology Study

Tissue Pathology/Group		Group Size	0	1 ppm Ba	10 ppm Ba	100 ppm Ba	250 ppm Ba
Adrenal							
(1) Focal Hyperplasia							
Male	36 weeks	12	1	0	0	2	2*
Male	68 weeks	10	1	3	2	4	–
Female	46 weeks	12	1	–	–	–	2
(2) Focal Hemorrhage							
Male	36 weeks	12	0	0	0	0	0*
Male	68 weeks	10	0	0	0	1	–
Female	46 weeks	12	1	–	–	–	0

*11 rather than 12 in this group.

comparable among control and treated groups. Similarly there were no differences in packed hematocrit.

Table 1 lists the incidence of adrenal finding by dosage and duration of exposure. Other examples of the random nature of the histology finding can be found in heart pathology (Table 2) and kidney pathology (Table 3). Of the tissues tested only the eye (Table 4) demonstrated what might be considered a dose-related trend, but then only if different duration exposure groups are combined. The lesion was characterized by focal absence of the outer layers of the retina, most often at the posterior segment of the globe and was not associated with any other ocular pathology.

TABLE 2
Ba Histology Study

Tissue Pathology/Group		Group Size	0	1 ppm Ba	10 ppm Ba	100 ppm Ba	250 ppm Ba
Heart							
Focal Myocarditis							
Male	36 weeks	12	4	6	4	3	2*
Male	68 weeks	10	0	0	0	0	–
Female	46 weeks	12	0	–	–	–	1

*11 rather than 12 rats in this group.

TABLE 3
Ba Histology Study

Tissue Pathology/Group		Group Size	0	1 ppm Ba	10 ppm Ba	100 ppm Ba	250 ppm Ba
Kidney							
(1) Chronic Nephropathy							
Male	36 weeks	12	4	3	7	4	4*
Male	68 weeks	10	9	9	7	6	–
Female	46 weeks	12	0	–	–	–	0
(2) Focal Mineralization							
Male	36 weeks	12	2	0	2	0	0*
Male	68 weeks	10	1	0	0	0	–
Female	46 weeks	12	2	–	–	–	2

*11 rather than 12 rats in this group.

Electrocardiographic Results

A representative electrocardiogram from a control rat, demonstrating normal sinus rhythm, is depicted in Figure 1. Eleven seconds after an I.V. injection of 5 μg/kg L-norepinephrine, a 2:1 heart block is demonstrated due to reflex vagal inhibition of the A V node (type 1 A V Blockade). By 110 seconds post I.V. injection, normal sinus rhythm is restored (Figure 1). This dosage of N.E. was considered to be the maximum tolerated dosage for the purposes of this experimentation.

Electrocardiographic data was collected at zero time and then again when all animals had returned to sinus rhythm (4 minutes). Table 5 data demonstrates normal reflex bradycardia in control animals at 4 minutes. Ba dosed rats (250 ppm Ba in drinking water) demonstrated significantly exaggerated bradycardia

TABLE 4
Ba Histology Study

Tissue Pathology/Group		Group Size	0	1 ppm Ba	10 ppm Ba	100 ppm Ba	250 ppm Ba
Eye							
Retinal Dystrophy							
Male	36 weeks	12	0	0	0	5	0*
Male	68 weeks	10	1	2	2	2	–
Female	46 weeks	12	0	–	–	–	7

*11 rather than 12 rats in this group.

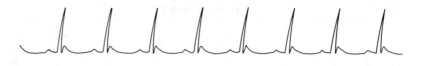

Control

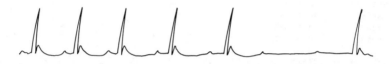

11 seconds post I.V. 5 μg/kg norepinephrine injection.

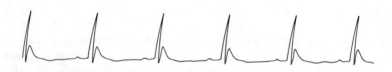

110 seconds post I.V. 5 μg/kg norepinephrine injection.

FIGURE 1. Electrocardiograms of anesthetized (50 mg/kg Nembutal) Sprague Dawley rat before, 11, and 110 seconds after a 5 μg/kg I.V. injection of L-norepinephrine (Levophed).

at 4 minutes post N.E. injection. By 60 minutes, control animal heart rate was still depressed; however, Ba exposed animals had almost fully regained their normal heart rate.

PR, QS, QT, and ST interval durations were measured at 0, 4, and 60 minutes post I.V. norepinephrine injection in control and Ba exposed animals (Table 6). There were no significant differences between control and Ba exposed animals in any parameters measured. There was a tendency toward an increased ST interval at 4 minutes in Ba exposed animals. This corresponds with the period of exaggerated bradycardia (Table 5).

Peak amplitudes were measured at 0, 4, and 60 minutes in control and Ba exposed animals (Table 7). There were no significant differences in any peaks measured, at any time period, regardless of Ba exposure.

TABLE 5

Parameters	Time After N.E. Injection	Control	Barium
Heart Rate	0 minutes	349 ± 7	339 ± 19
(BPM SEM)	4 minutes	309 ± 11	267 ± 51 P < 0.05
	60 minutes	310 ± 12	327 ± 12
Heart Rate Difference			
Time (0 - 4 minutes)		40 ± 16	72 ± 16
Time (0 - 60 minutes)		39 ± 17	12 ± 25

Blood Pressure Studies

Normotensive SD rats which were exposed to Ba in distilled drinking water or in physiologic saline drinking water demonstrated no Ba related changes in blood pressure (Figure 2). While there are variances in blood pressure, no trend is established either by varying Ba concentration in drinking water or by varying Ba concentration in saline.

Uninephrectomized SD rats also received Ba in drinking water derived from distilled water or 0.9 % saline (Figure 3). Ba concentration in drinking water was 1, 10, 100, or 1000 ppm. Again blood pressure fluctuates but no hypertensive trend is established.

Differences in response to Ba were recorded during the first week from salt sensitive rats receiving 1 ppm Ba in 0.9 % NaCl and during the first 2 weeks of exposure in salt sensitive rats receiving 10 ppm Ba in 0.9 % NaCl. These rats

TABLE 6

Parameters	Time After N.E. Injection	Control	Barium
PR Interval	0 minutes	51.6 ± 2.0	52.1 ± 1.5
(Msec ± SEM)	4 minutes	51.4 ± 2.8	53.8 ± 1.7
	60 minutes	52.5 ± 2.1	54.4 ± 1.7
QRS Duration	0 minutes	11.9 ± 0.7	11.9 ± 0.8
(Msec ± SEM)	4 minutes	17.3 ± 0.9	16.0 ± 1.1
	60 minutes	13.5 ± 0.5	12.3 ± 0.9
QT Interval	0 minutes	69.6 ± 3.2	73.1 ± 4.5
(Msec ± SEM)	4 minutes	79.8 ± 4.5	86.0 ± 4.9
	60 minutes	71.3 ± 3.4	68.7 ± 3.4
ST Interval	0 minutes	57.7 ± 3.1	61.2 ± 5.0
(Msec)	4 minutes	62.5 ± 4.4	70.0 ± 5.5
	60 minutes	57.8 ± 3.3	56.1 ± 3.8

TABLE 7

Parameters	N.E. Injection	Control	Barium
P Amplitude	0 minutes	0.14 ± 0.02	0.13 ± 0.02
(Mill.volts ± SEM)	4 minutes	0.13 ± 0.01	0.11 ± 0.02
	60 minutes	0.13 ± 0.2	0.12 ± 0.02
Q Amplitude	0 minutes	0.02 ± 0.01	-0.01 ± 0.02
(Mill.volts ± SEM)	4 minutes	-0.02 ± 0.01	0.00 ± 0.02
	60 minutes	-0.01 ± 0.02	0.01 ± 0.02
R Ampliture	0 minutes	2.55 ± 0.30	2.90 ± 0.16
	4 minutes	2.21 ± 0.28	2.19 ± 0.42
	60 minutes	2.70 ± 0.23	2.64 ± 0.30
S Amplitude	0 minutes	-0.81 ± 0.16	-0.72 ± 0.19
	4 minutes	-0.85 ± 0.20	-0.47 ± 0.17
	60 minutes	-0.82 ± 0.19	-0.68 ± 0.19
T Amplitude	0 minutes	0.21 ± 0.07	0.18 ± 0.07
	4 minutes	0.20 ± 0.07	, 0.27 ± 0.10
	60 minutes	0.29 ± 0.10	0.21 ± 0.09

demonstrated blood pressure well above normal, 160 mmHg and 150 mmHg, respectively (Figure 4). Much like the other groups in all other respects there was a fluctuation in blood pressure but no Ba related trend in hypertension was recorded.

Electron micrographic studies conducted on the kidney of all rats in the blood pressure studies demonstrated no histopathologic changes in arteriolar vessel walls or in tubules of the nephrons. However, structural changes were seen in the glomeruli from animals receiving sustained high levels of Ba (1000 ppm). These changes were not restricted to one group or another, but were seen in all groups receiving 1000 ppm Ba. Fused podocyte process and thickening of the capillary basement membrane are demonstrated in Figure 5. Myelin figures can also be seen in Bowman's space (the urine collecting area of the glomerulus) (Figure 6).

DISCUSSION

A drinking water standard of 1 ppm Ba has been promulgated by the U.S. Public Health Service (1962) and the U.S. Environmental Protection Agency (1975). Since then Calabrese (1978) reported on several potable water supplies containing Ba in excess of the drinking water standard. These studies have been initiated in order to help determine the health effects of various concentrations of Ba in drinking water.

Both the histopathology and the electrocardiogram studies reported here suffer from a methodologic problem. The Purina Rat Chow used in these contains 12 ppm Ba. Calculations based upon food consumption per kg body weight data indicate a background Ba level of 1 mg/kg/day for the rats used in

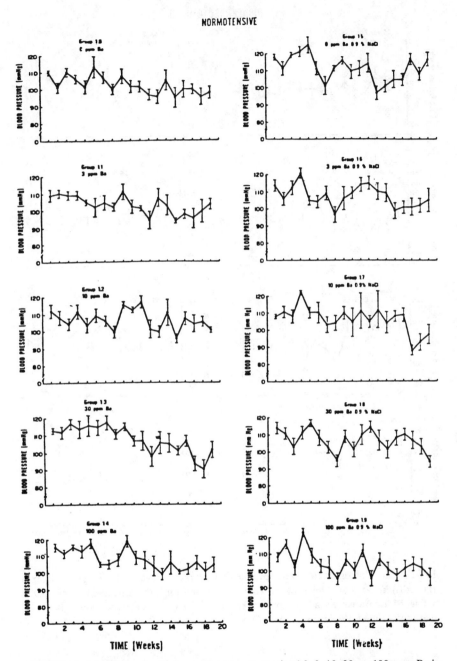

FIGURE 2. Normotensive Sprague Dawley rats received 0, 3, 10, 30, or 100 ppm Ba in drinking water. The drinking water was made from either distilled water or 0.9 % saline. Blood pressure readings were taken weekly for 20 weeks by the standard tail cuff method in unanesthetized rats (N = 6).

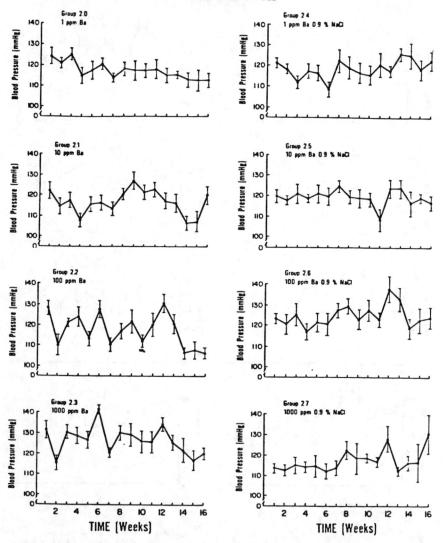

FIGURE 3. Uninephrectomized Sprague Dawley rats received 1, 10, 100, or 1000 ppm Ba in drinking water. The drinking water was made from either distilled water or 0.9 % saline. Blood pressure readings were taken weekly for 16 weeks by the standard tail cuff method in unanesthetized rats (N = 6).

these two studies. Calculations of drinking water consumption per kg body weight indicate an exposure rate of 1.5 mg/kg/day from water at the exposure level of 10 ppm Ba in drinking water. The blood pressure and electron microscope study does not suffer as the Tekland diet was used which yields a Ba background of 0.5 μg Ba/kg/day.

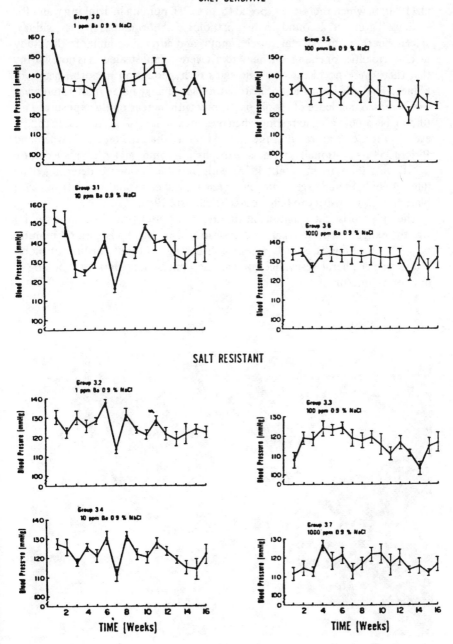

FIGURE 4. Salt sensitive (Dahl) and salt resistant (Dahl control) Sprague Dawley rats received 1, 10, 100, or 1000 ppm Ba in drinking water. The drinking water was made from 0.9 % NaCl. Blood pressure readings were made by the standard tail cuff method in unanesthetized rats (N = 6).

The histology study reported here compares with a similar study by Tardiff et al. (1980) in which rats were exposed to up to 250 ppm Ba in drinking water for 90 days. Tardiff et al. found no histopathologic abnormalities in liver, kidney, spleen, heart, brain, skeletal muscle, femur, and adrenals. Similar to this study no abnormalities or changes in hematocrit were demonstrated. It is noteworthy that there were no histopathologic signs of hypertension in aorta, heart, or kidney. The only indication of histopathologic change noted in this study was the increased incidence of retinal dystrophy with increasing Ba exposure. This finding became more interesting when one notes that Ba concentrates in rodent eyes, but it is concentrated in the choroid rather than the retina (Sowden and Pirie, 1958). Additionally, retinal dystrophy is a common degenerative disease in SD rats (Schardein et al., 1975) with variable incidence determined by intensity of light and cage composition (clear plastic or stainless steel) and cage placement with respect to light source (Bellhorn, 1980).

The only statistically significant finding in the electrocardiographic studies was the exaggerated bradycardia demonstrated by Ba exposed rats 4 minutes post I.V. injection of 5 μg L-norepinephrine/kg. Without concurrent blood pressure, peripheral resistance, or cardiac contractility data this finding is difficult to interpret.

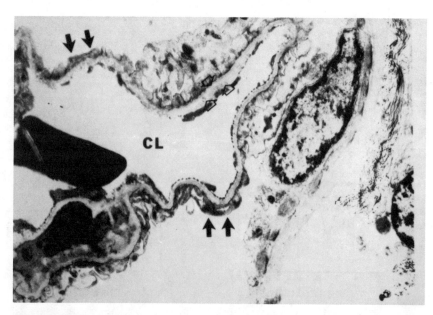

FIGURE 5. An electron micrograph of a glomerular capillary derived from a rat exposed to 1000 ppm Ba in drinking water for 16 weeks. Fused podocyte process (solid arrows) and a thickening basement membrane (open arrows) can be seen in this micrograph. The black object is an erythrocyte within the capillary lumen (CL) (Mag 5000 $\times$, 3″ $\times$ 4 1/2″ print).

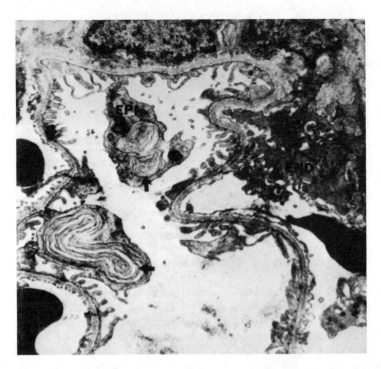

FIGURE 6. An electron micrograph of an epivascular space (Epi) (Bowman's Space) within the glomerulus. Myelin figure demonstrated within the podocyte process (solid arrows). Endovascular space (End) and erythrocytes (black objects) are also depicted. Rat treatment was the same as in Figure 5. (Mag 5000 ×, 3″ × 4 1/2″ print).

There were no significant trends toward hypertension in any of the rats given as much as 1000 ppm Ba for 16 weeks. The transient increase in blood pressure demonstrated by the Dahl salt sensitive rats in the low Ba dose groups is a normal response to the insult of the 0.9 % NaCl included in the drinking water. One is tempted to speculate as to why the high dose Ba salt sensitive rats did not also respond normally to the saline insult.

Possibly the most alarming result of the studies was the podocyte process fusion, basement membrane thickening and myelin figure formation in podocyte process demonstrated in 1000 ppm Ba exposed rats. These are all signs of impending or existing renal disease associated with inefficient glomerular filtration and hypertension.

This paper reports the results of three separate approaches to investigate the health effects of chronic drinking water Ba. Histopathologic studies of 35 tissues, electrocardiographic and blood pressure studies, and electron microscopic studies of renal morphology were conducted. Results indicate the need for further consideration of (1) a possible link between Ba and retinal dystrophy, (2) Ba linked transient exaggerated bradycardia in response to L-norepinephrine challenge, and (3) electron microscopic renal pathology due to high dose Ba exposure.

ACKNOWLEDGEMENTS

I would like to thank Dan McCullin, Monica Terkar, and Isaac Washington for their help in gathering food and water consumption data. I would like to acknowledge Experimental Pathology Laboratory Inc. (North Carolina) whose pathologist conducted the light microscopic examination of the chronically treated animals. My appreciation to Pat Underwood who has patiently typed and proofed this manuscript.

The research described in this article has been reviewed by the Health Effects Research Laboratory and approved for publication. Mention of trade names or commercial products does not constitute endorsement or recommendation for use.

REFERENCES

BELLHORN, R.W. (1980). Lightning in the animal environment. Lab. Animal Sci. **30**:440–450.

CALABRESE, E.J. (1978). Excessive barium and radium-226 in Illinois drinking water. *J. Environmental Health* **39**:366–369.

CHERNICK, W.S. (1971). The ions: Potassium, calcium, magnesium, fluoride, iodide and others. In: *Drills Pharmacology in Medicine,* 4th ed. DaPalma, JR. (ed.), p. 949.

HAMMOND, P.B. and BELILES, R.P. (1980). Metals. In: *Toxicology: The Basic Science of Poisons.* J. Doull, C.D. Klassen and M.O. Amdur (eds.). Macmillan, New York, pp. 409–467.

McCAULEY, P.T. and WASHINGTON, I.S. (1983). Barium bioavailability as the chloride, sulfate, or carbonate salt in the rat. Drug and Chemical Toxicology **6**:209–217.

MILLER, R.G., FEATHERSTONE, J.B.D., CURZAN, N.E.J., MILLS, T.S. and SHIELDS, C.P. (1985). Barium in teeth as indicator of body burden. In: *Inorganics in Drinking Water and Cardiovascular Disease,* Princeton Scientific Publishers, Princeton.

NATIONAL INSTITUTE OF OCCUPATIONAL SAFETY AND HEALTH REGISTRY OF TOXIC EFFECTS OF CHEMICAL SUBSTANCES. (1976). U.S. Dept. H.H.S., Washington, DC, 6th ed., p. 148.

SCHARDEIN, J.L., LUCAS, J.A. and FITZGERALD, J.E. (1975). Retinal dystrophy in Sprague-Dawley Rats. Lab. Animal Sci. **25**:323–326.

SHANBAKY, I.O., BOROWITZ, J.L. and KESSLER, W.V. (1978). Mechanisms of cadmium- and barium-induced adrenal catecholamine release. Toxicol. Appl. Pharmacol. **44**:99–105.

SOWDEN, E. and PIRIE, A. (1958). Barium and strontium concentrations in eye tissue. Biochem. J. **70**:716–717.

TARDIFF, R.G., ROBINSON, M. and ULMER, N.S. (1980). Subchronic oral toxicity of $BaCl_2$ in rats. J. of Environmental Pathol. Toxicol. **4**:267–275.

U.S. ENVIRONMENTAL PROTECTION AGENCY. (1975). Water Programs; National Interim Primary Drinking Water Regulations, Federal Register **40**(248): 59566–59588.

U.S. PUBLIC HEALTH SERVICE DRINKING WATER STANDARDS. (1962). Revised ed., U.S. Dept. of Health and Human Services, Public Health Service, Washington, DC.

CHAPTER XIX

BARIUM IN TEETH AS INDICATOR OF BODY BURDEN

Robert G. Miller,* John D.B. Featherstone,† Martin E.J. Curzon,†
Tammy S. Mills,* and Carole P. Shields†
*U.S. Environmental Protection Agency,
Health Effects Research Laboratory,
Toxicology and Microbiology Division,
Chemical and Statistical Support Branch,
Cincinnati, Ohio

†Eastman Dental Center,
Department of Oral Biology,
Rochester, New York

ABSTRACT

A study was conducted to determine the biological availability of naturally occurring barium in a municipal drinking water by the analysis of barium in deciduous teeth of children. The grade school children of two Illinois towns were chosen for this study. The towns were chosen based upon the barium content of their drinking water supply, geographic proximity, population, ethnic composition, and socioeconomic status of its residents. The high barium town had an average drinking water level of 10 mg/L and a mean of 36 μg Ba/g Ca in teeth of life-long residents drinking city water compared to teeth levels of 7 μg Ba/g Ca in the children of the low level barium town which had a drinking water concentration of 0.2 mg/L barium.

INTRODUCTION

Barium (Ba), an alkaline earth element, occurs in the earth's crust at relatively high concentrations. However evidence thus far indicates that barium is not essential for life. Little is known of the biological function of barium in calcified or soft tissues even though it is found in the tissues of most living things. The most common geologic stratum containing barium is barite or $BaSo_4$, which is the main source of the element for industrial use. The extensive industrial use of the element has meant that man is exposed to increasing concentrations of barium.

Municipal drinking waters in the USA contain barium ranging from 1.7–380 μg/L according to a report by Durfor et al. (1964). However, the average drinking water source accounts for only about 9% of average daily intake of barium which according to Schroeder et al. (1972) is approximately 1.0 mg/day. The bulk of barium intake is from food except where waters are particularly hard, containing barium at high concentrations.

The Safe Drinking Water Act of 1974 set a maximum contaminant level (MCL) for barium at 1 mg/L. It was suggested by Healy et al. (1963) that dietary differences in barium intake are reflected in contents of bone, enamel and dentin. Schroeder et al. (1972) indicated that clearance of barium in the urine of test subjects was only 9% and 5% of that of calcium and strontium respectively, indicating a preferential excretion of strontium. The absorption of barium compounds from the gut appeared to be poor both from water and food.

The oral toxicity of barium seems to depend upon the compound ingested. In a study of barium bioavailability, McCauley et al. (1983) found that in tubular fed rats the barium absorption rates were nearly identical with the use of barium chloride and barium sulfate, the carbonate was half as much for the first hour. Reeves (1979) reported that in rare instances of acute barium toxicity the mechanism of action of barium is based upon its physiological antagonism to potassium.

According to Kajola et al. (1979), symptoms following acute ingestion are vomiting, diarrhea, hypertension and hypokalemia. There have been no morbidity data presented that indicate any adverse health effects consistently associated with barium. Very few studies involving low dose barium ingestion have taken the absorbability of barium into account. Therefore this study was designed to determine whether or not the ingested barium via drinking water is absorbed.

Bauer et al. (1975) indicate that barium is a bone seeker and not retained by serum; therefore, assessment of body burden or intake can best be accomplished by analysis of calcified tissues such as bones and teeth. Since deciduous teeth were readily accessible, these were used as markers of barium exposure similar to Needleman et al. (1979) who used elevated dentine lead level as a marker for lead exposure. According to a report by Curzon et al. (1983), barium normally occurs in enamel of teeth at the 10–100 μg/gm levels.

Experimental Design. Through the review of the data reported by Brenniman et al. (1979), two communities were selected for this study based on levels of barium in the finished drinking water and the stability of this level over time, geographic proximity, population, ethnic composition and socioeconomic status.

West Dundee, Illinois was selected as the high barium community. The drinking water is obtained from one main well and contained 8.7–11.4 mg/L barium, and is aerated, fluoridated and chlorinated. In 1980 the total population of West Dundee was 3,551. In the selection of a control community where the drinking water supply contained low levels of barium it was necessary to match a range of population size from 2,500 to 4,500 in order to prevent a size too small to obtain the required number of nonexposed teeth. The control communities were to be within 10–100 miles of West Dundee as a practical distance which would allow the control of tooth collection in both communities to be done by one person and far enough apart to eliminate the probability of substantial contamination of the control population.

Based on these dual criteria of size and location, twelve communities were initially selected.

West Dundee has a non-white population of (1.2%) which further dictated that the control community be predominantly composed of white residents. Two control communities were eliminated using this criterion.

The socio-economic status of residents of the remaining 10 prospective communities were compared to West Dundee by median family income and occupational categories.

After analysis of all available data taken from the 1980 census and based upon population, location, ethnic composition, and socio-economic status, the city of Marengo, Illinois was selected as the control community. Descriptive characteristics of the two communities are in Table 1.

Within both study communities, the target population was children in all elementary grades. Parental consent forms and questionnaires were collected from each participant. An agreement was made with the communities' public and parochial school systems to carry out the project.

Sample Collection. Exfoliated deciduous teeth were collected from the grade school children throughout the 1982–83 school year by a dental hygienist. As the teeth were collected, each tooth was placed inside a separate envelope, sealed, and the child's name, age, sex, and community residence written on the outside of the envelope. A record of each tooth was also maintained on the parental consent forms. The envelopes containing the teeth were sent to our laboratory where they were blind coded and sent forward to be analyzed for barium and calcium. Throughout the study, drinking water of each community was collected and preserved according to the EPA Handbook for Sampling and Sample Preservation of Water and Wastewater (1982) and analyzed for barium.

Analytical Methods and Quality Control. All identifiable teeth samples received were prepared for analysis by removal of root (if present) and treated with 2 ml of 10 percent (v/v) HCl for one week. For calcium analysis an aliquot

TABLE I.
Characteristics of the Two Study Communities

Community	Population	Miles Apart	Median Family Income	Percent Nonwhite
West Dundee	3551	25	22,996	1.2%
Marengo	4361	25	22,538	5.1%

(5 or 10 μl) of the dissolved enamel was diluted with 1200 ppm KCl solution to surpress ionization. Measurements were made by use of the flame atomic absorption spectrophotometry technique of Perkin–Elmer (1983) using nitrous oxide/acetylene fuel at a wavelength of 422.4 nm. The sensitivity for calcium is 0.05 mg/L for 1 percent absorption with a linear range up to 5 ppm with reproducibility of $\pm$ 1 percent. Each group of 10 samples was compared to a blank and a 2 ppm calcium standard analyzed before and after unknown analyses. Each reported measurement of calcium is a mean of ten analytical readings for that analysis. Recoveries for spiked solutions of calcium ranged from 95–105%.

Barium analyses were measured using flameless atomic absorption techniques of Perkin–Elmer (1983). Detection limit for each 20 μl aliquot of sample was 0.04 μg/L and linear to 200 μg/L. Each analysis was performed in duplicate with $\pm$ 5% reproducibility. Each set of 5 unknowns were compared to a blank and standards (4.0 μg/L) analyzed before and after each group. Recoveries for spiked solutions of barium ranged from 100–102%. Barium analysis of the community drinking water samples were performed by the flame atomic absorption spectrophotometry technique of Perkin–Elmer (1983).

Calculations. The ratio of the barium to calcium concentrations in the filtrate for each tooth was determined. This is a method of objectively determining the replacement of calcium in enamel with barium and also eliminates the impossible job of separating enamel (containing the barium) from dentin in primary teeth.

Upon completion of the analysis and submission of the data, the results of each sample were then identified as to town origin. Inspection of questionnaires showed that some samples were not from natives of either community. The final separation of the 291 teeth fell into 5 categories (A) West Dundee natives (N = 102), (B) West Dundee immigrants (N = 63), (C) Marengo natives (N = 112), (D) Marengo immigrants (N = 1), (E) Samples not analyzed because they were permanent teeth or had gross amalgam (N = 13). In addition to Categories D & E, 16 teeth from the other categories were not used in the statistical analysis because pertinent information (i.e., age, home water supply) was missing. There were 106 subjects whose teeth data (total teeth = 261) were used in the analysis.

The subjects contributed varying numbers of teeth during the course of the study, but in all residence categories 75–85% of the subjects contributed 3 or fewer teeth. For this reason, the range of the Ba/Ca ratio values for each subject was used to investigate the within subject variability. The median range for West Dundee subjects was twice that for the West Dundee non-natives and 4 times that for the Marengo residents. The values were 22.6, 13.4, and 5.6 respectively. Since the subjects contributed varying numbers of teeth, a summary measure was needed for each student as the response variable in the statistical analysis. There was no difference between the mean and median μg Ba/gm Ca ratios for a given individual. Thus, to investigate if an association existed with barium in drinking water, it was determined that the mean ratio was an adequate indicator of the subject's body burden of barium.

In addition to residence category and type of home water supply, age, sex and

TABLE II.

Concentrations of Barium, Calcium and Other Elements
in the Drinking Waters of the Study Communities

Analysis Date	West Dundee (ppm)					Marengo (ppm)				
	Ca	Mg	Sr	F	Ba	Ca	Mg	Sr	F	Ba
Sept 1982	51.9	–	3.09	1.0	9.9	76.2	33.7	0.11	0.4	0.10
Nov 1982	55.1	20.1	2.20	0.5	11.4	74.8	33.4	0.12	0.4	0.50
Dec 1982	54.6	20.3	2.08	0.5	11.4	–	–	–	–	–
Feb 1983	–	–	–	–	9.0	–	–	–	–	0.10
May 1983	–	–	–	–	8.7	–	–	–	–	<0.10

length of residence in W. Dundee for non-natives were identified as potential confounders in the data analysis.

RESULTS

As an indicator of continued exposure to high and low levels of barium, Table II shows the stability of the Barium content of the studied communities' drinking water supplies (detection limit 0.10 mg/L).

The association of the concentration ratio of Ba/Ca in teeth with the potential confounders were considered individually in separate analysis. In Table III, comparisons were made of the Ba/Ca ratio between the sexes. In every residence category, the females had higher average ratios than the males. An analysis of variance for each residence category found no significant difference in the Ba/Ca ratio between the sexes in the West Dundee non-natives and the Marengo categories ($p > 0.30$), but a marginally significant difference was found in the West Dundee category ($p < 0.06$). The average ratio for females was 39.7 μg Ba/gm Ca compared to 22.6 for the males. Since the small number of males ($n = 5$) in the West Dundee non-native category and this borderline sex difference could possibly make differences in the Ba/Ca ratio between the residence categories, females and males were considered separately in a supplemental analysis.

A correlation between age and Ba/Ca ratio for each residence category showed no significant relationship (Table IV). Also, no significant relationship

TABLE III.
Comparison of Sex and Ba/Ca Ratio in the Residence Categories

Sex	Residence – Mean μg Ba/gm Ca Ratio					
	West Dundee	N	West Dundee Non-Native	N	Marengo	N
Female	39.7	19	14.5	16	7.7	19
Male	22.6	25	6.4	5	6.9	22

TABLE IV.
Comparison of Age and Ba/Ca Ratio in the Residence Categories

	Residence – Mean µg Ba/gm Ca Ratio					
Age	West Dundee	N	West Dundee Non-Native	N	Marengo	N
5	28.7	4	–	–	4.4	1
6	25.3	6	49.3	1	11.5	4
7	26.2	16	11.7	9	4.1	9
8	47.8	5	15.3	4	13.5	7
9	33.2	1	–	–	7.9	4
10	20.9	7	8.7	3	5.4	6
11	45.3	4	5.9	3	5.7	9
12	–	–	–	–	0.1	1
13	–	–	3.9	1	–	–
14	33.5	1	–	–	–	–
(p)	0.22	(>0.10)	−0.40	(>0.07)	−0.24	(>0.10)

was found between length of residence or age of immigration for non-natives of West Dundee and the Ba/Ca ratio. In Table V for each residence category, comparisons were made between the mean Ba/Ca ratio for each age and sex with no major differences indicated.

A two factor analysis of variance and Tukey's multiple comparison procedure were used to compare the Ba/Ca ratio among the 3 residence categories and between the 2 types of water supplies. A log transformation was used to stabilize the variance among the responses, a necessary condition for the statistical analysis. Table VI shows that the mean Ba/Ca ratio in the West Dundee residents was twice that of the non-native West Dundee residents and four times more than those living in the control community, Marengo (p < 0.05). The difference between the mean Ba/Ca ratios of the non-natives of West Dundee and the Marengo residents was not statistically significant (p > 0.05). In addition, because of the borderline significance between the sexes for West Dundee, females and males drinking city water were considered separately. For females, the same results as the overall analysis were found (West Dundee significantly higher than both Marengo and West Dundee nonnative). For males, the West Dundee residents were significantly higher than the Marengo residents, but not higher than the West Dundee nonnatives. The West Dundee residents drinking city water at home had a significantly higher Ba/Ca ratio than West Dundee residents drinking private well water at home (p < 0.01, Table VII). No significant difference among the residence categories was found when those drinking well water were considered separately.

TABLE V.
Comparison of Sexes Within Each Residence Category
and Ba/Ca Ratio With Each Age Group

| | Residence – Mean μg Ba/gm Ca Ratio | | | | | | | | | |
| | West Dundee | | | West Dundee Non-Native | | | | Marengo | | |
Age	Female	N	Male	N	Female	N	Male	N	Female	N	Male	N
5	51.8	2	5.6	2	-	-	-	-	4.4	1	-	-
6	26.8	4	22.3	2	49.3	1	-	-	14.9	3	1.6	1
7	44.2	4	20.2	12	11.7	9	-	-	2.9	2	4.5	7
8	59.8	3	29.8	2	16.2	3	11.4	1	12.9	3	14.0	4
9	33.2	1	-	-	-	-	-	-	8.0	3	7.9	1
10	21.1	2	20.8	5	9.7	2	6.6	1	4.4	4	7.4	2
11	38.9	2	51.7	2	7.8	1	5.0	2	3.6	3	6.7	6
12	-	-	-	-	-	-	-	-	-	-	0.1	1
13	-	-	-	-	-	-	3.9	1	-	-	-	-
14	33.5	1	-	-	-	-	-	-	-	-	-	-

Although information was received through each child's questionnaire concerning the use of water softeners, a formal statistical evaluation of that data would be erroneous because of additional information needed (i.e., water softener on hot or cold or both water systems). However, by examining the means of the tooth enamel Ba/Ca ratio for the city water drinkers, the Ba/Ca ratio of West Dundee residents (N = 10) with water softeners was 32.0 μg Ba/g Ca or three times that of Marengo residents (N = 16) with water softeners at 10.6 μg Ba/g Ca.

TABLE VI.
The Ba/Ca Ratio of Deciduous Teeth Enamel in the Study Communities

| | | μg Ba/gm Ca Ratio | | | |
Residence Category	N	Min	Med	Max	Mean
West Dundee	44	0.2	22.9	156.5	29.98
West Dundee (non-native)	21	1.9	8.65	49.3	12.56
Marengo	41	0.1	5.15	32.5	7.25

TABLE VII.
Comparisons of μg Ba/gm Ca Ratio of Deciduous Teeth Enamel of Residents Using Different Water Supplies

Water Supply	Residence					
	West Dundee		West Dundee Non-Native		Marengo	
	μg Ba/gm Ca	N	μg Ba/gm Ca	N	μg Ba/gm Ca	N
Well	10.79	10	7.47	3	6.42	6
City	35.62	34	13.41	18	7.39	35

CONCLUSION

Both male and female residents of West Dundee, the high barium exposure community, had significantly higher Ba/Ca ratios than those residents of the low barium exposure community. In addition, the West Dundee females had significantly higher Ba/Ca ratios than those of non-native West Dundee females. These differences were only seen in those subjects whose home water was supplied by the city.

The evidence from this study indicates that exposure to higher levels of barium via the drinking water source can result in a higher body burden of barium as measured in deciduous teeth. Because of the large variability of Ba/Ca ratios within a subject, a sampling of one tooth per child might not provide a reliable estimate of their body burden of barium. Further studies are needed to evaluate the differences between males and females and gather information on the critical exposure period.

ACKNOWLEDGEMENTS

The tooth collection and analyses were performed by Eastman Dental Center, Rochester, N.Y. under EPA Contract #68-03-3097. The authors thank Rebecca Osborne and Dan Greathouse for their contribution in the initial planning of this study and Melda Hirth and Keith Kelty for the preparation of the manuscript.

The research described in this paper has been peer and administratively reviewed by the U.S. Environmental Protection Agency and approved for publication. Mention of trade names or commercial products does not constitute endorsement or recommendation for use.

REFERENCES

BAUER, G.C.H., CARISSON, A. and LINDQUIST, B. (1957). Metabolism of Ba[140] in Man. *Acta Orthop. Scand.* **26**:241–54.

BRENNIMAN, G.R., KAJOLA, W.H., LEVY, P.S., CARNOW, B.W., NAMEKATA, T. and BRECK, E.C. (1979). Health Effects of Human Exposure to Barium in Drinking Water, EPA-600/1-79-003, U.S. Environmental Protection Agency, Cincinnati, Ohio.

CURZON, M.E.I. and FEATHERSTONE, J.D.B. (1983). Chemical Composition of Enamel: Handbook of Experimental Aspects of Oral Biochemistry, Chemical Rubber Co., Cleveland, Ohio, pp. 123–135.

DURFOR, C.D. and BECKER, E. (1964). Public Water Supplies of the 100 Largest Cities in the United States: Geological Survey Water Supply, Paper #1812, U.S. Government Printing Office, Washington, DC, p. 78.

HEALY, W.B. and LUDWIG, T.G. (1963). Molybdenum in Teeth. *New Zealand J. Dent. Res.* **42**:130.

KOJOLA, W.H., BRENNIMAN, G.R. and CARNOW, B.W. (1979). A review of environmental characteristics and health effects of barium in public water supplies. Rev. Env. Health, **1**:79–95.

McCAULEY, P.T. and WASHINGTON, I.S. (1983). Barium Bioavailability as the chloride, sulfate, or carbonate salt in the rat. *Drug and Chemical Toxicology* **6**:209–217.

NEEDLEMAN, H.L., GUNNOE, G., LEVITON, A., REED, R., PERESIE, H., MAHER, C. and BARRETT, P. (1979). Deficits in phychologic and classroom performance of children with elevated dentine lead levels. *New England J. Med.* **300**(13):599–695.

PERKIN–ELMER CORPORATION. (1983a). Analytical Methods for Atomic Absorption Spectrophotometry. Perkin–Elmer Methods Manual, Norwalk, CT.

PERKIN–ELMER CORPORATION. (1983b). Analytical Methods for Furnace Atomic Absorption Spectrophotometry. Perkin–Elmer Methods Manual, Norwalk, CT.

REEVES, A. (1980). Barium. In: *Handbook on the Toxicology of Metals,* L. Friberg et al. (eds.), Elsevier, New York, pp. 321–328.

SCHROEDER, H.A., TYPTON, M. and NASON, A.P. (1972). Trace metals in man: strontium and barium. *J. Chron. Dis.* **25**:491–517.

U.S. EPA. (1982). Handbook for Sampling and Sample Preservation of Water and Wastewater, EPA-600/4-82-029, U.S. Environmental Protection Agency, Cincinnati, OH.

CHAPTER XX

BARIUM–INDUCED HYPERTENSION

**H. Mitchell Perry, Elizabeth F. Perry,
Margaret W. Erlanger and Stephen J. Kopp**
*Veterans Administration Medical Center
and the Hypertension Division,
Department of Internal Medicine,
Washington University School of Medicine,
St. Louis, Missouri*

ABSTRACT

Because high barium concentrations (2 to 10 ppm) in human drinking water have been reported to be associated with elevated cardiovascular mortality, hypertension was sought in rats chronically exposed for 1 to 16 months to drinking water containing 1, 10, and 100 ppm barium.

From weaning, female Long-Evans rats were kept in a "low contamination" environment and fed a diet low in trace metals. Their drinking water was deionized and then fortified with five essential trace metals, and 0, 1, 10, or 100 ppm barium was added. Barium produced no change in growth rate, and no evidence of toxicity was recognized.

Indirect systolic pressure of unanesthetized rats was measured in triplicate at 1, 2, 4, 8, 12, and 16 months. Average systolic pressure increased after exposure to 100 ppm barium for one month and after exposure to 10 ppm barium for 8 months. (Average increases at 8, 12, and 16 months for these concentrations were 16 ± 1 mm Hg, with $p < 0.001$, and 6 ± 1 mm Hg, with $p < 0.025$, respectively).

Limited and preliminary physiologic and biochemical studies on animals exposed to 100 ppm barium for 16 months revealed (1) depressed cardiac contractility and conduction, and (2) decreased high energy phosphate and phosphorylation potential as measured by ^{31}P-NMR spectroscopy.

In conclusion, chronic exposure of rats to 10 or 100 ppm barium in water can induce increases in blood pressure. After 16 months, the higher exposure induced other functional and metabolic changes in the heart. Although the induced increases in rat blood pressure were modest, comparable mild hypertension in man would have major health implications.

INTRODUCTION

An increase in mortality rates was reported from communities in Illinois with high levels of barium in drinking water. A population of about 25,000 which was exposed to 2 to 10 mg of barium per liter (ppm) of drinking water was compared with a demographically similar population of 50,000 with low barium exposure (< 0.2 ppm). In the "high barium" areas, total deaths, after correction for the age and sex composition of the population, were higher by 10% and heart disease deaths by 15% than in "low barium" areas. Both of these differences were statistically significant, with $p < 0.05$ (Brenniman et al., 1979). In a subsequent study involving much smaller populations, the blood pressures of people living in high and low barium areas were compared. No differences were found in the incidence of hypertension or in the average level of diastolic pressure; however, less than 2,500 individuals were examined (Brenniman et al., 1981).

This preliminary paper reports some of the significant effects observed in rats that were exposed to three widely differing doses of barium in drinking water for up to 16 months. The weights of individual rats were measured and their systolic pressures were indirectly determined without anesthesia after six different intervals of barium exposure (1, 2, 4, 8, 12, and 16 months). Animals were sacrificed after three different exposure intervals (after 1, 4, and 16 months); weights of heart, liver, kidney, adrenals, and aorta were measured in these animals; and calcium, magnesium, potassium and sodium content of all but the adrenals and of plasma were measured. Barium was measured likewise at four months (except in the aorta) and at 16 months. In addition, further physiologic and biochemical studies were done on hearts of rats with the highest and longest barium exposure. Only the most significant results are reported here. The experimental plan is indicated in Table 1.

METHODS

A total of 195 female weanling Long-Evans rats were divided into three similar populations of 65 rats each; these populations were designated "1 month," "4 month," and "16 month" populations. In each population, there were three barium exposure groups, each initially containing at least 13 animals, and a control group of 26 animals. The three exposure groups received 1, 10, and 100 ppm barium (as the chloride) in their drinking water, which was fortified with five essential metals: 1 ppm Mo, 1 ppm Co, 5 ppm Cu, 10 ppm Mn, and 50 ppm Zn. All animals received our standard rye-based diet which contained 1.5 ppm barium and low concentrations of other trace metals, as previously described (Perry, H.M. et al., 1982, Perry, H.M. et al., 1977). Each group of 13 animals was housed in a large stainless steel cage which was maintained in our standard, very low contamination environment, with a 12-hour "light-dark cycle" and a constant temperature of 21° C. A total of 26 animals received the same fortified water without the barium and were housed in two cages under conditions identical to the barium-exposed animals; how-

TABLE 1.
Plan of Experiment

Barium Exposure For	1	2	4	8	12	16	Months
Individual Weight	✓	✓	✓	✓	✓	✓	At least 12 rats in 1, 10 & 100 ppm Ba
Systolic Pressure	✓	✓	✓	✓	✓	✓	groups & > 20 controls
Organ Weights	✓	✓				✓	At least 12 rats sacrificed per Ba group
Metal Concentrations	✓	✓				✓	& > 20 controls
Conductivity and Contractility Studies						✓	Hearts of 11 rats with 16 mos exposure to
^{31}P–NMR Analysis of Phosphate Metabolites						✓	100 ppm Ba & 16 controls

Three initial populations of 65 rats each were used: 26 were controls (only 21 were tested) and groups of 13 each were exposed to 1, 10, and 100 ppm Ba. Population 1 was sacrificed at one month, immediately after systolic pressure was measured. Population 2 was sacrificed at four months, having had their pressures measured at two and four months. Population 3 was sacrificed at 16 months, having had their pressures measured at 8, 12, and 16 months.

ever only 21 of these rats were actually used as controls; the remainder were used solely to keep numbers of animals in all cages comparable. Except for routine cage cleaning and testing, animals were not removed from their cages or disturbed. Food and water intakes were approximated for the first week of each month throughout the experiment.

Individual weights and systolic pressures were measured only at 1 month for the "1 month" population, at 2 and 4 months for the "4 month" population, and at 8, 12, and 16 months for the "16 month" population. Systolic pressure was measured by the indirect tail cuff procedure in trained unanesthetized animals which had been previously warmed to 39° C for 10 minutes. After the final weight and blood pressure measurements, heparinized blood was collected for total catecholamines and metal analyses by cardiac puncture of rats anesthetized with intraperitoneal injections of 35 mg/kg sodium pentobarbital. Blood for catecholamine analysis was cooled to 4° C, immediately separated, and the plasma frozen until assay by the HPLC and electro-chemical detection technique (Greenfield et al., 1975). Heart, liver, kidney, aorta, and adrenal were removed and weighed; aliquots of the first four of these tissues and plasma were frozen and assayed for metal concentration. Calcium, magnesium, potassium, and sodium were measured by atomic absorption spectrography, and barium was measured by inductibly coupled plasma atomic emission spectrography.

In the 16 month population only, cardiac measurements were made in anesthetized rats given 0 or 100 ppm barium. These measurements included peak left ventricular pressure, ventricular activation time, cardiac conduction times from His bundle electrographic and electrocardiographic analysis (Kopp, S.J., et al., 1980). Heart extracts prepared as previously described were analyzed for tissue metabolite concentrations (Kopp et al., 1978).

The blood pressure measurements were submitted to a two-way (length x intensity of barium exposure) analysis of variance. Least square mean comparisons were used to compare average blood pressures across treatments within time periods (1-tail tests) (Rimm et al., 1980).

RESULTS

The cumulative barium intakes from food and water over the 16 month period were estimated to be 16 mg for a control rat, 28 mg for a rat exposed to 1 ppm barium; 134 mg for a 10 ppm exposure rat; and 1200 mg for a 100 ppm exposure rat.

There were no significant differences in average weight (i.e., growth rate) between the control group and any of the barium exposure groups, and there were no other obvious evidences of toxicity.

A significant pressor effect averaging 12 mm Hg was observed in the 100 ppm barium group after only 1 month of exposure ($p < 0.001$). A significant increase in average pressure for 100 ppm barium over control rats was consistently present at all subsequent measurements (for both the 4 months and the 16 months populations); moreover the average difference between barium and control rats gradually rose to 16 mm Hg after 16 months of exposure. Ten ppm of barium also induced a pressor effect, but the effect was less marked ($p < 0.025$), and did not occur until after eight months of exposure. The data tabulated in Table 3 are *increases* in average blood pressure of barium-exposed rats compared to the average blood pressure of 21 control animals from the same populations.

At no time did any group of barium-exposed rats differ significantly from the control animals in average weight of aorta, heart, liver, kidneys, or adrenals.

After four months of exposure, statistically significant increase in tissue barium was only observed in the kidneys of rats exposed to 100 ppm barium. After 16 months, all tissues of 100 ppm animals had significant increases as did the kidneys of 10 ppm animals (Table 4).

The average concentrations of calcium, magnesium, potassium, and sodium in heart, liver, kidney, aorta, and plasma were determined after 1, 4, and 16 months of exposure to the three concentrations of barium. Kidney calcium

TABLE 2.
Average Cumulative Barium Intake from Food and Water

	1	2	4	8	12	16 Months
Control	0.9	1.8	3.6	7.2	11	16
1 ppm Ba	1.3	2.8	5.9	12	18	28
10 ppm Ba	5.4	12	27	55	87	134
100 ppm Ba	46	107	234	487	771	1198

Average cumulative intake (mg of barium per rat). The intake of control animals was entirely from food. All rats had this intake which in the barium exposed group was augmented by the barium added to the drinking water.

TABLE 3.
Barium-Induced Hypertension in Rats

ppm Ba	1 Mo	2 Mo	4 Mo	8 Mo	12 Mo	16 Mo
1	1	-1	1	2	1	1
10	3	1	5	6*	7*	4*
100	12**	6*	12**	15**	16**	16**

Average increase in systolic pressure (13 rats), in mm Hg, measured against the control average (21 rats) for each period. See text for details. Asterisks indicate statistical significance of the increase, one asterisk indicates $p < 0.01$ and two asterisks indicate $p < 0.001$.

concentrations were consistently lower in barium-exposed animals than in control rats in both 10 and 100 ppm barium groups at 4 and 16 months, but the effect was significant only in the 10 ppm barium group at 16 months ($p < 0.025$). No statistically significant differences were found for magnesium, potassium or sodium.

There were no significant barium-induced differences or suggestive trends in the measured catecholamine concentrations.

Exploratory studies revealed physiologic and biochemical effects on the heart of the rats with the highest and longest barium exposure: 100 ppm for 16 months; no other exposure groups were studied. The notable barium-induced *in vivo* changes in myocardial contractility were: (1) reduction in peak left intraventricular pressure; (2) changes in rate of pressure development; (3) slower contractile element shortening velocity. In addition there was significant prolongation of PR and AH intervals, as demonstrated by ECG and Hiss Bundle electrogram. Details of these changes have been presented elsewhere (Kopp et al., 1984).

Perchloric acid extracts of myocardium were assayed by ^{31}P-NMR spectrography for 20 phosphatic metabolites. Barium reduced ATP and phosphocrea-

TABLE 4.
Average Barium Concentrations in Organs After 16 Months

	Heart	Liver	Kidneys	Aorta
0 ppm Ba	0.010	0.007	0.022	0.12
1 ppm Ba	0.006	0.005	0.020	0.17
10 ppm Ba	0.014	0.008	0.092*	0.24
100 ppm Ba	0.105**	0.08*	1.39**	1.80**

Values are μg barium per gm of wet tissue. Note: The 16 month aortic average excludes one high outlier of 3.6 $\mu g/g$. Asterisks indicate statistical significance of the increased barium concentration; one indicates $p < 0.05$ and two $p < 0.01$.

TABLE 5.

**Change in Probability of Coronary Heart Disease in Men During 6 Years
With Systolic Pressure Increase From 120 to 135 mm Hg
(Without Cigarettes, LVE, or Glucose Intolerance)**

	40 Yrs	50 Yrs	60 Yrs
Increase in CHD*	0.3%	0.8%	1.3%

*1% incidence = 100,000 men/10 million hypertensives

Legend: Increase in new coronary heart disease (CHD) for men in three age groups during 6 years of followup as a function of an increase in systolic pressure from 120 to 135 mm Hg. These data are from the Framingham Study and hence are limited to whites. They assume moderate total cholesterol (235 mg %) and no cigarette smoking, no left ventricular enlargement (LVE) by EKG, and no glucose intolerance. The absolute increases in CHD rates would be larger if any of these additional risk factors were present.

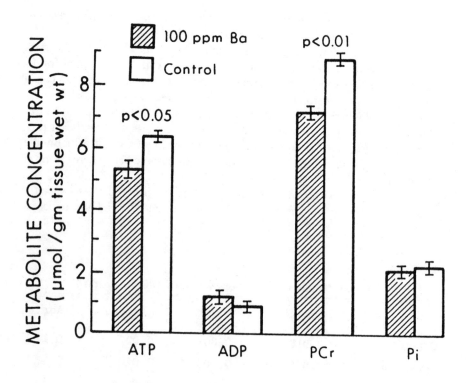

FIGURE 1. Barium-induced changes in ATP, ADP, phosphocreatine (PCr) and inorganic phosphate (Pi). These are preliminary data on perchloric acid extracts of myocardium from rats exposed to 100 ppm barium for 16 months.

tine (Figure 1) and therefore the high energy phosphate available to muscle contraction. This was reflected in a reduced phosphorylation potential (ATP/ADP × Pi).

DISCUSSION

Barium has long been recognized as causing contraction of smooth muscle, including that in blood vessels. Therefore it is not surprising to find that chronic barium exposure can induce hypertension. Prior attempts to show that barium feeding induces a prolonged pressor effect in intact animals have failed, although vasoconstrictor effects have been demonstrated in isolated aortic strips (Perry, H.M. et al., 1967).

Long-term ingestion of three different heavy metals, barium, cadmium and lead—widely distributed in nature—can cause similar elevations in the systolic pressure of rats (Perry, H.M. et al., 1978; Perry, H.M. et al., 1977). These elevations in pressure are not associated with any recognized toxic manifestations or with any decrease in the growth rates of young rats; moreover the generally accepted toxic exposure levels are much higher than the pressor levels. It is noteworthy that these pressure elevations in animals have been induced by exposures—somewhat above perhaps, but comparable to—the environmental exposures of large numbers of Americans.

Although the basis of their pressor effects has not been defined, all three metals produced somewhat similar changes in the pattern of energy-related, phosphate-containing compounds in the heart (Perry, H.M. et al., 1983; Kopp et al., 1980). Various mechanisms by which trace metals might induce hypertension have been suggested for cadmium and lead. The most likely four would seem to be (a) sodium retention (Perry, H.M. et al., 1981); (b) direct vasoconstriction (Perry, H.M. et al., 1975; Perry, H.M. et al., 1967a); (c) stimulation of the renin-angiotensin system (Perry, H.M. et al., 1973; Victery et al., 1982); and (c) increase in cardiac output (Perry, H.M. et al., 1967b). A direct vasoconstrictor effect seems likely in the case of barium; this might well involve competition with calcium. Sodium retention seems very probably the mechanism in the case of cadmium, although there may well be some direct vasoconstriction. The data are less clear in the case of lead.

Thus, based on life-long but low-level feeding experiments in animals, three heavy metals seem to be possible contributors to human hypertension and hence to human cardiovascular disease. All three metals can certainly elevate blood pressure in animals—and do so in low concentrations to which many Americans are continuously exposed. The question is whether any of these metals actually raise blood pressure in human beings; and, if so, is the increase, which averages only 15 mm Hg in rats, of potential clinical significance?

We cannot answer the first question although recent NHANES data seem to show a strong positive correlation between blood lead and blood pressure levels (Harlan et al., 1985). In answer to the second, however, it is worth emphasizing that an average blood pressure increase of 15 mm Hg would clearly be clinically significant in man. For instance, according to the Framingham Study, in the absence of other risk factors, an increase in systolic pressure from 120 to 135 mm Hg would increase the probability of coronary heart disease developing within 6 years by 0.3%, 0.6%, and 1.2% for men 35, 45, and 55 years old, respectively (Framingham Study, 1971, as shown in Table 5). Since there are at least ten million men with mild hypertension in the United States, a pressor effect of this magnitude could lead to thousands of new cases of coronary heart disease annually. Thus, within the limits of practicality, it seems worthwhile to restrict the intake of any substance which is a possible pressor agent in man.

ACKNOWLEDGEMENT

This research was supported by the United States Environmental Protection Agency.

REFERENCES

BRENNIMAN, G.R., KOJOLA, W.H., LEVEY, P.S., CARNOW, B.W. and NAMETAKA, T. (1981). High barium levels in public drinking water and its association with elevated blood pressure. Arch. Environ. Health **36**:28–32.

BRENNIMAN, G.R., NAMETAKA, T., KOJOLA, C.H., CARNOW, B.W. and LEVY, P.S. (1979). Cardiovascular disease death rates in communities with elevated levels of barium in drinking water. Environ. Res. **20**:318–324.

GREENFIELD, S., JONES, I.L., McGRADIN, H.M. and SMITH, P.B. (1975). Automatic multi-sample simultaneous multi-element analyses with an H.F. Plasma. Anal. Chem. Acta **74**:225–231.

FRAMINGHAM STUDY, 16-YEAR FOLLOWUP. (1971). Coronary heart disease, atherothrombotic brain infarction, intermittent claudication—a multivariate analysis of some factors related to their incidence. Sec. 27, pp. 1–42.

HARLAN, W.R., LANDIS, J.R., SCHMOUDER, R.L., GOLDSTEIN, N.G., HARLAN, L.C. (1985). Blood lead and blood pressure. JAMA **253**:530–534.

KOPP, S.J., BARANY, M., ERLANGER, M.W., PERRY, E.F. and PERRY, H.M., JR. (1980). The influence of chronic low-level cadmium and/or lead feeding on myocardial contractility related to phosphorylation of cardiac myofibrillar proteins. Toxicol. Appl. Pharmacol. **54**:48–56.

KOPP, S.J., FISCHER, V.W., ERLANGER, M.W., PERRY, E.F. and PERRY, H.M., JR. (1978). Electrocardiographical, biochemical, and morphological effects of chronic low level cadmium feeding on the rat heart. Proc. Soc. Exp. Biol. Med. **159**:339–345.

KOPP, S.J., PERRY, H.M., JR., FELIKSIK, J.M., ERLANGER, M. and PERRY, E.F. (Submitted for publication). Cardiovascular dysfunction and hypersensitivity to sodium pentobarbital induced by chronic, subacute barium chloride ingestion. Toxicol. and Appl. Pharmacol.

PERRY, H.M., JR. and ERLANGER, M.W. (1982). Effect of diet on increases in systolic pressure induced in rats by chronic cadmium feeding. J. Nutrition **112**:1983–1989.

PERRY, H.M., JR. and ERLANGER, M.W. (1973). Elevated circulating renin activity in rats following doses of cadmium known to induce hypertension. J. Lab. Clin. Med. **82**:399–405.

PERRY, H.M., JR. and ERLANGER, M.W. (1975). Mechanism of cadmium-induced hypertension. Trace Substances Environ. Health **9**:339–348.

PERRY, H.M., JR. and ERLANGER, M.W. (1978). Pressor effects of feeding cadmium and lead together. Trace Substances Environ. Health **12**:268–274.

PERRY, H.M., JR. and ERLANGER, M.W. (1981). Sodium retention in rats with cadmium-induced hypertension. Science Total Environment **22**:31–37.

PERRY, H.M., JR., ERLANGER, M.W. and PERRY, E.F. (1977). Elevated systolic pressures following chronic low-level cadmium feeding. Am. J. Physiol. **232**: H114–121.

PERRY, H.M., JR., ERLANGER, M., YUNICE, A. and PERRY, E.F. (1967b). Mechanisms of the hypertensive effect of intra-arterial cadmium and mercury in anesthetized rats. J. Lab. Clin. Med. **70**:963–972.

PERRY, H.M., JR., KOPP, S.J., ERLANGER, M.W. and PERRY, E.F. (1983). Cardiovascular effects of chronic barium ingestion. Trace Substances Environ. Health **16**:155–173.

PERRY, H.M., JR., SCHOEPFLE, E. and BOURGOIGNIE, J.J. (1967a). In vitro production and inhibition of aortic vasoconstriction by mercuric cadmium, and other metal ions. Proc. Soc. Exp. Biol. Med. **124**:485–490.

RIMM, A.A., HARTZ, A.J., KALBFLEISCH, J.H., ANDERSON, A.J. and HOFFMAN, R.G. (1980). Basic Biostatistics in Medicine and Epidemiology. Prentice–Hall (Appleton–Century–Crofts), New York, pp. 207–228.

VICTERY, W., VANDER, A.J., SHULAK, H.M., SCHOEPS, P. and JULIUS, S. (1982). Lead hypertension and the renin-angiotensin system in rats. J. Lab. Clin. Med. **99**:354–362.

CHAPTER XXI

EPIDEMIOLOGICAL STUDY OF BARIUM IN ILLINOIS DRINKING WATER SUPPLIES

Gary R. Brenniman and Paul S. Levy
School of Public Health
University of Illiniois at Chicago
P.O. Box 6998, Chicago, Illinois 60680

ABSTRACT

This environmental epidemiology study was designed to determine if human mortality and morbidity rates were significantly different ($p < 0.05$) in populations ingesting elevated barium levels in their drinking water as compared to populations that ingest very little or no barium from their drinking water. Animal studies have shown that the principal effects of barium ingestion are on the heart, blood vessels and nerves.

Cardiovascular mortality rates for the years 1971–1975 were examined to determine if there were any differences between Illinois communities with barium concentrations ranging from 2.0–10 mg/l in their drinking water as compared to communities having drinking water concentrations of barium ranging from 0.2 mg/l or less. Results of this study indicated that communities with elevated barium concentrations in their drinking water had significantly higher mortality rates ($p < 0.05$) for "all cardiovascular disease" and "heart disease." Any inferences drawn about this finding must be interpreted with extreme caution because there was no method of controlling for removal of barium by home water softeners. In addition, some of the elevated barium communities had greater than 70% change in their population from 1960 to 1970.

From 1976–1977, a morbidity study was conducted with 1175 adults from West Dundee, Illinios and 1203 adults from McHenry, Illinois. West Dundee and McHenry have mean barium drinking water concentrations of 7.3 and 0.1 mg/l respectively. Age-specific mean systolic and diastolic blood pressure levels for adult males and females in West Dundee were compared to a control population of adult males and females from McHenry. No significant differences ($p < 0.05$) were found in adult male and female blood pressures between the high and low barium communities. Adjustment for duration of exposure, home water softeners, and high blood pressure medication did not have any effect on the findings. In addition, the prevalence rates for hypertension, stroke, heart disease and kidney disease in males and females from West Dundee were not significantly different ($p < 0.05$) from the prevalence rates for these respective diseases in males and females of McHenry.

The data from this study suggest that a mean drinking water barium concentration of 7.3 mg/l does not seem to have an adverse effect on adult blood pressures, and it does not seem to be associated with hypertension, stroke, and heart and kidney disease in adults. It is recommended that the National Interim Primary Drinking Water Regulation for barium (maximum contaminant level of 1. mg/l) be re-examined for other possible health effects.

INTRODUCTION

Human ingestion of 800-900 mg of barium chloride (550-600 mg as barium) has been shown to be a fatal dose (Sollman, 1957). Barium ingestion from acute human and animal exposures has characteristically resulted in stimulation of smooth, striated, and cardiac muscle (Goodman and Gilman, 1970; Smith et al., 1940; Roza and Berman, 1971; Diengott et al., 1964). Recorded symptoms from these acute exposures include salivation, vomiting, diarrhea, ventricular tachycardia, hypertension, hypokalemia, twitching, flaccid paralysis of skeletal muscle, respiratory muscle paralysis, and ventricular fibrillation. Chronic human health effects associated with exposure to low levels of barium in drinking water are not well defined.

Since there was no human health data available from chronic exposure to low levels of barium in drinking water, the current federal maximum contaminant level (MCL) of 1. mg/l barium has been developed utilizing an extrapolation from the threshold limit value (TLV) of 0.5 mg Ba/m^3 air (U.S. Environmental Protection Agency, 1976 and 1977; Stockinger and Woodward, 1958; American Conference of Governmental Industrial Hygienists, 1971). Besides confusion on the source and validity of the TLV for barium, the extrapolation used to develop the current MCL for barium in drinking water required several assumptions including an absorption factor of 0.75 for inhalation and 0.90 through the gastrointestinal tract, both of which are unsubstantiated (Larsen, 1979; Kojola et al., 1979).

Due to the paucity of data upon which to base a well-grounded standard for barium in drinking water, an epidemiological study was conducted in Illinois to determine whether human mortality and morbidity rates were significantly different ($p \leq 0.05$) in populations ingesting greater than 1. mg/l barium in their drinking water as compared to control populations. Illinois has greater than 150,000 individuals who are exposed to drinking water barium concentrations greater than 1. mg/l (Illinois Institute for Environmental Quality, 1974). These barium concentrations are found in deep rock or drift walls, and are the result of the natural leaching of barium from the surrounding geological strata into ground water (Gilkeson et al., 1978).

232

TABLE 1

Population Characteristics of Persons Living in Northern Illinois Communities
with Elevated Versus Low Barium in Their Drinking Water
(U.S. Bureaus of the Census, 1973).

General Population Characteristics	Elevated Barium Communities (≥ 2-10 mg/ℓ)	Low Barium Communities (≤ 0.2 mg/ℓ)
Population	25,433	46,905
Males	12,488	22,621
Females	12,945	24,284
% Negro and other races	0.5	1.7
% Under 18 years old	39.1	35.8
% 65 years old and over	7.2	9.9
Persons per household*	3.5	3.1
Median school years completed*	12.5	12.2
Mean income*	15,305	13,654
Median age*	26.5	29.7

* Averages of four high barium communities (Algonquin, Crystal Lake, Lake Zurich, and West Dundee) and seven low barium communities (Antioch, Batavia, Fox Lake, Geneva, Harvard, Libertyville and Marengo).

METHODOLOGY

Mortality Study. Mortality rates for cardiovascular diseases, as classified by the U.S. Department of Health, Education and Welfare (1968), were retrospectively determined for the years 1971-1975 from Illinois State Death Certificates. Statistical comparisons of age-adjusted cardiovascular mortality rates were made between communities with drinking water barium concentrations ranging from $\geq$ 2.0-10 mg/l and communities with up to 0.2 mg/l barium. Barium was the only contaminant found to exceed U.S. Environmental Protection Agency (1977) drinking water regulations in any of the public drinking water supplies studied.

The Illinois communities selected for the study were chosen from the northern part of the state and were matched for demographic and socioeconomic status (SES) characteristics (Table 1). Although communities with high rates of population change, industrialization, and geographical difference were excluded to minimize cardiovascular effects from other confounding variables, the communities of Algonquin and Crystal Lake, with about 75% change in

TABLE 2

Comparison of Age and Sex-Adjusted Mortality Rates Per 1,000,000 Persons for Cardiovascular Disease in Communities with Barium Concentrations Ranging from 2-10 mg/l and Those in Communities with Barium Concentrations 0.2 mg/l or less, 1971-75

	Elevated Barium Communites			Low Barium Communities			
	# of Deaths		Mortality Rates	# of Deaths		Mortality Rates	Mortality Ratio
Category	Males	Females	(A)	Males	Females	(B)	(A)/(B)
All Cardiovascular Disease	335	290	651.1	720	634	573.4	1.136*
a. Heart Disease	269	206	493.9	569	451	432.0	1.143*
1. Arteriosclerosis	259	199	476.8	543	434	413.8	1.152*
2. Other	10	7	17.1	26	17	18.2	0.940
b. Cerebrovascular Disease	45	62	113.1	91	137	96.5	1.172
c. General Arteriosclerosis	8	8	16.7	23	20	18.2	0.918
d. Hypertension without mention of heart	2	7	9.4	6	6	5.1	1.843
e. Other Circulatory Disease	11	7	18.0	31	20	21.6	0.833
All Causes	638	520	1148.2	1335	1109	1036.8	1.107*
Population (1970)	12,488	12,945		22,621	24,284		
Total Person Years	62,440	64,725		113,105	121,420		

* P ≤ 0.05 (for males and females combined) (Mantel and Haenszel, 1959).

population between 1960 and 1970, were kept in the study because there were no other elevated barium communities which could have served as a satisfactory replacement.

The elevated and low barium communities listed in Table 1 were screened for mortality attributable to cardiovascular diseases using the 1971-1975 Illinois Death Certificate tapes. A mortality rate by cause was computed for specific age groups of a target population using standard population information for each group (U.S. Bureau of the Census, 1973; Brenniman et al., 1979). In this manner, the average annual age-adjusted mortality rates for a target population were calculated using a direct method of computation (Barclay, 1958).

Morbidity Study. West Dundee and McHenry, Illinois were selected for the morbidity study because of similar demographic and SES characteristics, and a 70 fold greater barium concentration in West Dundee's drinking water (a mean of 7.3 mg/l versus a mean of 0.1 mg/l). Barium was the only contaminant found in either community which exceeded U.S. Environmental Protection Agency (1977) regulations. This study was conducted to examine differences in blood pressure levels and prevalence rates for hypertension, stroke, and heart and renal disease in males and females between these two communities.

There were 1,175 and 1,203 adult males and females respectively from West Dundee and McHenry who participated in the study. Subjects were selected by taking a random sample of blocks within each community, listing every household within each block, and including every person 18 years of age or older in each listed household as an eligible subject.

All subjects who participated in the study had their blood pressures taken and were administered a health questionnaire. Three blood pressures of each participant were taken over a period of about 20 minutes with a calibrated

Sphygmostat Model B-250 electronic blood pressure apparatus. All blood pressures in both communities were taken by four trained female survey workers with the individuals seated and their left arm resting on a table. The health questionnaire was developed with the objective of obtaining data on such variables as sex, age, weight, height, smoking habits, family history, occupation, medication, and cardiovascular, cerebrovascular and renal disease.

All data were collected from a cluster sample, and more than one person per household could appear in the sample. The sample design was self-weighting because very individual 18 years old and older in each community had the same chance of being selected in the sample. As a consequence, analysis of variance was used to determine if mean blood pressures in males and females between communities were significantly different ($p \leq 0.05$). The statistical method used was appropriate for unequal cell sizes (Snedecor and Cochran, 1967).

Prevalence rates for hypertension, stroke, and heart and kidney disease were analyzed using the signed rank test for age-specific rates and the weighted Z test for total population rates (Fleiss, 1973). When a particular prevalence rate was found to be higher but not significantly different ($p > 0.05$), the Mantel-Haenszel test was run to determine if there was a significant difference in actual numbers of the disease (Mantel and Haenszel, 1959).

TABLE 3

Systolic and Diastolic Blood Pressure Among White Persons 18-75+ Years of Age who Live in West Dundee or McHenry, Illinois, 1976-77

Blood Pressure Age (Years)	West Dundee						McHenry					
	Male			Female			Male			Female		
	No. Cases	Mean	SD[†]	No. Cases	Mean	SD[†]	No. Cases	Mean	SD[†]	No. Cases	Mean	SD[†]
Systolic												
18–24	77	123.3	13.9	114	104.6	10.2	54	120.2	12.5	53	106.1	10.6
25–34	122	123.9	13.2	147	106.5	12.3	77	122.2	12.6	111	106.4	11.9
35–44	92	123.9	16.7	133	111.6	15.0	74	124.1	15.2	88	111.3	17.0
45–54	89	127.9	16.2	91	121.3	17.5	75	129.7	15.3	90	116.3	18.6
55–64	69	131.3	21.4	75	128.1	21.1	77	135.6	17.8	136	129.5	22.3
65–74	29	139.1	20.1	60	138.1	21.0	128	140.7	21.0	137	136.2	20.4
75+	28	149.8	20.3	49	151.6	23.4	47	144.8	22.0	56	146.1	21.3
Total Pop.*	506	129.7	17.8	669	120.7	21.5	532	129.8	19.2	671	119.6	22.8
Diastolic												
18–24	77	73.9	10.7	114	70.1	7.9	54	71.5	10.9	53	72.9	6.7
25–34	122	76.8	10.7	147	73.4	9.9	77	78.4	10.4	111	74.6	11.0
35–44	92	82.7	10.4	133	77.3	11.5	74	82.6	11.1	88	79.6	11.6
45–54	89	84.0	11.3	91	83.5	11.1	75	85.8	11.4	90	81.5	14.1
55–64	69	82.7	13.1	75	84.4	14.9	77	86.1	12.7	136	87.0	15.1
65–74	29	82.1	13.8	60	85.8	14.5	128	85.8	13.4	137	86.6	14.7
75+	28	80.4	10.1	49	88.0	14.6	47	81.7	12.5	56	83.4	16.5
Total Pop.*	506	80.4	11.8	669	79.7	13.1	532	81.8	12.7	671	80.6	14.4

* Total sex specific means are age-adjusted to the total sample size for each sex.
† SD = Standard Deviation.

RESULTS AND DISCUSSION

Mortality Study. Mortality rates for cardiovascular diseases in communities with barium drinking water concentrations ranging from 2-10 mg/l were compared to mortality rates for cardiovascular diseases in communities with barium drinking water concentrations of 0.2 mg/l or less (Table 2). Mortality rates in the elevated barium communities were significantly higher (p $\leq$ 0.05) for male and female mortality combined for "all cardiovascular disease," "heart disease (arteriosclerosis)," and "all causes." Generally, the 65 and older age group accounted for the largest difference between observed and expected deaths. In addition, although "hypertension without mention of heart" had the highest mortality ratio (1.843), it lacked statistical significance, because of the small number of recorded deaths. As a consequence, this ratio is too unstable for any conclusions or inferences to be drawn.

Furthermore, any inferences drawn from higher mortality rates in the elevated barium communities must be treated with extreme caution because of potentially confounding variables that could not be controlled in this retrospective epidemiology study. For instance, there was no way to control for home water softeners in this study. Since these softeners remove such divalent metallic cations as barium, calcium and magnesium, and increase sodium concentrations, any inferences drawn from the findings of this study could possibly be due to the softened water and not the barium.

Another confounding variable was that two of the elevated barium communities had a substantial increase in population between 1960 and 1970. Therefore, the possibility exists that mortality rates in the elevated barium communities based on 1970 census population figures could be higher than the actual mortality rates for the years 1971-1975.

Finally, there was no way of controlling for length of time that an individual lived in a community. Therefore, mortality attributed to cardiovascular disease for people living in the elevated barium communities a relatively short period of time probably cannot be highly associated with the barium.

Morbidity Study. No significant differences (p > 0.05) were found when West Dundee male and female mean systolic and diastolic blood pressures were compared similarly to blood pressures of McHenry males and females (Table 3). Since no significant differences were found in blood pressures between communities for the total population sample, a subpopulation of individuals who do not have home water softeners, are not taking high blood pressure medication, and have resided more than 10 years in their respective community was analyzed statistically. Water softeners, medication, and duration of exposure could possibly be masking a blood pressure effect. However, when these three factors were taken into consideration, no significant differences were found (Table 4). In addition, such factors as smoking and obesity were found to have no relationship to this finding.

The prevalence rates for hypertension, stroke, and heart and kidney disease in males and females from West Dundee were not significantly different (p > 0.05) from the prevalence rates for these respective diseases of males and females

TABLE 4

Systolic and Diastolic Blood Pressure Among White Persons 18-75+ Years of Age, Who Do Not Have Water Softeners, Are Not Taking High Blood Pressure Medication and Have Lived Greater than 10 Years in West Dundee or McHenry, Illinois, 1976-77.

Blood Pressure Age (Years)	West Dundee						McHenry					
	Male			Female			Male			Female		
	No. Cases	Mean	SD[†]	No. Cases	Mean	SD[†]	No. Cases	Mean	SD[†]	No. Cases	Mean	SD[†]
Systolic												
18-24	12	122.7	12.1	8	105.6	14.2	16	122.1	12.1	16	106.2	11.2
25-34	8	127.8	18.6	7	109.3	14.1	6	122.8	9.3	13	106.6	12.8
35-44	16	124.5	16.9	23	111.6	14.2	11	123.9	12.5	16	114.9	20.5
45-54	14	137.2	17.0	25	120.2	17.6	14	126.0	14.0	20	117.9	17.4
55-64	17	143.4	28.4	19	126.4	19.4	10	138.3	20.1	12	132.7	17.0
65-74	6	139.0	15.7	14	129.9	12.9	7	145.4	26.5	9	131.3	19.6
75+	12	152.2	19.0	20	150.9	25.4	7	138.0	21.9	7	151.1	16.2
Total Pop.*	85	134.6	21.6	116	121.8	22.6	71	129.9	17.8	93	122.9	20.7
Diastolic												
18-24	12	74.2	8.2	8	72.0	11.7	16	72.6	11.4	16	71.9	7.0
25-34	8	82.9	12.5	7	76.9	4.2	6	74.3	10.2	13	75.6	13.9
35-44	16			23	78.8	12.5	11	86.8	10.8	16	82.8	13.3
45-54	14	86.5	8.1	25	82.3	9.9	14	83.9	14.8	20	83.9	16.7
55-64	17	87.0	15.1	19	80.7	10.1	10	87.7	15.8	12	92.4	13.4
65-74	6	81.3	9.3	14	82.8	9.2	7	86.7	8.5	9	81.7	7.7
75+	12	79.2	11.1	20	90.5	16.3	7	79.7	11.1	7	89.8	15.9
Total Pop.*	85	82.1	12.0	116	80.8	12.3	71	81.9	13.4	93	83.3	14.4

* Total sex specific means are age-adjusted to the total sample size for each sex.
† SD = Standard Deviation.

living in McHenry (Table 5-8). Although the rates for stroke for males in age groups 65 and older were higher in West Dundee than a similar population group in McHenry (Table 6), there also was no significant difference (p > 0.05) in actual numbers of this disease between these West Dundee and McHenry males.

TABLE 5

Prevalence Rates of Definite Hypertension for Persons 18-75+ Years of Age Who Live in West Dundee or McHenry, Illinois, 1976-77.

Definite Hypertension[†] and Age (Years)	West Dundee				McHenry			
	Male		Female		Male		Female	
	Pop. Size	Rate/100 Pop.	Pop. Size	Rate/100 Pop.	Pop. Size	Rate/100 Pop.	Pop. Size	Rate/100 Pop.
18-24	77	5.2	114	0.0	54	3.7	53	0.0
25-34	122	7.4	147	2.7	77	5.2	111	1.8
35-44	92	12.0	133	6.0	74	13.5	88	11.4
45-54	89	15.7	91	17.6	75	18.7	90	13.3
55-64	69	14.5	75	20.0	77	23.4	136	27.9
65-74	29	31.0	60	21.7	128	28.9	137	29.2
75+	28	21.4	49	44.9	47	38.3	56	32.1
Total Pop.*	506	14.8	669	13.7	532	17.0	671	15.3

† Systolic blood pressure of at least 160 mmHg or diastolic blood pressure of at least 95 mmHg.
* Total population rates are age-sex adjusted to the total sample size.

TABLE 6

Prevalence Rates of White Persons 18-75+ Years of Age, Who Have Had a Stroke Diagnosed by a Physician and Live in West Dundee or McHenry, Illinois, 1976-77.

| Stroke and Age (Years) | West Dundee | | | | McHenry | | | |
| | Male | | Female | | Male | | Female | |
	Pop. Size	Rate/100 Pop.	Pop. Size	Rate/100 Pop.	Pop. Size	Rate/100 Pop.	Pop. Size	Rate/100 Pop.
18–24	77	0.0	114	0.0	54	1.9	53	0.0
25–34	122	0.0	147	0.0	77	0.0	111	0.0
35–44	92	0.0	133	1.5	74	0.0	88	0.0
45–54	89	0.0	91	1.1	75	1.3	90	1.1
55–64	69	2.9	75	2.7	77	6.5	136	3.7
65–74	29	13.8	60	8.5	128	5.5	137	8.0
75+	28	17.9	49	4.1	47	6.4	56	8.9
Total Pop.*	506	3.8	669	2.4	532	2.7	671	2.6

* Total population rates are age–sex adjusted to the total sample size.

CONCLUSIONS

1. Although some cardiovascular mortality rates were significantly higher (p $\leq$ 0.05) in the elevated barium communities, any inferences drawn about these findings must be treated with extreme caution because of potentially confounding variables.

2. Adult blood pressures do not seem to be adversely affected when drinking water containing in excess of 7 mg/l barium is ingested.

3. No significant differences (p $>$ 0.05) were found for adult males and females in either West Dundee or McHenry with respect to the prevalence of hypertension, stroke, and heart and kidney disease.

4. The drinking water standard for barium of 1. mg/l should be reexamined for other possible health effects in adults as well as for health effects in children.

TABLE 7

Prevalence Rates of White Persons 18-75+ Years of Age, Who Have Had Heart Disease Diagnosed by a Physician and Live in West Dundee or McHenry, Illinois, 1976-77.

| Heart Disease and Age (Years) | West Dundee | | | | McHenry | | | |
| | Male | | Female | | Male | | Female | |
	Pop. Size	Rate/100 Pop.	Pop. Size	Rate/100 Pop.	Pop. Size	Rate/100 Pop.	Pop. Size	Rate/100 Pop.
18–24	77	0.0	114	0.0	54	0.0	53	0.0
25–34	122	0.0	147	0.0	77	0.0	111	0.0
35–44	92	3.3	133	1.5	74	0.0	88	2.3
45–54	89	3.4	91	4.4	75	6.7	90	4.4
55–64	69	4.3	75	4.0	77	13.0	136	9.6
65–74	29	13.8	60	5.0	128	15.6	137	8.0
75+	28	21.4	49	8.2	47	14.9	56	16.1
Total Pop.*	506	5.3	669	2.8	532	6.3	671	4.9

* Total population rates are age–sex adjusted to the total sample size.

TABLE 8

Prevalence Rates of White Persons 18-75+ Years of Age, Who Have Had Kidney Disease Diagnosed by a Physician and Live in West Dundee or McHenry, Illinois, 1976-77.

| Kidney Disease and Age (Years) | West Dundee | | | | McHenry | | | |
| | Male | | Female | | Male | | Female | |
	Pop. Size	Rate/100 Pop.	Pop. Size	Rate/100 Pop.	Pop. Size	Rate/100 Pop.	Pop. Size	Rate/100 Pop.
18-24	77	5.2	114	21.1	54	1.9	53	9.4
24-34	122	7.4	147	21.8	77	9.1	111	16.2
35-44	92	4.3	133	9.0	74	6.8	88	13.6
45-54	89	13.5	91	16.5	75	10.7	90	20.0
55-64	69	7.2	75	10.7	77	10.4	136	8.8
65-74	29	6.9	60	10.0	128	10.9	137	18.2
75+	28	3.7	49	14.3	47	14.9	56	12.5
Total Pop.*	506	7.3	669	14.9	532	8.9	671	14.3

* Total population rates are age-sex adjusted to the total sample size.

ACKNOWLEDGEMENTS

This work has been funded in part by the United States Environmental Protection Agency under grant R803918 to the University of Illinois at Chicago. It has been subject to the Agency's review and it has been approved for publication as an EPA document. Mention of trade names of commercial products does not constitute endorsement or recommendation for use. Permission to use Illinois mortality tapes was given by the State of Illinois Department of Public Health. The University of Illinois Survey Research Laboratory at Chicago assisted with questionnaire development. Computer services used in this research were provided by the University of Illinois at Chicago.

This paper summarizes the following three publications:

1. BRENNIMAN, G.R., KOJOLA, W.H., LEVY, P.S., CARNOW, B.W., NAMEKATA, T. and BRECK, E.C. (1979). *Health Effects of Human Exposure to Barium in Drinking Water,* EPA-600/1-79-003. U.S. Environmental Protection Agency, Cincinnati, Ohio.
2. BRENNIMAN, G.R., NAMEKATA, T., KOJOLA, W.H., CARNOW, B.W. and LEVY, P.S. (1979). Cardiovascular Disease Death Rates in Communities with Elevated Levels of Barium in Drinking Water. *Environ. Res.* **20**:318-324.
3. BRENNIMAN, G.R., KOJOLA, W.H., LEVY, P.S., CARNOW, B.W. and NAMEKATA, T. (1981). High Barium Levels in Public Drinking Water and Its Association with Elevated Blood Pressure. *Arch. Environ. Hlth.* **36**(1):28-32.

REFERENCES

AMERICAN CONFERENCE OF GOVERNMENTAL INDUSTRIAL HYGIEN-ISTS. (1971). Documentation of the Threshold Limit Values. 3rd ed., Cincinnati, Ohio.

BARCLAY, G.W. (1958). Techniques of Population Anaylsis. John Wiley and Sons, New York.

BRENNIMAN, G.R., KOJOLA, W.H., LEVY, P.S., CARNOW, B.W., NAME-KATA, T. and BRECK, E.C. (1979). Health Effects of Human Exposure to Barium in Drinking Water. EPA-600/1-79-003, U.S. Environmental Protection Agency, Cincinnnati.

DIENGOTT, D., ROZA, O., LEVY, N. and MUAMMAR, S. (1964). Hypokalemia in Barium Poisoning. Lancet 2:343–344.

FLEISS, J. (1973). Statistical Methods for Rates and Proportions. John Wiley and Sons, New York.

GILKESON, R., SPECHT, S., CARTWRIGHT, K. and GRIFFIN, R. (1978). Geologic Studies to Identify the Source for High Level of Radium and Barium in Illinois Groundwater Supplies. Illinois State Geological Survey, Urbana, Illinois.

GOODMAN, L.S. and GILMAN, A. (1970). The Pharmacological Basis of Therapeutics. The MacMillan Co., New York.

ILLINOIS INSTITUTE FOR ENVIRONMENTAL QUALTIY. (1974). Advisory Report on Health Effects of Barium in Water, HEQ Document No. EHRC-12, Chicago, Illinois.

KOJOLA, W.H., BRENNIMAN, G.R. and CARNOW, B.W. (1979). A Review of Environmental Characteristics and Health Effects of Barium in Public Water Supplies. Rev. Environ. Hlth. 3(1):79–95.

LARSEN, R.P. (1979) Statement of Robert P. Larsen, Ph.D. Hearing Before the Subcommittee on Health and the Environment, Serial No. 98–81, pp. 105–117. Prepared for the U.S. House of Representatives, Committee on Interstate and Foreign Commerce.

MANTEL, N. and HAENSZEL, W. (1959). Statistical Aspects of the Analysis of Data From Retrospective Studies of Disease. J. Nat. Cancer Inst. 23:719–748.

ROZA, O. and BERMAN, L.B. (1971). The Pathophysiology of Barium: Hypokalemic and Cardiovascular Effects. J. Pharmacol. Exp. Ther. 177:433–439.

SMITH, P.K., WINKLER, A.W. and HOFF, H.E. (1940). Cardiovascular Changes Following the Intravenous Administration of Barium Chloride. J. Pharmacol. Exp. Ther. 68:113–122.

SNEDECOR, G.W. and COCHRAN, W.G. (1967). Statistical Methods. The Iowa State University Press, Ames, Iowa.

SOLLMAN, T.A. (1957). A Manual of Pharmacology. W.B. Saunders Co., Philadelphia.

STOCKINGER, H.E. and WOODWARD, R.L. (1958). Toxicologic Methods for Establishing Drinking Water Standards. J. Am. Water Works Assn. 50:515–529.

U.S. BUREAU OF THE CENSUS. (1973). Census of Population, 1970, Vol. 1, Washington, D.C.

U.S. DEPARTMENT HEALTH EDUCATION AND WELFARE. (1968). International Classification of Diseases, Adapted, 8th Revision, Pub. No. 1693. Public Health Service, Washington, D.C.

U.S. ENVIRONMENTAL PROTECTION AGENCY. (1977). National Interim Primary Drinking Water Regulations, EPA—570/9-76-003, Washington, D.C.

U.S. ENVIRONMENTAL PROTECTION AGENCY. (1976). Quality Criteria for Water. EPA-440/9-76-023, Washington, D.C.

DISCUSSION II

Moderator: Are there any questions regarding this session?

Ohanian: Yes, I have a couple of questions. The first one is addressed to Dr. Kopp. Steve, in Dahl hypertension-sensitive and resistant rats, intra-arterial administration of cadmium produced diphasic responses. Specifically, an initial depressor response followed by a pressor response. We speculated that the pressor response was associated with an assumed cardiovascular reflex mechanism. Don't you think that you are observing a similar phenomenon in your rats?

Kopp: All of the graphs presented depict effects during the period subsequent to stabilization of the pressor or depressor responses to administered cadmium. Generally speaking, I have always attributed the general fall in blood pressure to a direct effect of cadmium on the heart. Under these circumstances, cadmium tends to cause a marked depression of myocardial contractile function.

Ohanian: Agreed.

Kopp: And what we may be looking at with respect to the change in blood pressure—the actual pressor response—may be an effect mediated sympathetically. Perhaps preferential alpha and beta receptor blockade may prove useful in further characterizing the mechanistic basis for this purpose.

Ohanian: The next question is addressed to Drs. McCauley and Douglas. Weanling Dahl rats are more susceptible to hypertension induced by various environmental insults than older or adult rats. Furthermore, the onset of hypertension is significantly delayed in adult rats. If you go back to your slide showing various blood pressures, you will notice a slight elevation of blood pressure in rats exposed to 3 ppm barium for 16 weeks. Unfortunately, you ended the study at this crucial point. Also, the fluctuations in blood pressures could be atrributed to sudden changes in temperature, humidity, etc. I suggest very strongly that you repeat this study with weanling Dahl rats since these rats are valuable tools for the investigation of metal-induced hypertension and its complications.

Douglas: Ed, you are absolutely right about the age at which we started. We did not start with weaning. We did not carry them beyond sixteen weeks. And, as you well know, there are a number of things that can raise the blood pressure in these Dahl rats. With regard to barium and hypertension I want to cast a negative vote as far as cause-and-effect. We have taken all our blood pressures on the unanesthetized animal. We have given barium to normal animals. We have given barium to uninephrectomized animals, barium plus salt to uninephrectomized animals, barium plus salt to normal animals. We have given barium to the Dahl rats but didn't carry them beyond sixteen weeks. We have given it to them at weening. We have even given barium to spontaneously hypertensive rats. It had no effect on the development of blood pressure. We gave barium in doses of 1, 10, 100, and 1000 ppm to more than 400 different rats on different occasions. We have never seen an effect on blood pressure. We only carried our animals 16 weeks. Dr. Perry carried his 16 months I believe. I think that is the reason for the difference in our results.

Ohanian: I am afraid that the hypertensinogenic effect of 3 ppm barium is noticeable at week 16. You should have prolonged the study instead of terminating it at this juncture.

Douglas: I don't know. I guess we should really bring the slide back out. Are you basing this entirely on one week?

Ohanian: Ben, I am just convinced that we are looking at the onset of barium-induced hypertension in this model of rats at week 16.

McCauley: Did you have a comment?

Douglas: I can't comment on what happens beyond this sixteen week period because that is as far as we carried the study. We'll be right within that period. With regard to Dr. Perry's data, he carried his on for I believe sixteen months. Is that correct? But still, at that time he had systolic blood pressures that had increased 10 to 15 millimeters mercury, which is not that drastic an increase in blood pressure for sixteen months in an animal that has a life expectancy of thirty-six months.

Perry: We do indeed observe a cadmium-induced increase in systolic pressure of 15 to 20 mm Hg. Three comments seem in order: 1) This increase is small when compared to other types of induced hypertension; however, it is an average of all exposed animals so that some animals have much larger increases. Thus, as is true for human populations, some animals are hypertensive and some are not; moreover, a few are markedly hypertensive. 2) Extrapolating from the Framingham data, an increase of 15 mm Hg for man would be highly significant; it would well double the risk of cardiovascular morbidity. Finally, the tenor of the discussion yesterday clearly indicated that an average increase of 2 or 3 mm Hg would be considered significant for a population of human beings.

Douglas: Do you use the tail cuff method?

Perry:	Yes, we use the tail cuff method. We routinely measure three pressures in 5 to 10 minutes under very closely standardized conditions and used the median of these three readings. Does the vertical line on your slides indicate standard deviation or standard error?
Douglas:	Standard errors.
Perry:	If it is standard error, there certainly appear to be statistically significant week-to-week differences in pressures. It is difficult to know how to interpret statistically significant but apparently random variations, with one group being high one week and another being high the next week. Our rats do not show significant up and down differences from week-to-week, rather we see consistent changes that persist over long periods and seem to present an interpretable pattern.
Douglas:	I don't either.
Perry:	But we plain don't see that. What we have is a hypertensive response it is persistent, it stays.
Douglas:	There is something else that bothered me on your high barium dose slide. It seems that those animals started off with a higher blood pressure. Was that the very first pressure or a control pressure?
Perry:	We did not measure pressures on barium-fed animals before they began barium exposures. Thus, they were already on barium at the time the first pressure was measured; we have not routinely obtained pressures on 40 gm weanling rats. At the time of the first pressure measurement, i.e., 1 month after weaning, the 100 ppm barium groups had a significantly higher pressure than the control rats and a significant difference was present at all 6 times the pressure was measured—and this was true despite the fact that there were 3 different populations of rats. Otherwise there were no significant differences between groups. Our animals are randomly assigned to exposure groups at weaning, and we have relied on consistent differences between metal-exposed and control animals to indicate a metal-induced effect. It seems unreasonable to expect that small differences between two groups of weanling animals will have significance for adult animals after 16 months of exposure.
Douglas:	Ordinarily, in our colony of animals that are sixteen months old, we do not really consider systolic pressure of 125 and 130 to be hypertension.
Perry:	Our control systolic pressure averaged 100 mm Hg for anesthetized and 110 mm Hg for unanesthetized animals with a standard

deviation of 10 mm Hg for both. Let me reemphasize that these values are consistent, i.e., are found in population after population of similar animals that are similarly treated. Any statistically significant increase above that value is considered an elevation in blood pressure.

Douglas: In your normal colony of rats, does their systolic pressure increase with age? Ours do.

Perry: There is little if any increase in pressure up to 18 months. From 18 to 24 months there is a considerable increase in pressure with 24 month animals having average unanesthetized systolic pressures of almost 131. (Perry, H.M., et al., Am. J. of Physiol. **232**:H114, 1977).

Revis: I would just like to ask Mitch Perry a question. I noticed that in your...the MDR for the rat. Do you know what it is, Mitch?

Perry: We have never attempted to determine the minimal daily requirement of calcium for the strain of rats we use or for our rye-based diet. Our diet contains 0.38% calcium. This amount of calcium under our routine laboratory conditions is enough to permit normal growth in our Long-Evans rats, i.e., there are no differences in growth when we feed our diet of Purina Lab Chow fed to litter mate rats. (Perry, H.M., et al., J. of Nut. **112**:1983, 1982).

Revis: On your slide was 0.38 percent. The reason why I ask that question is because we find in the rat that Purina Chow makes a chow which has 0.7 percent calcium. If you reduce the calcium down to 0.4 percent the animal is in a negative calcium balance. The reason why I ask Mitch this question is because I think he showed in his slide that the calcium concentration was 0.38 percent. So one would anticipate an increase, for example, in barium absorption. I don't know what the calcium level was in the diets that we used by Dr. Douglas and Dr. McCauley, but this may explain why there were differences between these two studies.

Perry: Although I did not know the minimum daily requirement, Bernhart referred to high and low calcium diets as containing 1.4 and 0.1% calcium respectively. (F.W. Bernhart, et al., J. of Nut. **98**:443, 1969).

Revis: Mitch, one of the things that again have been discussed here today with regard to cadmium is the importance of calcium. And the fact that some investigators have not been able to reproduce the results of Shorter and Rousell. I think one of these factors may be the level of calcium that is in the diet. I think this is an error that deserves further consideration. I do point out again that your level of 0.3 percent would suggest a deficiency state.

Perry: Certainly the amount of calcium in the diet is important, but our diets is not deficient, i.e., it permits normal growth in our rats from weaning to adulthood! (See above.) It is possible, however, that a diet deficient in calcium might affect cadmium-induced "hypertension." Another possible cause of failure to induce hypertension by cadmium-feeding is that the control animals get the small amount of cadmium needed to induce an increase in pressure; hence there is no difference between cadmium-fed and control pressures. In this context anything we do to contaminate, i.e., add cadmium to, the environment, food or water, causes an increase in the control systolic pressure. Thus, our low contamination environment and our low-cadmium diet are very important in getting the sort of effects that we get. It seems very likely to us that some of the failures to reproduce cadmium-induced hypertension have occurred in situations where there has been a possibility of cadmium contamination of the control groups. For instance, experiments that we have done with Purina Rat Chow, which contains about 10 times as much cadmium as our low-cadmium diet, indicate that the control value slowly rises to something very close to the pressures associated with cadmium-induced "hypertension." We interpret this to mean that the control animals fed Purina Rat Chow are getting enough cadmium to induce hypertension. Seven of 13 reports, i.e., more than half of the reported attempts to induce hypertension with cadmium, have been successful and the 3 of 6 failures occurred when cadmium was present in food. (Perry, H.M., et al., J. of Nut. **112**:1983, 1982).

Ohanian: I would like to stress that 1 ppm cadmium produced hypertension in Dahl whereas 10 ppm cadmium failed to do so. It could very well be that the mechanism of barium-induced hypertension is similar to that of cadmium. High levels of barium might turn off the release of the hypertensinogenic factor in Dahl rats.

Perry: On that slide, it seems to me that if those vertical lines are standard errors then we really must have unexplained statistically significant variations in pressure.

Douglas: We see this type of variation of pressure in animals which receive cadmium or, as in this situation, with the Dahl rats which are getting sodium. Perhaps we started it not as we should have— when they were weaned—but at a later age. There is fluctuation. There is variation. We see variation in blood pressure of normal rats. Not to this extreme. Not to this degree. I can see the point that perhaps the Dahl rats would have gotten hypertensive had we carried them on. But I stand by my other statement that barium has no effect on SHR in normal rats or in uninephrectomized-plus-sodium when treated for 16 weeks. And we have done it on over 400 animals.

Perry: It may have no effect under your conditions. If it had effects of the magnitude that we consistently see, however, it would be very difficult to observe in the presence of the considerable week-to-week fluction you see. The small consistent differences that we report would be very difficult to recognize in the face of large random variations. I will emphasize again that our animals had normal growth curves, and that there was no evidence of a deficiency of calcium. The addition of barium does not alter growth rates, and the rats look normal. Moreover, we do have tissue calcium levels which are the same with or without barium-feeding.

Douglas: 0.38% Ca is a little below the minimum daily requirement. We give a level of 0.47% Ca which we consider the marginal minimum daily requirement. If we want to go above the MDR, we will give 0.72% Ca.

Perry: What I am saying is that when we give higher amounts we can demonstrate no difference. I would think, as far as I can tell, this is not below the minimum daily requirement, being as rats grow normally, have no abnormalities that I can pick up, and have normal tissue concentrations.

Revis: When you say tissue, are you talking about bone?

Perry: No, I am not talking about bone, I am talking about paren-chymatous tissue.

Revis: You wouldn't expect tissue calcium concentrations to change in hypocalcemic states?

Perry: No, I would agree. But you would expect that there would be some diminution in growth rate. And you just don't find it.

Ohanian: I don't think that you will get hypocalcemia with 0.38 percent.

Perry: That is the amount. I am not saying that you get hypocalcemia. What I am saying is that you get a negative calcium balance. OK? That is observed.

McCauley: You will have the parathyroid hormone being secreted. That is about 60% of MDR for calcium. Hydroxy vitamin D levels will also be elevated.

Perry: Actually, we don't. We have looked at that.

Kopp: If I could comment. You are looking at calcium only in isolation. I think that you have to take into consideration factors such as magnesium in the diet, potassium in the diet, sodium in the diet, because they all interact. I think just looking at calcium alone might not be the answer. Calcium bioavailability would seem to be an equally important factor that should be considered rather than concentrating solely on dietary calcium levels. I think one of the points that Dr. Perry has been making is that Ben's rats' pressures vary. In order to have a variable response you might require an animal with normal calcium on the diet. The point turned around is, in a hypocalcemic state, are these animals capable of varying the way that we've seen blood pressure vary in human exposure in Dr. Calabrese's study yesterday?

Revis: I think Dr. Perry has done studies—and maybe, Mitch, you can comment on them better than I can—but he has done them with child diets as well as with other diets. And he still doesn't see the kind of variations that you are seeing.

Perry: Well, I don't think it is a function of diet at all.

Douglas: These pressures you see are not for all of the animals we have done. Those are just for the Dahl rats. My goodness, no! we have done normal SHR and a host of other types. Incidentally, we got our information for our MDR on Ca out of the National Institute of Health Handbook of Requirements for Lab Animals.

Moderator: I think we ought to change the mode of question. We have a question from this other fellow.

Respondent: It is only a small change. I was just thinking of the effect of the sort of fiber, the level of fiber has on the absorption availability of divalent cation and what effect that has on blood pressure.

Perry: There is fiber in our diet. I don't know how much. However, even if I did, would you know what the fiber content for a rat diet should be?

Cotruvo: I have a general question. If we design a clinical study with barium, what would be the maximum level that we would want to give to human volunteers?

Perry: I think that the maximum dose of barium that one could use in a human study is the amount of barium which occurs in water to which human beings are noramlly exposed. In other words, if one went to a "high barium" location and obtained high barium water there, one could probably get the appropriate committee approvals to give it to human volunteers. To add any more barium would be very difficult to defend as being ethical.

Respondent: We have Dr. Brenniman's study looking at 10 ppm of barium. That is above the maximum of what you see. And they didn't really. It might be tough to see an effect in a clinical study only using 10 ppm.

Perry:	But I suspect, tough or not, you will find it impractical to use any higher levels. Otherwise, you might have to go with Dr. Masironi to New Guinea.
Moderator:	Do we have national information on the barium content of our diet?
McCauley:	Yes. Schroeder published something on that line. It is very low actually. I think half a milligram per kilogram per day is what to expect.... Marine species tend to concentrate barium.
Respondent:	The other question is what relationship do your blood pressure levels in the two groups have to Hanes data?
Brenniman:	Do you mean how do blood pressures in the two communities compare with national averages?
Respondent:	Right.
Brenniman:	They might—and I have to doublecheck this—they might be slightly higher. I don't know if it would be significantly higher. But I think they are a little bit higher than the national average. I could get that information for you.
Respondent:	I can tell that in Hanes, the 18 to 75 standardized pressure was 83.4-83 point something—83.4 for the diastolic pressure. I don't know the systolic.
Brenniman:	I don't know the Hanes systolic standard for pressure either. However, back to your questions about how much we could feed humans. I agree with Dr. Perry that you might find a human experimentation problem in going above what you find some population is being exposed to in their food and water.
Respondent:	If you are only getting 10 percent of your barium from the drinking water, other people will have barium from their food.
Respondent:	About 600 micrograms per day.
Perry:	You could then use high barium food plus high barium water up to the maximum exposure that some reasonable population might have.
Brenniman:	So it might be very controlled. Give them a low barium diet and increase the amount of barium in the water and/or the diet and compare the two groups.
Perry:	It is probably pertinent to comment that the availability of barium—or any other metal—may be very different in food and water, with that combined in food often being considered less available.
Moderator:	O.K. Are there any other questions? I would just like to briefly

summarize today's events. I think we have demonstrated an effect of soft water on cardiovascular disease development, which is independent of high sodium content of drinking water; perhaps we have been looking at the wrong parameter. There are obviously many complex factors involved here. We can't discount the effect of lowered calcium levels on any of the various parameters. I think there also might be a possibility that the water's hardness is altering the absorption of different dietary components or possibly altering the biliary excretion of heavy metals. There are other factors that would be involved; I think that other studies should be designed to try and differentiate some of these different effects. I would like to thank you all for coming today. Thank you for your comments and we'll see you tomorrow.

CHAPTER XXII

THE EFFECT OF COOKING WITH WATER HAVING ELEVATED SODIUM LEVELS UPON THE CONCENTRATION OF SODIUM AND POTASSIUM IN VEGETABLES

Carol A. Rowan* and Edward J. Calabrese†
*Office of Research and Standards
Massachusetts Department of
Environmental Quality Engineering,
Boston, Massachusetts

†Division of Public Health
University of Massachusetts,
Amherst, Massachusetts

ABSTRACT

This study compared the sodium and potassium levels in three naturally low sodium vegetables (cabbage, potato and squash) cooked in water with sodium typical of a range of existing water supplies (i.e., 0, 100, and 250 mg/L). In addition, sodium and potassium retention in vegetables as a result of adding salt (NaCl) during the cooking process was tested. The results indicated that sodium levels are markedly increased in a dose-dependent manner for each vegetable studied, while potassium levels were not consistently affected by the sodium concentration of the cooking water.

INTRODUCTION

The United States Environmental Protection Agency (EPA) has promulgated primary drinking water standards for a number of inorganic and organic substances posing a threat to human health. Their approach to the derivation of drinking water standards has been to consider, where possible, multimedia exposures to an element, that is, exposures from air, water, and food as analyzed in market basket surveys. However, in only a few instances (National Academy of Sciences, 1977; PHS, 1962) has the effect of cooking with increased levels of an element in water been taken into account in the derivation of the standard.

Experimentation on the effect of cooking with increased levels of an element in tap water has shown that this route of exposure is of importance as certain tested foods have the ability to substantially concentrate elements such as lead and fluorine (Moore et al., 1978; Martin, 1951). It has also been experimentally determined that during cooking in different water types (i.e., hard and soft waters) certain essential elements may be leached from the foods to different extents (Schlettwein–Gsell and Mommsen Straub, 1973).

Of importance is that the chemical composition of the water affects the chemical composition of the food and that increased ingestion of harmful elements from this type of exposure are not quantified for many substances. Since market basket surveys do not include the effect of cooking and uptake of elements from the water into the food, whether the drinking water standards have adequately assessed the total exposure of elements to the human population is questionable.

The primary objective of this study was to measure the sodium content of vegetables cooked with water containing increasing levels of sodium typical of existing water supplies and common cooking methods in order to determine if elevated levels of sodium in drinking water contribute in an insidious manner to the total daily gastrointestinal exposure in sodium. In addition, two common cooking techniques (i.e., fully- and half-covering the vegetables with the water) were also studied to determine factors influencing the uptake of sodium into the food. A preliminary report of these investigations was reported earlier (Rowan and Calabrese, 1981).

METHODS

Low sodium vegetables were chosen for the study based upon values reported in the U.S. Department of Agriculture Handbook (1975) Number 456, and the American Heart Association's low sodium diet requirements (1957). The vegetables tested were cabbage (*Brassica capitata,* L), butternut squash (*Curcubita maxima*) and potato (*Solanum tuberosum,* L), which were obtained fresh from the same garden. After discarding the outer layers of the cabbage, the heads were uniformly washed with minimal amounts of deionized-distilled water. The squash and potatoes were peeled and briefly rinsed to remove all surface particles. The cabbage was chopped to uniform one inch pieces, and the squash and potato were cubed to one inch pieces.

The cooking water was prepared for each sodium level by diluting the stock solution of sodium chloride (1000 mg Na/L) with deionized-distilled water. The concentrations tested were 0, 100, and 250 mg Na/L. A fourth sodium level was prepared by making a 100 mg Na/L solution to which one teaspoon (tsp.) of salt was added. Since one tsp. of salt has from 2000 to 2200 mg of sodium (Cooper and Heap, 1967), 2 grams of sodium ion (in the form of NaCl) were added, after being weighed on a Mettler Balance.

The common cooking methods were tested, fully covering and half-covering the vegetables. The volume of water required to fully cover the cabbage was 2000 mls; the squash, 500 mls; and the potato, 500 mls. Half-covering utilized half of these volumes. For the half-covered method at the fourth concentration, only 1/2 tsp. of salt, or 1 gram of sodium, was added to the water so that the concentrations of the fully and half-covered methods would be comparable.

The cooking was conducted in duplicate in 4 quart aluminum pans with tightly fitting covers. Five hundred grams of each vegetable were added to the boiling water, and the cooking time for each vegetable began when the water reached 100° C (cabbage, 12 minutes; squash, 25 minutes; and potato, 22 minutes). When the vegetables were cooked half-covered, it was necessary to turn them so that each piece was exposed to the water.

After cooking, the vegetables were weighed and dried to a constant weight in an oven at 29° C. They were then ground with an agate mortar and pestle and were stored in polyethylene bottles in a dessicator.

Raw portions of the vegetables were also dried, ground and stored for analysis.

Inorganic measurements were conducted by dry ashing the vegetables followed by analysis of sodium and potassium using a modified combination of the methods recommended by Perkin Elmer (1971) and the Association of Official Analytical Chemists (1980). Testing was conducted to determine the accuracy of the dry ashing technique for sodium and potassium analysis, and the results are published elsewhere (Rowan et al., 1982).

The samples to be analyzed were redried at 29° C for 24 hours before analysis. One gram of the finely ground sample was weighed on the Mettler Balance and was placed into a nickel crucible partially covered with a nickel lid. The crucibles were placed in the muffle furnace at 300° C for partial oxidation, and then the temperature was raised to 500° C for progressive oxidation. The samples were ashed for three hours. The white ash was dissolved in 5.0 mls of 20% HCL and was warmed on a hotplate for 30 minutes. Deionized-distilled water was used to rinse the lid, and the sample was filtered and diluted to a volume suitable for the working range of the instrument. Six replicates were conducted per sample.

Analysis of sodium and potassium was conducted by atomic absorption spectrophotometry with a flame apparatus. A Perkin–Elmer Model 103 with a Model 56 recorder was used. The method of standard additions was conducted on each vegetable matrix to determine if elements present in the samples were causing interferences in the absorption signal.

Statistical analysis involved an analysis of variance, and significance was calculated by conducting Tukey's Method of Multiple Comparisons.

TABLE 1.

Concentration of Sodium and Potassium in Uncooked Vegetables
(mg/500 g product)

Vegetable	Sodium	Potassium
Cabbage	9.6	1106.0
Squash	1.3	1365.4
Potato	4.6	1741.9

TABLE 2.
Sodium Content of Vegetables Cooked Fully-Covered
with Water Containing Increasing Sodium Concentration
(mg/500 g product)

Vegetable	Uncooked Value	Initial Sodium Concentration (mg/L)			
		0	100	250	ADDED*
Cabbage	9.6	4.0	61.4**	144.9**	499.1**
Squash	1.3	1.1	26.3**	65.1**	1048.8**
Potato	4.6	4.2	30.8**	73.8**	1040.1**

*ADDED: Concentration of cooking water; cabbage, 1100 mg Na/L; squash and potato, 4100 mg Na/L.

**Results are statistically significant from the uncooked and from the zero sodium cooking level, $p < 0.01$.

RESULTS

General Findings

The concentrations of sodium and potassium for each uncooked vegetable are shown in Table 1. As shown and as normal for most vegetables, the potassium content is much higher than the sodium values (U.S. Dept. of Agriculture, 1975).

The results indicate that for each vegetable and for each cooking technique (i.e., full- or half-covered), there was a progressively greater sodium retention at each greater level of sodium in the cooking water (Tables 2 and 3). With the sole exception of the difference between the 0 and 100 mg Na/L half-covered potato group which was statistically significant at the 0.05 level, all differences were statistically significant at the 0.01 level. It is interesting to note that the increases in sodium content as a result of cooking were proportional to the amount of sodium in the water of either cooking technique. (Table 4).

The potassium content of each vegetable was found to be consistently reduced after cooking, and all the results were statistically significant at the 0.01 level for each cooking technique. More potassium was leached from the vegetable during the full method (Tables 5 and 6). While a consistent pattern of potassium content for each vegetable cooked at the different sodium levels did not occur, it was observed that with the exception of four results (i.e., fully covered potato cooked at 100, 250 and 1100 mg Na/L and cabbage, half-covered at 250 mg Na/L) the potassium level in the vegetables was higher when sodium was in the water.

Intermethod Effects

Cabbage. When no sodium was in the water, the cooking methods did not produce results which were statistically different ($p > 0.01$); the cooking method had no significantly different effect upon leaching of sodium from the plant (Tables 2 and 3). At every other level of sodium in the cooking water, there were

TABLE 3.
Sodium Content of Vegetables Half-Covered
with Water Containing Increasing Sodium Concentration
(mg/500 g product)

Vegetable	Uncooked Value	Initial Sodium Concentration (mg/L)			
		0	100	250	ADDED*
Cabbage	9.6	5.3	45.3**	117.8**	455.8**
Squash	1.3	1.1	17.5**	39.9**	759.3**
Potato	4.6	4.2	23.4***	53.2**	764.8**

*ADDED: Concentration of cooking water; cabbage, 1100 mg Na/L; squash and potato, 4100 mg Na/L.

**Results are statistically significant from the uncooked and from the zero sodium cooking level, $p < 0.01$.

***Results are statistically significant from the uncooked and from the zero sodium cooking level, $p < 0.05$.

significantly different results between the methods ($p < 0.01$) with larger sodium values consistently occurring in the fully-covered method.

Comparison of the changes in potassium concentration in cabbage between the methods revealed that for each sodium level there were significantly different results between the methods ($p < 0.01$). When the cabbage was only half-covered, less potassium was leached out at each sodium level (Tables 5 and 6).

Squash. When no sodium was in the cooking water and when 100 ppm sodium was tested, the levels of sodium taken into the squash were not significantly different between the methods ($p > 0.01$). However, when the sodium levels increased to 250 and 4100 ppm, the uptake into squash when cooked fully covered was significantly larger ($p < 0.01$) than the half-covered method (Tables 2 and 3).

The potassium values for squash were significantly different ($p < 0.01$) at each level of sodium in the cooking water between each method, with the

TABLE 4.
Percentage of Sodium in the Vegetable after
Cooking Compared to the Amount Added
(mg found/mg added)

Vegetable	Cooking Method	Initial Sodium Concentration (mg/L)		
		100 mg/L	250 mg/L	ADDED*
Cabbage	Full	25.9	27.0	22.0
	Half	35.7	43.3	40.6
Squash	Full	50.1	51.1	51.1
	Half	65.2	61.8	74.0
Potato	Full	52.4	55.4	50.5
	Half	75.0	77.7	74.2

*ADDED: Concentration of cooking water; cabbage, 1100 mg Na/L; squash and potato, 4100 mg Na/L.

potassium content consistently being higher for the half-covered method (Tables 5 and 6).

Potato. Results for the sodium content of potato after cooking at 0, 100, and 250 ppm did not produce significantly different results between the cooking methods. At 4100 ppm, there was a significantly greater level of sodium retention for the fully covered method ($p < 0.01$) (Tables 2 and 3).

The potassium content produced by each cooking method was significantly greater at each sodium level ($p < 0.01$) for the half-covered method than the fully covered method (Tables 5 and 6).

The effect of the cooking method can also be considered by comparing sodium retention to the amount of sodium added to the cooking water. As shown in Table 4, while the increases in sodium content as a result of cooking were proportional to the amount added, the half-covered method produced higher percentage uptakes. Thus, it appears that effect of the half-covered method is to take up sodium more efficiently in the vegetable on a percentage basis; however, uptake based on absolute values are higher for the fully covered method, probably because there is more sodium in the water.

DISCUSSION

The results indicated that three low sodium vegetables take up statistically significantly ($p < 0.01$) greater amounts of sodium when cooked in a typical manner in water with elevated but not uncommon levels of sodium. A survey of 2100 water supplies providing drinking water to approximately 50% of the U.S. population showed that approximately 9 percent had sodium ion concentrations ranging from 100–250 mg/L (National Academy of Sciences, 1977). In practical terms, a person consuming a one cup serving of each of these three vegetables per day which had been cooked in water with 100 or 250 mg Na/L would have ingested an additoinal 37 and 96 mg of sodium, respectively. While this is a modest additional sodium exposure for the average American who

TABLE 5.
Potassium Content of Vegetables Cooked Fully-Covered
with Water Containing Increasing Sodium Concentration
(mg/500 g product)

| Vegetable | Uncooked Value | Initial Sodium Concentration (mg/L) | | | |
		0	100	250	ADDED*
Cabbage	1106.6	325.6	432.5**	452.9**	430.2**
Squash	1365.4	907.0	949.3**	911.0	1016.3**
Potato	1741.9	1344.1	1248.6	1312.6	1154.7**

*ADDED: Concentration of cooking water; cabbage, 1100 mg Na/L; squash and potato, 4100 mg Na/L.

**Results are statistically significant from the uncooked and from the zero sodium cooking level, $p < 0.01$.

All results are statistically significant from uncooked, $p < 0.01$.

TABLE 6.

Potassium Content of Vegetables Cooked Half-Covered
with Water Containing Increasing Sodium Concentration
(mg/500 g product)

Vegetable	Uncooked Value	Initial Sodium Concentration (mg/L)			ADDED*
		0	100	250	
Cabbage	1106.6	500.5	524.1	499.9	504.4
Squash	1365.4	962.8	1033.2**	1072.1**	1148.4**
Potato	1741.9	1517.2	1594.9	1522.4	1549.6

*ADDED: Concentration of cooking water; cabbage, 1100 mg Na/L; squash and potato, 4100 mg Na/L.

**Results are statistically significant from the uncooked and from the zero sodium cooking level, p < 0.01.

All results are statistically significant from uncooked, p < 0.01.

consumes 5–10 g Na/day (National Academy of Sciences, 1977), it does clearly indicate that drinking water may contribute more sodium than originally thought and that this may be of some concern to those following a sodium restricted diet.

In addition, with regard to the impact of the cooking practice of adding salt to the cooking water, the consumption of a serving of these three vegetables a day would increase the intake up to a gram of sodium.

The two cooking methods tested, one fully covering versus only half-covering the vegetables, demonstrated the increased sodium uptake to be generally greater on an absolute scale when more water was used. Therefore, the method by which individuals cook their food can also cause statistically significant different exposures, even when the same sodium concentrations are found in the water. Furthermore, when using a fully covered cooking method, higher dietary exposure to sodium along with a larger decrease in potassium occurs than when less water is used.

Of considerable interest is that the percentage of uptakes of sodium are directly proportional to the levels of sodium added to the water for each vegetable and cooking method. The observation makes it possible to estimate the contribution of sodium to the tested vegetables at other levels of sodium in water. The following equation permits this computation for each vegetable and cooking method:

Predicted Na Content of Vegetable = (Average % Increase) (mg Na in Cooking Water) + (Uncooked Na Value in Vegetable)

CONCLUSIONS

It was determined that the sodium content of selected low sodium vegetables can markedly increase as the concentration of sodium in the cooking water increases. These findings are of potential significance for persons following low sodium diets with respect to drinking water supplies and cooking practices.

Finally, the results reported here and the recent report of Moore et al. (1978) suggest that the uptake of heavy metals into foods cooked in drinking water with variable levels of these metals be evaluated and included as a component of the EPA methodology for determining multimedia exposure levels.

ACKNOWLEDGEMENTS

This paper was previously published in the *Journal of Environmental Science and Health* A16(2):125–137, 1981.

REFERENCES

AMERICAN HEART ASSOCIATION. (1957). Your 500 Milligram Diet. New York.

ASSOCIATION OF OFFICIAL ANALYTICAL CHEMISTS. (1980). Methods of Analysis. 13th Edition.

COOPER, G.R. and HEAP, B. (1967). Sodium in drinking water. II. Importance, problems, and potential applications of sodium-ion-restricted therapy. J. Am. Diet. Assoc. 50:37–41.

MARTIN, D.J. (1951). The Evanston dental caries study. VIII. Fluorine content of vegetables cooked in fluorine containing waters. J. Dental Res. 30(5):676–81.

MOORE, M.R., HUGHES, M.A. and GOLDBERG, D.J. (1978). Lead absorption in man from dietary sources. Int. Arch. Occ. Env. Hl. 44:81–90.

NATIONAL ACADEMY OF SCIENCES. (1977). Drinking Water and Health, Vol. 1. National Academy of Sciences, Washington, DC, pp. 401–403.

PERKIN ELMER. (1971). Analytical Methods for Atomic Absorption Spectrophotometry.

PHS. (1962). Silver. Public Health Service Drinking Water Standards. U.S. HEW PHS.

ROWAN, C.A. and CALABRESE, E.J. (1981). The effect of cooking with water having elevated sodium levels upon the concentration of sodium and potassium in vegetables. J. Environ. Sci. Hlth. A16(2):125–137.

ROWAN, C.A., ZAJICEK, O.T. and CALABRESE, E.J. (1982). Dry ashing vegetables for the determination of sodium and potassium by atomic absorption spectrophotometry. Analytical Chemistry 54:149–151.

SCHLETTWEIN–GSELL, D. and MOMMSEN–STRAUB, S. (1973). Spurent–elements in Lebensmitteiln. Hans Huber, Bern.

U.S. DEPARTMENT OF AGRICULTURE. (1975). Nutritive Value of American Foods in Common Units. Agricultural Handbook No. 456, Washington, DC.

CHAPTER XXIII

UPTAKE OF LEAD FROM WATER

Michael R. Moore
University Department of Medicine,
Gardiner Institute, Western Infirmary,
Glasgow, Scotland

ABSTRACT

The role that lead in domestic water supplies can play in the economy of environmental lead exposure in man is beyond dispute. A part of the equation linking the curvilinear relationship between blood lead and dietary lead is the accumulation of lead from water by foodstuffs during the cooking process. Foodstuffs normally cooked in an excess of water, such as pastas and vegetables, show a significant uptake of lead from the cooking solution whilst beverages which are prepared from vegetable material which is discarded, show a significant fall in lead concentration. The adsorption of lead by these materials is not linear. The rate of uptake is both time and concentration dependent.

These differences in the amount of lead made available for dietary absorption can in part explain the cube root relationship which exists between blood and water lead concentrations and which extends to water lead concentrations as low as 10 μg/l. This relationship contains no term linked to dietary lead intake but analysis of duplicate diet shows that the form of the relationship between blood lead and dietary lead intake is identical. This information now makes it possible to calculate accurately the acceptable limits that might be set on water lead concentrations using as a yardstick acceptable blood lead concentrations rather than arbitrary assignment of upper acceptable levels on non-biological measures.

INTRODUCTION

Scotland has the dubious dual distinction of the highest death rate from ischaemic heart disease (European Society for Cardiology, 1978), and the worst record for exposure to environmental lead in Europe (Commission of the European Communities, 1977; DOE, 1981; DOE, 1983). Whether these two are causally related remains a matter of conjecture, but it is clear that there exists a very necessary requirement to investigate potential vectors of environmental lead exposure in these circumstances.

The role that water may play in the economy of the exposure, absorption and retention of lead by humans is not often appreciated. There is little doubt that food plays the major role in exposure of humans to lead in normal domestic environments, but it has become clear as part of recent experimentation that solid diet lead concentrations are only one part of the equation linking dietary lead intake and body lead concentrations. Perhaps the most significant extra source of exposure to lead is from lead in water supplies.

The problem of such exposure is one that has been of particular importance in the environmental context of the West of Scotland. Water supplies there tend to be soft, acidic and consequently plumbosolvent (Moore, 1983). These supplies contain little or no lead at source but, when transmitted through domestic plumbing systems containing lead, can dissolve quite remarkable quantities of this metal. It might be thought that few plumbing systems in modern dwellings contain lead but it must not be forgotten that lead solder is still used extensively to join copper piping, and that the use of lead pipe was only discontinued in Scotland in 1969.

Although emphasis on health effects of lead has concentrated lately on the emotive subjects of infant development, behaviour and intelligence, many other organ systems other than the nervous system are affected by lead (Mahaffey, 1985). In particular, pronounced effects upon the cardiovascular system have been found. Animal studies show an unequivocal change in cardiac ultrastructure and function (Moore et al., 1975). These functional changes include depressed phosphorylation of cardiac contractile proteins and lowered intracardiac conduction (Kopp et al., 1980a, b), and increased vulnerability to catecholamine induced arrhythmias (Williams et al., 1977). In humans similar changes have yet to be reported, but there is more than a little evidence that hypertension and lead are causally related (Beevers et al., 1976, 1980; Pirkle et al., 1985), and that equivalent effects on the heart may be found for humans as have been found already for animals (Williams et al., 1983).

It is for these health related reasons that knowledge of the processes of exposure to lead in water must be better understood (Royal Commission on Environmental Pollution, 1983). This present paper investigates domestic water usage and relates this to the uptake of lead both by humans and by the food that they eat.

METHODS

In these experiments, three different types of vegetables were chosen to represent the three different forms used as food: carrots, of root vegetables; cabbage, leaf and shoot vegetables; and peas, of seed vegetables. All were grown on the same plot of land which had a soil lead content of 9.5 μmol/Kg dry weight. All of the vegetables were prepared before use by washing in distilled water and discarding any bruised or damaged parts. Carrots were then peeled, washed and cut into 5 mm thick slices and trimmed to discs of diameter 20 mm. Cabbage leaves were stacked after washing in distilled water and a 25 mm punch used to prepare discs of leaves. These discs were sorted to remove any through which thick veins passed in order to ensure homogeneity. Peas were podded and sorted into a group of uniform size, small and large ones being discarded. In addition to the vegetables, a pasta, macaroni, was also studied as being representative of a foodstuff which was always cooked in water.

In the studies of the relationship between blood lead and water lead, blood samples were collected into 5 ml polystyrene EDTA tubes from the kettle in the kitchen. All the tubes used came from batches which had been checked for lead contamination before use.

Cooking Procedures. All glassware used in these studies was washed overnight in 50% v/v nitric acid solution. Lead chloride solution (10 μmol/L) was made up in double distilled water "spiked" with carrier free ^{203}Pb chloride (prepared by The MRC Cyclotron Unit, Hammersmith Hospital, London) to give a concentration of 6.2 MBg ^{203}Pb/L. This stock solution was used to prepare solutions of lead of concentrations of 0.1, 1, 2 and 5 μmol/L. 500 ml of these solutions was put into a 1 litre beaker, covered with a watchglass, and brought to the boil on an electric hotplate—another beaker, prepared similarly; was left cold. When the solution was boiling freely, 50 g aliquots of vegetable or pasta were put into both boiling and cold water. Individual samples of the material were removed at time points up to 30 minutes from both hot and cold beakers, blotted dry, rinsed three times in double distilled wter, dried again and placed in a weighed polystyrene tube for gamma counting (Wallac) and reweighed.

The samples were counted at the ^{203}Pb principal peak of 280 KeV and at subsidiary peaks of 400 and 680 KeV. Following counting, the materials in the tubes were freeze-dried to constant weight, and lead measurement made on the dried material. Results were expressed as the percentage uptake of radioactive lead per gram of wet weight sample and as the ratio of counts per gram of dry weight samples to the counts per ml. of cooking solution.

Blood and Water Lead Comparisons. These studies were carried out over the period 1979 to 1983. The blood analyses were made on a group of young women who had children between the ages of 10 weeks and five years. In total 568 of these mothers were examined for both blood lead concentration and concentration of lead in the water in their kitchen kettle. Previous studies had established that this represented the most satisfactory means of obtaining a representative domestic water sample (Moore et al., 1979; DOE, 1982).

Lead measurement was carried out by electrothermal atomic absorption spectrophotometry with deuterium background correction (Perkin Elmer 306 with HGA 72) at the lead absorption line of 217 nm using argon gas to purge the system, or latterly at 283 nm (Perkin Elmer 703 with HGA 500).

Blood samples were diluted 1 to 5 with 0.1% Triton $\times$ 100 solution prepared with double distilled water. Twenty microlitres of this solution were pipetted into the furnace, dried at 100° C for 20 seconds, ashed at 450° C for a further 20 seconds and atomised at a peak temperature of 2040° C for 4 seconds to complete the analysis. Checks on accuracy and precision were made by participation in Quality Control Schemes and by a 10% exchange of samples with other accredited laboratories. Lead concentrations in the food samples were measured similarly after digestion in concentrated nitric/perchloric acid, heating to dryness in a muffle furnace at 300° C and redissolution in 1 mol/litre hydrochloric acid. Water lead analysis was carried out on water which had been acidified with 1M hydrochloric acid.

RESULTS

Food Lead Uptake. For each of the foodstuffs examined here there was a significant uptake of lead during the cooking process which was greatly in excess of any lead uptake by the same foodstuff from cold water. The longer the food was cooked the greater was this uptake as is shown here for peas (Table 1).

Very similar relationships were found for each of the other vegetables and macaroni. When cabbage was cooked in water containing different concentrations of sodium chloride, there was some diminution in uptake in parallel with the rise in salt concentration (Table 2). This would be consistent with competition for binding sites by sodium and lead ions. Such binding is not unlimited. As the lead concentration in solution rose, so the relative rise in food lead concentration fell. This could be explained by saturation of binding sites at higher lead concentrations with a consequent non-linearity in the relationship between lead uptake and solution lead concentration.

In practical terms it was of interest to examine the changes in cooked food lead concentration when that food had been prepared in solutions of varying lead concentration in a manner similar to that which would be used in the home.

Table 3 shows that in all cases, as the solution lead concentration rises the relative lead uptake increases. The concentrations of lead in the water here were chosen to approximate standards in use in the world today for lead in water (50 $\mu g/L$ - 0.24 μM and 100 $\mu g/L$ - 0.48 μM). Even at the lower of these limits the uptake of lead virtually doubled the foodstuff lead concentration although salt was present to modify uptake. The relative uptake varies but was obviously greatest for macaroni and least for peas.

Blood/Water Lead Relationship. For the 568 mothers examined in this part of the study a least squares linear regression was found to provide a satisfactory description of the relationships between blood and water lead. Its failing was that it indicated an excessively high intercept on the blood lead axis where water lead concentrations were zero. The best fit relationship was found to be non-linear with blood lead varying as the cube root of the kettle water lead concentration.

$$\text{Blood lead } (\mu M) = 0.27 - 0.76 \, [\text{water lead } (\mu M)]^{1/3}$$

with coefficient of correlation r = 0.77 (Fig. 1).

DISCUSSION

The significant but non-linear uptake of lead into foodstuffs during cooking which by extrapolation must reflect some part of the non-linear association

TABLE 1
Uptake of Lead into Peas During Cooking in Aqueous Lead Solutions

INITIAL DOUBLE DISTILLED WATER SOLUTION LEAD CONCENTRATION (µM)

Time (m)	0.1		1.0		2.0		3.0		5.0	
	%	ratio	%	ratio	%	ratio	%	ratio	%	ratio
1	157	6	106	4	128	5	110	4	68	3
2	233	10	196	8	226	9	134	5	81	3
5	616	26	465	20	378	16	818	24	204	9
10	1007	46	429	20	513	23	509	23	370	17
20	1486	74	1971	53	742	37	529	29	355	18
30	1967	109	1031	55	956	53	776	39	471	27
30 min cold	187	6	125	4	182	6	106	3	98	3

% uptake/g wet weight and ratio of counts/g dry weight to counts per ml solution

between water lead exposure and blood lead concentrations might have been expected. Previous studies have shown that there is some accumulation of lead by foodstuffs from water supplies (Heusghem et al., 1973; Berlin et al., 1977; Moore et al., 1979; Smart et al., 1981), although the exact relationship was not defined. The hardness of the water supply was of little consequence in the uptake (Smart et al., 1981) but sodium chloride concentrations appeared to diminish the relative uptake of the lead from solution as did length of cooking time.

TABLE 2
Uptake of Lead from Solution (1 µM) into Cabbage at Varying Saline Concentrations

SALINE CONCENTRATION (mM)

Time (m)	0		76		150		300	
	%	Ratio	%	Ratio	%	Ratio	%	Ratio
1	109	11	95	9	48	8	21	2
2	918	102	411	42	136	15	70	8
10	3052	521	801	126	354	47	192	34
20	5744	887	1133	299	523	165	355	52
30	7862	1512	4215	621	1980	409	988	221

% - % uptake/g wet weight cabbage
Ratio - Ratio of counts/g dry weight cabbage to counts/ml solution

Water regained by the foodstuffs during cooking will obviously enhance uptake but only relative to the quantity of solution retained. The available surface area will also be of importance (Moore et al., 1979). The amount of lead retained by the foodstuffs was therefore greatest in the one sold dessicated, macaroni, and least in the vegetable with the smallest surface area, peas. The question of lead concentrations of beverages has been considered (Moore et al., 1979; Smart et al., 1981). Effectively, any beverage which is prepared from vegetable matter (coffee or tea) loses lead from solution to the vegetable matter but gains lead by leaching from the vegetable matter. The balance in these circumstances is entirely contingent upon the solution and vegetable matter lead concentrations, but usually results in a net loss of lead from the solution.

In previous studies, a significant regression was observed between kettle water lead and domestic tap water lead concentrations (Wigle and Charlebois, 1978; Moore et al., 1979). The use, therefore, of kettle water lead as an index of

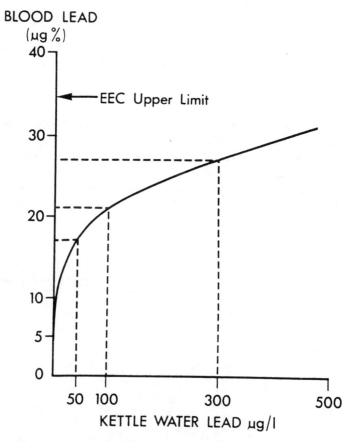

FIGURE 1. The cube root relationship between blood and water lead. This graph intercepts the blood lead axis at 0.27 μM (5.5 μg%). The upper limit for blood lead according to the directive of the Commission of the European Communities is 1.69 μM (35 μg%).

TABLE 3

Lead Concentrations in Vegetables and Pasta Cooked in Two Concentrations of Lead/Saline Solution (0.25 and 0.5 μM)

(Mean + SD umol/KG dry weight)

		SALINE	SALINE + LEAD (0.25 μM)	SALINE + LEAD (0.5 μM)
CABBAGE	0	44.1+2.8	-	-
	30m	43.6+5.4	94.0+10.3	148+12.1
CARROT	0	20.0+3.6	-	-
	30m	21.1+4.9	42.6+ 7.7	78.7+ 6.9
MACARONI	0	17.0+1.8	-	-
	30m	16.9+2.2	67.0+ 3.1	111.0+ 3.9
PEA	0	21.2+2.3	-	-
	30m	21.0+4.0	37.5+ 6.3	52.4+ 7.4

(SALINE CONCENTRATION 75mM)

TABLE 4

A Balance Sheet of Lead Exposure in an Urban Resident in Great Britain

SUBJECT: Adult female, 60 Kg - aged 30 years

EXPOSURE:
Blood Lead	0.75 μmol/L
Water Lead	0.25 μmol/L
Air Lead	5 nmol/m^3
Food Lead	705 nmol/day

This includes
i.   63 nmol from the air
ii. 246 nmol from water (25 nmol from cooking)
iii. 80 - 160 nmol from canned food

ABSORPTION

% Absorption from gut: 15%
Uptake from GI tract - 106 nmol/d
% Absorption from lungs: 40%
Uptake from lungs 29 nmol/d

TOTAL UPTAKE - 135 nmol/d

EXCRETION

Urinary excretion - 77 nmol/day
Endogenous faecal excretion - 18 nmol/day

TOTAL EXCRETION - 95 nmol/d

BALANCE 40 nmol/d (as bone storage)

water lead exposure is apposite, principally because such water is truly representative of the water used in a household for alimentary purposes, either in beverage preparation or in the cooking of foodstuffs. It furthermore provides an integrated measure of exposure, taking in potentially harmful household practices, such as use of hot water supplies in the preparation of food. This practice is harmful since the plumbosolvency of hot water is much greater than that of cold water. It must not be forgotten that domestic water lead problems have their provenance in the home and leaden plumbing therein and not in the water supplies at source, which are usually free of lead. Of the many factors implicated in water lead uptake, only two relate to the water at source. These are acidity and hardness. Important domestic factors include temperature of the water and the presence of lead in various forms in the plumbing, such as soldered joints in copper piping (Wong and Berrang, 1976; Moore, 1977; Lyon and Lenihan, 1977); hot galvanised steel piping (Burgmann et al., 1978) and lead-filled plastic piping (WHO, 1973), other than the use of lead itself for piping and storage tanks.

The cube root relationship between lead and blood and lead in water has now been shown to have parallels in uptake from diet (DOE, 1982; Sherlock et al., 1982), and uptake from the air (Chamberlain, 1983a). This implies that there are central physiological mechanisms which help to limit lead absorption at higher concentrations. Into the equation linking dietary exposure and absorption, terms must be built to cover the relative bioavailability of lead in foodstuffs and the fact that lead accumulation by foodstuffs is not linear. There is, for example, some evidence that an increase in vegetable lead concentrations does not make any difference to mean blood lead concentrations in a population eating these vegetables (Wijn et al., 1983). In this particular instance the increase in lead was due to fallout from the air in a high traffic density region. Since Chamberlain (1983b) calculated that 63 nmoles per day would come from this source in the average adult diet, it is perhaps surprising that no change was found.

In these circumstances it is interesting to make some calculations of the importance of water lead exposure in the economy of lead balance in an average human. The example chosen here is an adult female aged 30 who lives in Glasgow, smokes 20 cigarettes a day and drinks modest quantities of wine. Assumptions made about this subject are that she has a blood volume of 5 litres and breathes $15m^3$ of air daily. Mean air lead is taken as 5 nmoles/m^3 for 24 hour exposure and absorption through the lungs as 40%. This gives an intake from the air of 21.5% in agreement with experimental studies (Fachetti et al., 1982). The alimentary absorption of lead is calculated as 106 nmole per day based on an intake of 705 nmol (DHSS, 1980), and 15% absorption from the gut (Moore et al., 1979). Canned food accounts for 6.3% of intake and supplies between 20 and 40% of dietary intake (MAFF, 1983). Water lead concentration is taken as 0.25 μM. The contribution from the cooking addition of lead from water is calculated as being 10% where water lead is around 0.25 μmol/L (15% where water lead is around 0.5 nmol/L). Thus, for this water lead exposure, assuming a mean daily intake of around 900 ml, the total contribution from water supplies to alimentary lead exposure is 246 nmol/d, 35% of exposure (Smart et al., 1981). This is a very substantial addition, at a very modest level of water lead exposure. The final figures making up the balance sheet are the blood lead concentration calculated from the cube root equation which is 0.75 μmol/L: IRCP reference man has a body lead burden of 580 μmol (IRCP, 1975): urinary excretion of lead is 77 nmol daily (Harrison and Laxen, 1981) and that the endogenous faecal excretion is 18 nmol daily based on a faecal to urinary excretion ratio of 0.23 (Moore, 1985). The net gain in this calculation, 40 nmol/day, accords well with the observation that 43 nmol/day of lead is stored in bone (Barry, 1975).

These figures serve to illustrate the importance of even modest levels of water lead exposure. At higher levels of exposure proportionately more lead would come from water. Where water lead concentrations exceed 0.48 μM, more than half of the total lead intake comes from water (Sherlock et al., 1982). In circumstances where there is no contribution of water lead, the resultant blood lead of 0.27 μmol/L shows the remarkable improvement achievable. In practice, such improvements have been demonstrated by treatment of water with lime to increase pH and to reduce plumbosolvency (Moore et al., 1982; Sherlock et al., 1984; Richards and Moore, 1984). There are obviously very small margins of safety in these figures. Indeed, for a water lead concentration as high as 0.48 μM, blood lead concentrations would not conform with the requirements of the European Community reference levels (Commission of the EEC, 1977) and even at 0.24 μM, there is only a limited margin of safety (Lacey et al., 1985). This work points to the requirements for a more satisfactory means of preparing concordant reference levels in which the establishment of exposure standards is based upon measurable biological change and which allow a satisfactory margin of safety with respect to these changes. Equations, such as that between blood and water lead, would allow this to be done.

REFERENCES

BARRY, P.S.I. (1975). A comparison of concentrations of lead in human tissues. British Journal of Industrial Medicine **32**:119–139.
BEEVERS, D.G., ERSKINE, E., ROBERTSON, M., BEATTIE, A.D., CAMPBELL, B.C., GOLDBERG, A., MOORE, M.R. and HAWTHORN, V.M. (1976). Blood lead and hypertension. Lancet **ii**:1–3.
BEEVERS, D.G., CRUICKSHANK, J.K., YEOMAN, W.B., CARTER, G.F., GOLDBERG, A. and MOORE, M.R. (1980). Blood lead and cadmium in human hypertension. Journal of Environmental Pathology and Toxicology 3:251–260.
BERLIN, A., AMAVIS, R. and LANGEVIN, M. (1977). Research on lead in drinking water in Europe (in relation to the possible uptake of lead by man). WHO Working group on the health hazards from drinking water, London.
BURGMANN, G., FRIEHE, W. and SCHWENK, W. (1978). Chemical corrosion and hygienic aspects of the use of hot galvanised threaded pipes in domestic plumbing for drinking water. Corrosion Prevention—Control **25**:7–17.
CHAMBERLAIN, A.C. (1983). Effect of airborne lead on blood lead. Atmospheric Environment **17**:677–692.
CHAMBERLAIN, A.C. (1983). Fallout of lead and uptake by crops. Atmospheric Environment **17**:693–706.

COMMISSION OF THE EUROPEAN COMMUNITIES. (1977). Council directive of 29 March 1977 on biological screening of the population for lead (77/321/EEC). Official Journal of the European Communities 20:10–17.

DEPARTMENT OF THE ENVIRONMENT. (1981). European Community Screening programme for Lead—U.K. results for 1979–80. Pollution Report No. 10, HMSO, London.

DEPARTMENT OF THE ENVIRONMENT. (1982). The Glasgow Duplicate Diet Study (1979/80). A joint survey for the Department of the Environment and the Ministry of Agriculture, Fisheries and Food. Pollution Report No. 11, HMSO, London.

DEPARTMENT OF THE ENVIRONMENT. (1983). European Community Screening programme for lead. United Kingdom results for 1981. Pollution Report No. 18, HMSO, London.

DEPARTMENT OF HEALTH AND SOCIAL SECURITY. (1980). Lead and Health, HMSO, London.

EUROPEAN SOCIETY OF CARDIOLOGY. (1978). Preventing coronary heart disease. R.C. De Boecx, eds., Van Gorcum, Amsterdam.

FACCHETTI, S., GEISS, F., GAGLIONE, P., COLOMBO, A., GARIBALDI, G., SPALLANZANI, G. and GILLI, G. (1982). Isotopic lead experiment. Commision of the European Communities, Luxembourg.

HARRISON, R.M. and LAXEN, D.P.H. (1981). Lead Pollution: Causes and Control, Chapman and Hall, London.

HEUSGHEM, C. and DE GRAEVE, J. (1973). Etude de l'importance de la contamination alimentaire par le plomb dans l'Est de la Belgique. Cebedeau 354:204–206.

INTERNATIONAL COMMISSION ON RADIOLOGICAL PROTECTION. (1975). Task group report on a reference mean. IRCP Publication 23, Pergammon Press, Oxford.

KOPP, S.J., PERRY, H.M., GLONEK, T., ERLANGER, M., PERRY, E.F., BARANY, M. and D'ARGROSA, L.S. (1980). Cardiac physiologic metabolic changes after chronic low level heavy metal feeding. Journal of Physiology 239:H22–H30.

KOPP, S.J. and BARANY, M. (1980). Influence of isoproterenol and calcium on cadmium or lead induced negative inotropy related to cardiac myofibrillar protein phosphorylation in perfused rat heart. Toxicology and Applied Pharmacology 55:8–17.

KOPP, S.J., BARANY, M., ERLANGER, M., and PERRY, H.M. (1980). The influence of chronic low level cadmium and/or lead feeding on myocardial contractility related to phosphorylation of cardiac myofibrillar proteins. Toxicology and Applied Pharmacology 54:48–56.

LACEY, R.F., MOORE, M.R. and RICHARDS, W.N. (1985). Lead in water, infant diet and blood. The Glasgow Duplicate Diet Study. The Science of the Total Environment 41:235–257.

LYON, T.D.B. and LENIHAN, J.M.A. (1977). Corrosion in solder jointed copper tubes resulting in lead contamination of drinking water. British Corrosion Journal 12:40–45.

MAHAFFEY, K.R. (ed.) (1985). Dietary and Environmental Lead: Human Health-Effects. Elsevier, Amsterdam. In press.

MINISTRY OF AGRICULTURE, FISHERIES AND FOOD. (1983). Food Additives and Contaminants Committee. Report on the review of metals in canned foods. FAC/REP/38. HMSO, London.

MOORE, M.R. (1983). Lead exposure and water plumbosolvency. In: *Lead versus Health*. M. Rutter and R.R. Jones, eds., Wiley, Chichester, 79–106.

MOORE, M.R. (1985). Levels of lead in humans, in *The Lead Debate*, R. Lansdown and W.N. Yule, eds., Croom Helm, Beckenham, in press.

MOORE, M.R., GOLDBERG, A., FYFE, W.M. and RICHARDS, W.N. (1981). Maternal lead levels after alteration to water supply. Lancet i:203–204.

MOORE, M.R., HUGHES, M.A. and GOLDBERG, D.J. (1979). Lead absorption in man from dietary sources. International Archives of Occupational Environmental Health 44:81–90.

MOORE, M.R., MEREDITH, P.A., GOLDBERG, A., CARR, K.E., TONER, P.G. and LAWRIE, T.D.V. (1975). Cardiac effects of lead in drinking water of rats. Clinical Science and Molecular Medicine 49:337–341.

MOORE, M.R., MEREDITH, P.A., CAMPBELL, B.C., GOLDBERG, A. and POCOCK, S.J. (1977). Contribution of lead in drinking water to blood-lead. Lancet ii:661–662.

MOORE, M.R., MEREDITH, P.A., WATSON, W.S. and CAMPBELL, B.C. (1979). The gastrointestinal absorption of 203 lead chloride in man. In: 13th Conference of Trace Substances in Environmental Health, D.D. Hemphill, ed., University of Missouri, Columbia, 368–373.

PIRKLE, J.L., SCHWARTZ, J., LANDIS, J.R. and HARLAN, W.R. (1985). The relationship between lead levels and blood pressure and its cardiovascular risk implications. Am J. Epidermiol 121:246–258.

RICHARDS, W.N. and MOORE, M.R. (1984). Plumbosolvency in Scotland—The problem, remedial action taken and health benefits observed. American Water Works Association Journal 76:60–67.

ROYAL COMMISSION ON ENVIRONMENTAL POLLUTION. (1983). 9th Report—Lead in the Environment, HMSO, London.

RUTTER, M. and RUSSELL–JONES, R. (1983). Sources and effects of low level lead exposure. In: *Lead versus Health*. Wiley, Chichester.

SHERLOCK, J., SMART, G., FORBES, G.I., MOORE, M.R., PATTERSON, W.J., RICHARDS, W.N. and WILSON, T.S. (1982). Assessment of lead intakes and dose-response for a population in Ayr exposed to a plumbosolvent water supply. Human Toxicology 1:115:112.

SHERLOCK, J.C., ASHBY, D., DELVES, H.T., FORBES, G.I., MOORE, M.R., PATTERSON, W.T., POCOCK, S.J., QUINN, M.J., RICHARDS, W.N. and WILSON, T.S. (1984). Reduction in exposure to lead from drinking water and its effect on blood lead concentration. Human Toxicology 3:383–392.

SMART, G., WARRINGTON, M. and EVANS, W.H. (1981). The contribution of lead in water to dietary lead intakes. Journal of Science, Food and Agriculture 32:129–133.

WIGLE, D.T. and CHARLEBOIS, E.J. (1978). Electric kettles as a source of human lead exposure. Archives of Environmental Health 33:72–78.

WIJN, M., DUIVES, P., HEVER, R. and BRUNEKREEF, B. (1983). Lead uptake from vegetables grown along highways. International Archives of Occupational and Environmental Health 52:263–270.

WILLIAMS, B.J., GRIFFITHS, W.H., ALBRECHT, C.M., PIRCH, J.H. and HEJTMANCIK, M.R. (1977). Effects of chronic lead treatment on some cardiovascular responses to norepinephrine in the rat. Toxicology and Applied Pharmacology 40:407–413.

269

WILLIAMS, B.J., MILTON, R., HEJTMANCIK, J.R. and ABREU, M. (1983). Cardiac effects of lead. Federation Proceedings **42**:2989-2993.

WONG, C.S. and BERRANG, P. (1976). Contamination of tap water by lead pipe and solder. Bulletin of Environmental Contamination and Toxicology **15**:530-534.

WORLD HEALTH ORGANISATION (1973). The hazards to health and ecological effects of arsenic, cadmium, lead, manganese and mercury. Report on a Working Group, Stockholm, p. 35.

CHAPTER XXIV

AVAILABILITY OF CADMIUM FROM FOODS AND WATER

Donald R. Buhler
Department of Agricultural Chemistry and
Environmental Health Sciences Center
Oregon State University
Corvallis, Oregon

ABSTRACT

In initial studies, male and female weanling Wistar rats were either fed semisynthetic diets or supplied with drinking water that contained 1, 3, 10, 50, 100, or 1000 ng Cd/g as [109]$CdCl_2$. Tissue Cd levels were then determined at 1, 2, 4, 8, and 12 weeks. No differences in the growth rate or organ weight were observed in the concentration range and time periods examined. There were no significant differences in total Cd body burden, percent of dose absorbed, or tissue Cd concentrations whether equivalent concentrations of Cd were supplied in the diet or in the drinking water. Kidneys accumulated the highest concentrations of Cd and the liver contained somewhat lower levels. The latter organ, however, accounted for 35–55% of the total body Cd burden (excluding the gastrointestinal tract) while kidney contained only 35–45% of the burden. Higher concentrations of Cd accumulated in the various tissues and organs with increasing dietary Cd levels and longer exposure times. However, the percent Cd absorbed by the rats on a given Cd regimen decreased with exposure time. Female rats accumulated Cd at a faster rate and absorbed a higher concentration of metal than did the male animals.

Rats were also fed diets containing freeze-dried carrot, lettuce, soybean, spinach, tomato, or wheat that had been grown on [109]$CdCl_2$ treated soil and supplied with [109]$CdCl_2$ spiked diets that contained nonradioactive plant material. At two weeks tissue Cd levels were quite comparable for a given plant source whether or not [109]Cd had been preincorporated in the plant or added to the diet. The relative distribution of Cd among the tissues was similar to that seen previously. However, tissue retention of Cd was significantly influenced by plant species, being lowest in animals fed wheat diets and highest in those receiving the tomato diets. Dietary differences in total oxalate and phytate contents may account for most of the observed differences in Cd accumulation by the rats. The amount and quality of protein in the diet and the presence of other cations in the drinking water were also found to influence the uptake of dietary Cd.

INTRODUCTION

Cadmium (Cd) is a highly toxic metal that is readily accumulated by both plants and animals (Friberg et al., 1974; Fulkerson and Goeller, 1973; Webb, 1979; Yost, 1984). Concern over the consequences of Cd pollution developed after chronic exposure to the metal of a rural population in Japan resulted in severe bone disease (Bernard and Lauwerys, 1984; Hallenbeck, 1984). Schroeder (1965) and others (Bernard and Lauwerys, 1984; Friberg et al., 1974; Hallenbeck, 1984; Webb, 1979) have all focused attention on the possible linkage between human hypertension and increased retention of Cd by the kidneys.

Although some Cd is absorbed via inhalation, especially in smokers (Ellis et al., 1979), food is considered to be the major source of non-occupational human exposure with intake via water generally thought to be of lesser importance (Fox, 1983; Friberg et al., 1974; Schroeder et al., 1967b; Sherlock, 1984; Webb, 1979; Yost, 1984). Estimates of dietary Cd intake in the U.S. range from 25 to 60 μg/day (Mahaffey et al., 1975). Water, however, may play a considerably greater role when Cd concentrations are naturally high (Horvath, 1972; Kopp, 1969) or are increased by the water distribution system (NAS, 1982; Schroeder et al., 1967b; Sharrett et al., 1982; Strain et al., 1975).

Recent evidence has shown that edible and other plants can accumulate substantial amounts of Cd from Cd-contaminated soils and that metal accumulation depends upon the plant species, soil composition, and Cd content of the soil (Bingham, 1979; Bingham et al., 1975; Davis, 1984; Haghiri, 1973; John, 1973, 1976; Root et al., 1975; Street et al., 1977; Turner, 1973). Various vegetable species, such as corn, tomato, radish, and Swiss chard, also efficiently concentrate Cd^{2+} from nutrient solutions (John, 1976; Page et al., 1972; Root et al., 1975; Turner, 1973).

Municipal sewage sludge is the end product resulting from the digestion and treatment of municipal wastes that may contain human excreta, residues from food processing, and a host of inorganic and organic constituents generated by industry. Disposal of the large quantities of municipal sewage sludge generated annually has led to its increasing utilization as a soil conditioner and a source of nutrients for agricultural crops. Sewage sludges typically contain high concentrations of various heavy metals (Davis, 1984; Furr et al., 1976a, 1976b, 1976c; Heffron et al., 1980), including Cd, with concentrations of this metal ranging between 1 to 1,500 μg Cd/g dry sludge (Page, 1974). When edible crops are then grown on soils treated with municipal sewage sludge, they accumulate high concentrations of Cd and other metals (Bingham et al., 1975; Browne et al., 1984; Davis, 1984; Furr et al., 1976a, 1976b; Jones et al., 1973; Linnman et al., 1973). Under these circumstances, leafy plants, such as lettuce, spinach, and turnip greens (tops), can accumulate Cd concentrations as high as 175 to 354

$\mu g/g$ tissue. Fruit and seed tissues of plants, including turnip tuber, tomato, wheat, radish, and squash, concentrate lesser amounts of the metal, ranging from 10 to 15 μg Cd/g tissue. The Cd content of soybeans and carrots reaches 30 $\mu g/g$ tissue while maximum levels in corn and rice are below 5 μg Cd/g tissue.

Because of the accumulation of high concentrations of toxic metals, especially Cd, in edible plants, the disposal of sewage or sewage-sludge on croplands or the use of high Cd fertilizers may pose a serious hazard to human or animal health. Similarly, crops grown on soils naturally high in Cd could also concentrate dangerously high levels of the metal. To assess the degree of hazard from such accumulations, however, it is first necessary to determine the biological availability of Cd^{2+} to animals fed diets containing various grains and vegetables. This project was, therefore, initiated to compare the absorption of ^{109}Cd by rats fed diets containing six species of edible plants grown on ^{109}Cd-treated soils, fed similar diets spiked with ^{109}Cd^{2+}, or supplied with ^{109}Cd^{2+} in their drinking water.

METHODS

Greenhouse crops of spinach (*Spinacia oleracea* L.), lettuce (*Lactuca sativa* L.), carrot (*Daucus carota* L.), soybean (*Glycine max* Merr.), tomato (*Lycopersicon esculentum* Mill.), and wheat (*Triticum aestivum* L.) were grown to maturity in plastic pots containing soil to which various concentrations of Cd^{2+} labeled with ^{109}Cd had been added, calculated on the basis of a predictive model (Browne et al., 1984) to yield comparable metal concentrations in the plants. At harvest, the edible portion of spinach (leaves), lettuce (head), carrot (root), soybean (bean), tomato (fruit), and wheat (grain) actually contained 18.1, 16.9, 6.4, 3.2, 5.2, and 1.6 μg Cd/g dry weight, respectively. Control plants were grown on untreated soil under similar conditions. The plant material was homogenized, freeze-dried, and the resulting powders used to formulate semi-synthetic diets similar to those used previously (Buhler et al., 1981). The general composition of the experimental diets is shown in Table 1. Four different types of diets were prepared.

The Diet 1 group of six diets contained the basal diet plus 10% of the different intrinsically ^{109}Cd-labeled plant powders; Diet 2 group (six diets) contained basal diet plus 10% of the different nonradioactive plant materials of the same species and varieties as with the Diet 1 group, but with ^{109}CdCl$_2$ added during mixing; Diet 3 (one diet) contained 66% cerelose and no plant material plus ^{109}CdCl$_2$ added at mixing; and Diet 4 (one diet) was a nonradioactive diet containing 10% whole wheat powder (flour). The diets were adjusted to contain approximately 0.24 μg ^{109}Cd/g diet (dry weight) through the mixing with appropriate amounts of radioactive and nonradioactive plant powders of low and intermediate Cd contents. The wheat powder diets, however, contained an average of 0.43 μg Cd/g diet. Additional diets were prepared as described in the Results section.

Groups of individually caged male and female weanling Sprague–Dawley rats were fed one of the four types of diets as previously described (Buhler et al., 1981). In some cases, groups of rats were also fed the nonradioactive Diet 4 and

TABLE 1.
Diet Composition.*

Casein	22
Cerelose	56
Freeze dried plant powder	10
Corn oil	5
Salts	4
Water or $^{109}CdCl_2$ solution	1
Vitamins†	1
Zinc mix‡	1
	100

*From Buhler et al. (1981).

†The following were added as a powder to the mixed diet (in mg/100 g diet): Thymine hydrochloride (0.4); riboflavin (0.8); pyridoxine hydrochloride (0.5); d-calcium pantothenate (0.4); inositol (20); menadione (0.4); folic acid (0.4); niacin (4.0); choline dihydrogen citrate (424); biotin (0.03); and B_{12} (0.02).

‡Zinc was added as zinc acetate (5 μg/g diet).

provided with distilled water containing $^{109}Cd^{2+}$ as $^{109}CdCl_2$ at a concentration of 3–1000 μg/L with or without addition of 100 mg/L Ca^{2+} as $CaCl_2$ or 20 mg/L Mg^{2+} as $MgCl_2$. Rats were initially fed an appropriate nonradioactive diet for a period of 14 days to establish diet acceptance. Food and distilled water were provided *ad libitum* and food and water intake were measured to determine ^{109}Cd ingestion. Food and radioactive water were removed one day prior to sacrifice, and after killing by CO_2 asphyxiation, various tissues and organs were removed, weighed, and counted. In most cases, liver and kidneys were the only tissues sampled since our previous research (Buhler et al., 1981) had shown that greater than 80% of the total body burden (excluding the gastrointestinal tract) was located in these tissues (Table 2).

The ^{109}Cd content of the plant powders, diets, drinking water, and tissue samples was determined by counting suitable aliquots in a Packard Auto-gamma spectrometer with appropriate correction for background and radioactive decay. The ^{109}Cd concentration of the tissues was determined from the radioactivity and the known specific activity of ^{109}Cd added to the diet since previous studies (Buhler et al., 1981) had shown an excellent correlation between Cd levels in tissues determined by atomic absorption analyses and those determined by measurement of radioactivity. After wet digestion, diets were also subjected to atomic absorption spectrometry to measure the Ca, Cd, Cu, Fe, and Zn contents. Total phytates were determined by the methods of Harland and Oberleas (1977) using the procedure of Lowry and Tinsley (1974) to measure the released phosphorous. Total oxalate in the extracts from phytate analyses was determined by gas chromatography after derivatization of dried aliquots and n-propionic acid anhydride in the presence of BF_3 (Lowry and Tinsley, 1984).

All statistical comparisons were performed either by the Statistical Interacting Programming System (SIPS) using the OSU campus computer or through the Compare program for the NIH PROPHET system.

RESULTS

In preliminary studies, groups of 4 rats (2 males and 2 females) fed a diet containing 56% cerelose and 10% whole wheat powder (flour) and supplied with drinking water containing 100 μg/L ^{109}Cd^{2+} as ^{109}CdCl$_2$ were killed at 1, 2, 4, 8, and 12 weeks (Buhler et al., 1981). The highest concentration of ^{109}Cd was found in the gastrointestinal tract (Table 2). Since these values were quite variable, they were not used in the estimation of total Cd absorption or body burden. Of the remaining tissues and organs, kidneys showed the highest Cd concentration and liver the next highest. Total amounts of ^{109}Cd were approximately the same in liver and kidney, accounting for well over 90% of the total body burden.

When groups of rats were fed the 10% wheat flour diet and supplied with drinking water containing 3–1000 μg/L ^{109}Cd^{2+} as ^{109}CdCl$_2$ or fed 10% wheat flour diets containing 1–1000 ng/g ^{109}Cd added at mixing, Cd bioaccumulation increased with time and was proportional to the Cd concentration in food or water (Fig. 1). The absorption of Cd was similar whether the ^{109}Cd was supplied in the water or in the food (Fig. 2).

Analogous results were obtained when diets containing spinach powder were compared. After feeding groups of 5 male and 5 female rats Diet 3 (66% cerelose with added ^{109}CdCl$_2$), high concentrations of ^{109}Cd were accumulated in kidney and all other tissues (Fig. 3). Inclusion of 10% spinach powder in the ^{109}CdCl$_2$ spiked diet (extrinsically labeled) markedly reduced uptake of the metal. Tissue ^{109}Cd accumulation was further decreased when an intrinsically labeled spinach diet was fed.

Diets prepared from the six plant materials and containing either plant bound ^{109}Cd (Diets 1) or added ^{109}CdCl$_2$ (Diets 2) were fed to male and female rats for a period of 14 days. The concentrations of ^{109}Cd in liver and kidneys are reported in Table 3 with the diets arranged in the order of decreasing bioavailability. Concentrations of metal accumulated by the rats varied significantly with the diet. Highest ^{109}Cd levels appeared in rats fed the tomato, carrot, and lettuce diets while the lowest concentrations were found in the spinach and wheat fed animals. Availability of the metal to the rats was similar whether or not the ^{109}Cd was supplied preincorporated into the plant material or added extrinsically to the diet. As reported in many previous studies (Webb, 1979), female rats concentrated significantly higher levels of ^{109}Cd than did the males. However, total renal and hepatic Cd contents failed to show a marked sex-linked difference (Table 4). Nevertheless, female rats retained a higher percentage of the ^{109}Cd ingested than did the male animals (Table 5). Generally, the percent ^{109}Cd retention was similar for both intrinsically and extrinsically labeled diets except in the case of the extrinsically labeled spinach diet where a much smaller proportion of the ingested ^{109}Cd appeared in the tissues.

To help identify the source of the variability in ^{109}Cd uptake, the compositions of the various diets were analyzed. There were no major differences in the mineral contents of the diets that could be correlated with the differential Cd bioavailability (Table 6). Mean concentrations of minerals in the semisynthetic diets were: Ca 0.67 (0.62–0.76), Cd 0.29 (0.19–0.41), Cu 4.5 (3.3–5.8), Fe 227

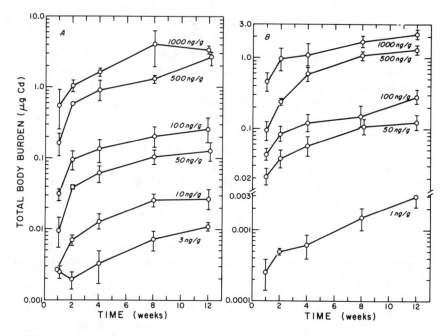

FIGURE 1. Cumulative body burden in rats supplied with ^{109}Cd in (A) water and (B) food. Mean ± S.D. of 4 animals. From Buhler et al. (1981).

TABLE 2.
Distribution of Cd in Tissues of Rats Supplied with
Water Containing 100 μg/L ^{109}Cd.*

Tissue	Cadmium concentration (ng/g)	% Body burden
Large intestine	258 ± 210	†
Caeca	202 ± 177	†
Stomach	118 ± 25	†
Small intestine	49 ± 46	†
Kidney	33 ± 12	43 ± 2.3
Liver	8.5 ± 3.4	43 ± 2.7
Pancreas	1.8 ± 1.2	0.56 ± 0.085
Spleen	0.70 ± 0.34	0.23 ± 0.025
Bone	0.35 ± 0.22	2.4 ± 1.5
Lung	0.24 ± 0.11	0.18 ± 0.014
Heart	0.28 ± 0.14	0.15 ± 0.010
Muscle	0.084 ± 0.043	5.1 ± 1.0
Red cells	0.078 ± 0.031	0.32 ± 0.047
Fat	0.070 ± 0.037	0.65 ± 0.062
Brain	0.030 ± 0.013	0.023 ± 0.0032
Plasma	0.0032 ± 0.017	0.0085 ± 0.0030

*Mean ± S.D. in 2 male and 2 female animals after 4 weeks of exposure.
†Not used in the estimation of body burden.

276

(173–276), and Zn 19 (14–28) $\mu g/g$ diet (dry weight), respectively. By contrast, there was an excellent correlation between [109]Cd accumulation and the oxalate or phytate contents of the diets (Table 6). Absorption of [109]Cd from spinach diets was poor and this was associated with a high oxalate content. Similarly, low [109]Cd uptake from soybean and wheat diets was related to high phytate content.

To determine if oxalate was actually capable of influencing dietary Cd uptake, we undertook an experiment in which rats were fed either Diet 3, Diet 3 to which was added 0.25% Ca oxalate (0.17% oxalate) or an extrinsically labeled spinach diet (Diet 2). Addition of Ca oxalate to the diet significantly reduced the accumulation of [109]Cd in rats as compared to the basal diet (Table 7). As observed previously (Fig. 3), absorption from the [109]Cd extrinsically labeled spinach diet was much less than from the basal ration. The reduced bioavailability of [109]Cd from the spinach diet appears to be associated with its higher (0.90%) oxalate content (Table 5).

Additional experiments examined the influence of other dietary variables. Groups of rats were fed nonradioactive diets containing 10% whole wheat flour (Diet 4) and supplied with distilled water containing 100 $\mu g/L$ [109]Cd^{2+} as [109]$CdCl_2$ or [109]Cd^{2+} drinking water that contained either 100 mg/L Ca^{2+} as $CaCl_2$ or 20 mg/L Mg^{2+} as $MgCl_2$. Absorption of [109]Cd from the water (Table 8) was similar to that previously reported (Buhler et al., 1981). Addition of 100 mg/L Ca^{2+} to the drinking water significantly increased [109]Cd uptake. Absorption of [109]Cd was also increased by addition of 20 mg/L Mg^{2+} to the drinking water.

TABLE 3.
Organ Concentrations of [109]Cd in Rats Fed Various Plant
Diets and Forms of [109]Cd

| | | [109]Cd Concentration (ng/g)[*] | | | |
| | | [109]Cd-plant | | Plant + [109]$CdCl_2$ | |
Plant species	Tissue	Male	Female	Male	Female
Tomato	Liver	8.9±3.3[a]	14.5± 4.4[a]	9.2± 2.3[a]	12.6± 2.5[a]
	Kidney	33.2±7.6[a]	47.6±17.5[a]	30.1±13.7[a]	39.1± 7.4[a]
Carrot	Liver	8.8±0.9[a]	10.3± 0.9[a]	5.5± 1.0[bc]	14.2± 8.1[a]
	Kidney	25.9±4.7[ab]	42.2±16.6[ac]	18.2± 1.6[ab]	31.1± 8.9[a]
Lettuce	Liver	8.1±1.4[a]	14.8± 3.6[a]	6.4± 1.4[ab]	14.8± 8.6[a]
	Kidney	21.9±5.2[b]	42.4±12.9[ab]	21.8± 5.3[ab]	32.9± 3.5[ab]
Soybean	Liver	6.3±2.1[ab]	11.3± 4.8[a]	6.8± 0.8[ab]	12.6± 5.2[a]
	Kidney	11.9±5.4[c]	21.8± 6.7[bc]	14.7± 8.9[ab]	26.2±13.3[afg]
Spinach	Liver	4.4±0.3[bc]	7.8± 0.9[a]	4.3± 1.6[bc]	6.4± 1.6[a]
	Kidney	18.5±1.9[bc]	19.6± 3.9[bc]	16.7± 6.2[ab]	18.2± 5.8[bceg]
Wheat	Liver	3.3±0.7[c]	7.8± 3.6[a]	3.4± 0.7[c]	5.8± 2.2[a]
	Kidney	14.4±1.1[c]	24.0±13.1[bc]	10.6± 1.1[b]	16.8± 4.7[cdf]

*Groups of 5 rats were fed diets for a 2 week period containing 10% dried plant material and approximately 0.24 μg [109]Cd/g diet, either intrinsically bound to the plant material or added to the diet as [109]$CdCl_2$. Means ± S.D. followed by the same letter for a given organ or diet do not differ significantly (P < 0.05).

TABLE 4.
**Total Accumulation of ^{109}Cd by Liver and Kidneys
of Rats Fed Various Plant Diets and Forms of ^{109}Cd.**

| Plant species | Liver + Kidney Cd (ng)* | | | |
| | ^{109}Cd-plant | | Plant + ^{109}CdCl$_2$ | |
	Male	Female	Male	Female
tomato	169±45[a]	187±36[abc]	163±46[ab]	150±35[a]
carrot	156±33[ab]	155±52[a]	108±13[ab]	133±38[acd]
lettuce	121±24[abe]	149±50[ab]	118±26[ab]	139±63[ab]
soybean	106±31[be]	101±29[ab]	99.9±36.6[a]	115±47[bde]
spinach	83.2±10.6[de]	73.7± 9.7[bc]	73.6±30.0[a]	67.0±17.7[bdf]
wheat	49.8±22.1[cd]	82.6±36.0[c]	50.9± 7.5	58.6±21.4[cef]

*Groups of 5 rats were fed diets for a 2 week period containing 10% dried plant material and approximately 0.24 µg ^{109}Cd/g diet, either intrinsically bound to the plant or added to the diet as ^{109}CdCl$_2$. Means ± S.D. followed by the same letter do not differ significantly (P < 0.05).

In other experiments, the effect of varying dietary protein levels and quality on ^{109}Cd accumulation has been examined in rats supplied with drinking water that contained 10 µg/L ^{109}Cd^{2+} as ^{109}CdCl$_2$. At eight weeks, total ^{109}Cd body burden was 26 ± 5 ng in rats fed a diet containing 22% casein but this was reduced to 9.1 ± 2.2 ng in animals receiving a 9.1% casein diet. Absorption of ^{109}Cd also decreased significantly when 16.5% α-protein or zein was substituted for an equivalent amount of casein in the diets.

DISCUSSION

The animal and limited human data all indicate that the absorption of dietary Cd^{2+} is low. Absorption of the metal in man is generally assumed to be between 3 and 8% of the dietary intake (Friberg et al., 1974; Webb, 1979), although greater variations (0.5 to 12%) have also been reported (Webb, 1979). Bioavailability of Cd to animals is frequently less than that reported for humans (Friberg et al., 1974; Webb, 1979). We have shown in previous studies (Buhler et al., 1981) employing ^{109}Cd, for example, that tissue absorption (excluding the gastrointestinal tract) by rats supplied low concentrations of Cd^{2+} averaged 0.10 to 0.22% over a 12-week experimental period. Percent retention in the animals of ^{109}Cd^{2+} added to food or water was similar (Figs. 1, 2) and, moreover, did not vary appreciably with increasing metal concentrations in the diet. The composition of the diet rather than the source of the Cd (water versus food) seems to be the primary factor in determining relative accumulation of the metal by animals (Buhler et al., 1981; Fox, 1983; Webb, 1979).

Limited studies have been conducted on the availability to animals of Cd naturally incorporated into edible plants. Furr et al. (1976c) fed Swiss chard, field-grown on soil treated with 100 dry tons per acre of municipal sewage

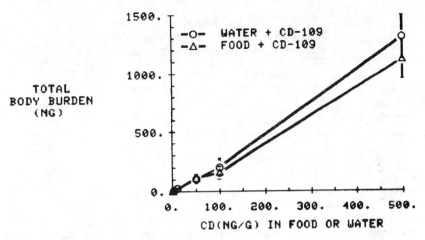

FIGURE 2. Bioaccumulation of [109]Cd in rat tissues and organs from food or water over a period of 8 weeks. From Buhler et al. (1981).

sludge, to guinea pigs for 28 days. While Cd levels in the kidneys were 71% increased over control values, no comparison was made to the availability of similar concentrations of Cd^{2+} added to a control diet or water. Consequently, the relative availability of naturally incorporated Cd^{2+} to the animals could not be assessed. Other studies have shown the accumulation of Cd in the kidneys and livers of mice fed lettuce grown on sewage sludge-amended soil (Chaney et al., 1978a), guinea pigs fed similarly grown lettuce (Chaney et al., 1978b), sheep fed similarly grown corn (Heffron et al., 1980), and meadow voles fed various crops grown on sludge treated soil (Baker et al., 1979; Williams et al., 1978). The accumulation of Cd was also observed to occur in livers and kidneys of rats fed lettuce grown hydroponically in the presence of Cd^{2+} (Welch et al., 1978; Welch and House, 1980). Several studies (Baker et al., 1979; Welch et al., 1978; Williams et al., 1978) also compared the availability of Cd from plants to that from comparable diets spiked with inorganic Cd^{2+} and showed that, for a given diet, the form of metal, whether intrinsically bound in the plant or added to the diet, had little influence on relative tissue accumulation of Cd by animals. Similar results were obtained in the present study when diets containing six different edible plant materials were fed to rats (Tables 3, 4, 5). The type of diet fed was the critical factor in controlling Cd bioavailability.

Absorption of Cd from the diet is known to be influenced by the composition of the diet (Fox, 1983; Friberg et al., 1974; Webb, 1979) and is thus likely to be more variable in man than in animals. For example, the Cd present in animal or plant foods can be bound in complexes that resist decomposition in the stomach and/or are absorbed differently than the free Cd^{2+} cations. Consequently, chelating agents, proteins or other ligands may play a role in Cd bioavailability (Fox, 1979, 1983; Webb, 1979). The availability of dietary Zn, for example, is influenced by the phytic acid (inositol hexaphosphate) content of the diet (Atwal et al., 1980; Cheryan, 1980; Erdman, 1979; Maga, 1982; O'Dell, 1969; O'Dell et al., 1972). When phytates are present in the diet, highly insoluble CaZn-phytate

TABLE 5.
**Percent Retention of ^{109}Cd in Liver and Kidneys
of Rats Fed Various Plant Diets and Forms of ^{109}Cd.***

Plant species	^{109}Cd-plant		Plant + ^{109}CdCl$_2$	
	Male	Female	Male	Female
Tomato	0.24	0.31	0.29	0.25
Carrot	0.17	0.32	0.14	0.27
Lettuce	0.19	0.38	0.14	0.28
Soybean	0.14	0.22	0.21	0.26
Spinach	0.13	0.16	0.03	0.06
Wheat	0.11	0.20	0.11	0.15

*Groups of 5 rats were fed diets for a 2 week period containing 10% dried plant material and approximately 0.24 μg ^{109}Cd/g diet, either intrinsically bound to the plant or added to the diet as ^{109}CdCl$_2$. Means ± S.D. followed by the same letter do not differ significantly (P < 0.05).

complexes can form, markedly reducing Zn absorption. Phytates also decrease the availability of dietary Fe to man (O'Dell, 1972).

In the present investigation, low ^{109}Cd absorption was found with diets containing soybean, spinach, and wheat powder (Tables 3, 4, 5). Since the soybean and wheat diets had high phytate contents (Table 6), the reduced ^{109}Cd bioavailability was presumably due to the formation of highly insoluble CaCd-phytate complexes analogous to those formed with Zn (Cheryan, 1980; Maga, 1982).

The low absorption of ^{109}Cd from spinach diets may be associated with their high oxalate content (Table 6). Oxalates, which are especially high in vegetables such as spinach, rhubarb, Swiss chard, and beets (Kohman, 1939), have been found to interfere with the absorption of other divalent metals by rats, including

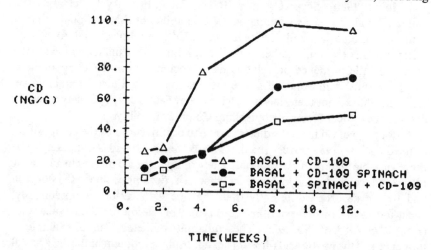

FIGURE 3. Accumulation of ^{109}Cd in kidneys of male and female rats fed basal diet plus ^{109}CdCl$_2$, 10% spinach diet plus ^{109}CdCl$_2$, and 10% ^{109}Cd-spinach diets.

TABLE 6.

Calcium, Cadmium, Zinc, Oxalate, and Phytate Contents of the Various Plant Diets in Relation to Hepatic ^{109}Cd Accumulation.

Plant species	Liver* Cd (ng/g)	Diet (μg/g)			Total oxalates (%)	Total phytates (%)
		Ca	Cd	Zn		
tomato	8.9 ± 3.3	0.65	0.22	14	0.01	0.00
carrot	8.8 ± 0.9	0.64	0.21	13	0.00	0.00
lettuce	8.1 ± 1.4	0.69	0.28	22	0.01	0.00
soybean	6.3 ± 2.1	0.77	0.24	16	0.01	0.17
spinach	4.4 ± 0.3	0.70	0.45	28	0.90	0.00
wheat	3.3 ± 0.7	0.75	0.19	19	0.01	0.11

*Mean ± S.D. of 5 male animals fed ^{109}Cd-plant (intrinsically labeled) diets.

Ca^{2+} (Hodgkinson and Zarembski, 1968) and Zn^{2+} (Welch et al., 1977). The 15 and 30% reduction in tissue ^{109}Cd concentrations in male and female rats, respectively, observed when 0.17% oxalate as Ca oxalate was included in the diet and ^{109}Cd^{2+} supplied in the drinking water (Table 7) is consistent with the probable inhibitory role of this chelator on Cd absorption from diets containing spinach or other plants that are high in oxalates.

The availability of ^{109}Cd^{2+} from drinking water was also decreased when the casein content of the experimental diet was reduced from 22 to 9.1% or when the casein was partially replaced by low quality proteins (α-protein or zein). The type of dietary protein and its concentration in the diet has previously been found by Fox (1979, 1983) to markedly influence Cd accumulation and toxicity.

Other nutritional factors can also affect the availability of Cd from the diet. Some reports, for example, have suggested that the mineral content of the diets could influence Cd absorption and/or toxicity (Fox, 1979; 1983; Friberg et al., 1974; Webb, 1979). Although some variability was seen in the Ca, Cd, Cn, Fe,

TABLE 7.

Effect of Dietary Oxalate on ^{109}Cd Accumulation in Rat Liver and Kidneys.*

Diet	Liver + Kidney Cd (ng)	
	Male	Female
basal + ^{109}CdCl$_2$	76.4 ± 4.0[a]	92.8 ± 25.4[a]
basal + ^{109}CdCl$_2$ + CaC$_2$O$_4$	65.1 ± 8.1[b]	64.8 ± 11.8[b]
basal + spinach + ^{109}CdCl$_2$	24.4 ± 5.2[c]	26.8 ± 4.6[c]

*Groups of 5 rats were supplied with diets containing 0.23 μg/g ^{109}CdCl$_2$, 0.25% CaC$_2$O$_4$ or 10% spinach powder for a period of two weeks. Means ± S.D. followed by the same letter do not significantly differ at the 5% level.

and Zn contents of the extrinsically and intrinsically labeled plant diets employed in present studies (Table 6), these differences in metal content could not be correlated with differences in tissue [109]Cd accumulation. King et al. (1979) also observed that feeding a diet containing 1200 μg/g supplemental Zn had no effect on tissue [109]Cd levels in rats dosed orally with [109]CdCl$_2$.

Cd has been implicated in human hypertension (Friberg et al., 1974; Hallenbeck, 1984; Schroeder, 1965; Webb, 1979) and many rat studies indicate that inclusion of Cd^{2+} in drinking water in the range of 0.1–20 μg/ml can produce elevated systolic and diastolic blood pressures and increased mortalities (Hallenbeck, 1984). The hardness of drinking water is thought to play a role both in Cd absorption and in the incidence of human cardiovascular disease (Hallenbeck, 1984). In a study on Swedish horses slaughtered for meat production, Elinder et al. (1980) found that a higher accumulation of Cd occurred in the kidneys of horses living in soft water areas. A strong negative correlation between the incidence of mortality in human cardiovascular disease and the degree of hardness of drinking water, specifically the sum of Ca and Mg concentrations, has focused attention on the possible protective action of these two elements (Arden, 1977). A reduced incidence of hypertension was also observed in female rats receiving Ca^{2+} in their drinking water (Schroeder et al., 1967a). Tissue deposition of Cd and associated toxicity is also enhanced by feeding diets low in Ca or by Ca deficiency (Larsson and Piscator, 1971; Washko and Cousins, 1976, 1977). However, other studies have shown that tissue Cd levels were not reduced when normal or elevated Ca diets were fed (Schroeder et al., 1967a; Washko and Cousins, 1976, 1977).

In our experiments, inclusion of 100 mg/L Ca^{2+} or 20 mg/L Mg^{2+} in drinking water containing 100 μg/L [109]Cd^{2+} markedly increased accumulation of the [109]Cd by rats (Table 8). While these results seem to be in disagreement with the findings of other investigators, rats in our experiment were fed nonradioactive diets containing 10% whole wheat flour, a diet with a 0.90% phytate content (Table 6). The bioaccumulation of Zn^{2+} has been found to be influenced by Ca when phytate containing diets are fed. The Ca^{2+} apparently competes with Zn^{2+} for phytate binding, thereby reducing the Zn^{2+} incorporated in insoluble CaZn-

TABLE 8.
Influence of Calcium and Magnesium on the Accumulation by Rats of [109]Cd from Drinking Water.*

Drinking water additive	Body burden (ng)	Percent absorption	Liver (ng/g)	Kidney (ng/g)
none	203 ± 94[a]	0.14 ± 0.06[a]	12 ± 6[a]	44 ± 23[a]
100 mg/L Ca[2+]	395 ± 152[a]	0.31 ± 0.10[b]	25 ± 8[a]	91 ± 30[a]
20 mg/L Mg[2+]	366 ± 178[a]	0.27 ± 0.15[b]	22 ± 13[a]	90 ± 63[a]

*Groups of 4 rats were supplied with 100 μg/L [109]Cd as [109]CdCl$_2$ in the drinking water for a period of 8 weeks. Some animals were also given water containing 100 ng/L Ca^{2+} as CaCl$_2$ or 20 mg/L Mg^{2+} as MgCl$_2$. Means ± S.D. followed by the same letter do not significantly differ at the 5% level.

phytate complexes, releasing the metal for absorption (Cheryan, 1980; Maga, 1982). It seems reasonable to suggest, therefore, that Ca^{2+} and Mg^{2+} acts in a similar way in our experiments, complexing with phytates present in the wheat flour, preventing the precipitation of $^{109}Cd^{2+}$ and making it more available to rats.

Numerous studies in experimental animals have shown that females bioaccumulate higher concentrations of Cd than do males (Friberg et al., 1974; Kello et al., 1979; Stonard and Webb, 1976; Webb, 1979). Tissue ^{109}Cd levels were also substantially higher in female rats in the present study (Table 3) than in males. While tissue ^{109}Cd concentrations were 60% higher in females than in males (Table 3), total organ content of the metal in females was only slightly greater than those of males (Table 4). Stonard and Webb (1976) have similarly concluded that, at equilibrium, hepatic and Cd contents in both sexes of rats are essentially the same. Large-scale epidemiological and clinical studies of the "Itai-itai" disease in Japan, however, indicate that only females on diets low in Ca and vitamin D suffer from this serious bone and kidney disease (Friberg et al., 1974).

The lower body retention of Cd in males could be the result of either a decreased intestinal absorption of Cd or its enhanced elimination. Females eat proportionally more food than males but this is insufficient to account for the observed differences in tissue Cd levels. Kello and co-workers (1979) have concluded, however, that the sexual differences in Cd retention are probably caused by differences in percent absorption between the sexes. Our data (Table 5) are supportive of the latter explanation.

The present study showed that the accumulation of ^{109}Cd in the livers and kidneys of rats fed diets containing 10% plant material was generally similar whether the ^{109}Cd was preincorporated into the plants (intrinsically labeled), added to the diet at mixing (extrinsically labeled) or supplied in the drinking water. Therefore, the composition of the diet appears to be the major factor in determining Cd bioavailability. In studies with six different edible plant materials, ^{109}Cd accumulation by rats varied markedly with the type of plant diet fed. Highest tissue levels occurred in rats fed tomato, carrot, or lettuce diets; a soybean diet yielded intermediate tissue concentrations; and the lowest tissue uptakes appeared in rats fed spinach and wheat diets. Suggestive evidence was obtained to implicate the occurrence of phytates and oxalates in plant material with the reduced bioavailability of Cd from soybean, spinach, or wheat diets. Whether or not phytates or other dietary constituents, capable of binding Cd and hence reducing its absorption, can offer protection against toxicity resulting from dietary or other Cd exposure remains to be established. Care must be exercised in interpreting such studies, however, since the present research has also indicated that minerals, such as Ca^{2+}, may be able to influence the binding of Cd to phytates and possibly to other dietary components, and thus modify the bioavailability of Cd.

ACKNOWLEDGEMENTS

The author is grateful to Dr. Jun-Lan Wang for her helpful suggestions and assistance in preparing this report. The many contributions of Dr. Ian J. Tinsley,

Dr. Jun-Lan Wang, Mr. Chris L. Browne, Mr. David C. Wright, Ms. Karen L. Smith, and Ms. Kristine Y–M. Wong to this research are also acknowledged. This work was supported by grants from the U.S. Environmental Protection Agency (R-803423) and the National Institutes of Health (ES-00210) and is issued as Oregon Agricultural Experiment Station Technical Paper No. 7329. Organization and analysis of data were carried out, in part, using the PROPHET system, a unique national resource sponsored by the NIH. Information about PROPHET, including how to apply for access, can be obtained from the Director, Chemical/Biological Information-Handling Program, Division of Research Resources, NIH, Bethesda, MD 20205.

REFERENCES

ARDEN, T.V. (1977). Cardiovascular Mortality: An Analysis of the Water Effect. National Academy of Sciences, Washington, D.C.

ATWAL, A.S., ESKIN, N.A.M., McDONALD, B.E. and VAISEY-GENSER, M. (1980). The effect of phytate on nitrogen utilization and zinc metabolism in young rats. Nutr. Rep. Inter. 21:257–267.

BAKER, D.E., AMACHER, M.C. and LEACH, R.M. (1979). Sewage sludge as a source of cadmium in soil-plant-animal systems. Environ. Health Perspect. 28:45–49.

BERNARD, A. and LAUWERYS, R. (1984). Cadmium in human population. Experentia 40:143–152.

BINGHAM, F.T. (1979). Bioavailability of cadmium to food crops in relation to heavy metal content of sludge-amended soil. Environ. Health Perspect. 28:39–43.

BINGHAM, F.T., PAGE, A.L., MAHLER, R.J. and GANJE, T.J. (1975). Growth and cadmium accumulation of plants grown on soil treated with cadmium enriched sewage sludge. J. Environ. Qual. 4:267–269.

BROWNE, C.L., WONG, Y.–M. and BUHLER, D.R. (1984). A predictive model for the accumulation of cadmium by container-grown plants. J. Environ. Qual. 13:184–188.

BUHLER, D.R., WRIGHT, D.C., SMITH, K.L. and TINSLEY, I.J. (1981). Cadmium absorption and tissue distribution in rats provided low concentrations of cadmium in food or drinking water. J. Toxicol. Environ. Health 8:185–197.

CHANEY, R.L., STOEWSAND, G.S., BACHE, C.A. and LISK, D.J. (1978a). Cadmium disposition and hepatic microsomal induction in mice fed lettuce grown on municipal sludge-amended soil. J. Agric. Food Chem. 26:992–994.

CHANEY, R.L., STOEWSAND, G.S., FURR, A.K., BACHE, C.A. and LISK, D.J. (1978b). Elemental content of tissues of guinea pigs fed swiss chard grown on municipal sludge-amended soil. J. Agric. Food Chem. 26:994–997.

CHERYAN, M. (1980). Phytic acid interactions in food systems. CRC Crit. Rev. Food Sci. and Nutr. 13:297–335.

DAVIS, R.D. (1984). Cadmium—a complex environmental problem. Part II. Cadmium in sludges used as fertilizer. Experientia 40:117–126.

ELINDER, C.-G., STENSTROM, T., PISCATOR, M. and LINNMAN, L. (1980). Water hardness in relation to cadmium accumulation and microscopic signs of cardiovascular disease in horses. Arch. Environ. Health 35:81–84.

ELLIS, K.J., VARTSKY, D., ZANZI, I., COHN, S.H. and YASAMURO, S. (1979). Cadmium: in vivo measurement in smokers and nonsmokers. Science 205:323–325.

ERDMAN, J.W. (1979). Oilseed phytates: nutritional implications. J. Am. Oil Chem. Soc. 56:736–741.

FOX, M.R.S. (1979). Nutritional influences on metal toxicity: cadmium as a model toxic element. Environ. Health Perspect. **29**:95–104.

FOX, M.R.S. (1983). Cadmium bioavailability. Fed. Proc. **42**:1726–1729.

FRIBERG, L., PISCATOR, M., NORBERG, G., and KJELLSTROM, T. (1974). Cadmium in the Environment, 2nd ed. CRC Press, Cleveland, Ohio.

FULKERSON, K. and GOELLER, H.E. (1973). Cadmium: The Dissipated Element, Pub. No. ORNL NSF EP21, Oak Ridge National Laboratory, Oak Ridge, Tennessee.

FURR, A.K., KELLEY, W.C., BACHE, C.A., GUTENMANN, W.H., and LISK, D.J. (1976a). Multielement absorption by crops grown in pots on municipal sludge-amended soil. J. Agric. Food Chem. **24**:889–892.

FURR, A.K., LAWRENCE, A.W., TONG, S.S.C., GRANDOLFO, M.C., HOF-STADER, R.A., BACHE, C.A., GUTENMANN, W.H., and LISK, D.J. (1976b). Multielement and chlorinated hydrocarbon analysis of municipal sludges of American cities. Environ. Sci. Technol. **10**:683–687.

FURR, A.K., STOEWSAND, G.S., BACHE, C.A. and LISK, D.J. (1976c). Study of guinea pigs fed Swiss chard grown on municipal sludge-amended soil. Arch. Environ. Health **31**:87–91.

HAGHIRI, F. (1973). Cadmium uptake by plants. J. Environ. Qual. **2**:93–95.

HALLENBECK, W.H. (1984). Human health effects of exposure to cadmium. Experientia **40**:136–142.

HARLAND, B.F. and OBERLEAS, D. (1977). A modified method for phytate analysis using an ion-exchange procedure: Application to textured vegetables. Cereal Chem. **54**:827–832.

HEFFRON, C.L., REID, J.T., ELFVING, D.C., STOEWSAND, G.S., HASCHEK, W.M., TELFORD, J.N., FURR, A.K., PARKINSON, T.F., BACHE, C.A., GUTENMANN, W.H., WSZOLEK, P.C. and LISK, D.J. (1980). Cadmium and zinc in growing sheep fed silage corn grown on municipal sludge amended soil. J. Agric. Food Chem. **28**:58–61.

HODGKINSON, A. and ZAREMBSKI, P.M. (1968). Oxalic acid metabolism in man: A review. Calc. Tiss. Res. **2**:115–132.

HORVATH, D.J. (1972). An overview of soil/plant/animal relationships with respect to utilization of trace elements. Ann. N.Y. Acad. Sci. **199**:82–94.

JOHN, M.K. (1973). Cadmium uptake by eight food crops as influenced by various soil levels of cadmium. Environ. Poll. **4**:7–15.

JOHN, M.K. (1976). Interrelationship between plant cadmium and uptake of some other elements from culture solution by oats and lettuce. Environ. Poll. **11**:85–95.

JONES, R.L., KINESLY, T.D. and ZIEGLER, E.L. (1973). Cadmium content of soybeans grown in sewage-sludge amended soil. J. Environ. Qual. **2**:351–353.

KELLO, D., DEKANIC, D., and KOSTIAL, K. (1979). Influence of sex and dietary calcium on intestinal cadmium absorption in rats. Arch. Environ. Health **34**:30–33.

KING, B.D., LASSITER, J.W., NEATHERY, M.W., GENTRY, R.P. and MILLER, W.J. (1979). Effect of dietary cadmium and zinc on tissue [109]Cd contents of orally dosed rats. Nutr. Rep. Inter. **19**:875–894.

KOHMAN, E.F. (1939). Oxalic acid in foods and its behaviour and fate in the diet. J. Nutr. **18**:233–246.

KOPP, J.R. (1969). The occurrence of trace elements in water. In *Trace Substances in Environmental Health,* D.D. Hemphell, ed., pp. 59–73. University of Missouri Press, Columbia, Missouri.

LARSSON, S.E. and PISCATOR, M. (1971). Effect of cadmium on skeletal tissue in normal and calcium-deficient rats. Israel J. Med. Sci. **7**:495–498.

LINNMAN, L., ANDERSSON, A., NILSSON, K.O., LIND, B., KJELLSTROM, T. and FRIBERG, L. (1973). Cadmium uptake by wheat from sewage sludge used as a plant nutrient source. Arch. Environ. Health **27**:45–47.

LOWRY, R.R. and TINSLEY, I.J. (1974). A simple sensitive method for lipid phosphorous. Lipids **9**:491–492.

LOWRY, R.R. and TINSLEY, I.J. (1984). Unpublished results.

MAGA, J.A. (1982). Phytate: Its chemistry, occurrence, food interactions, nutritional significance, and methods of analysis. J. Ag. Food Chem. **30**:1–9.

MAHAFFEY, K.R., CORNELIUSSEN, P.E., JELINEK, C.F. and FIORINO, J.A. (1975). Heavy metal exposure from food. Environ. Health Perspect. **12**:63–69.

NATIONAL ACADEMY OF SCIENCES. (1982). Drinking Water and Health, vol. 4, National Academy of Sciences, Washington, DC.

O'DELL, B.L. (1969). Effect of dietary components upon zinc availability. Amer. J. Clin. Nutr. **22**:1315–1322.

O'DELL, B.L. (1972). Dietary factors that affect biological availability of trace elements. Ann. N.Y. Acad. Sci. **199**:70–81.

O'DELL, B.L., BURPO, C.E. and SAVAGE, J.E. (1972). Evaluation of zinc availability in foodstuffs of plant and animal origin. J. Nutr. **102**:653–660.

PAGE, A.L. (1974). Fate and Effects of Trace Elements in Sewage Sludge When Applied to Agricultural Lands, EPA Report No. 670/2-74-005, Office of Research and Development, U.S. Environmental Protection Agency, Cincinnati, Ohio.

PAGE, A.L., BINGHAM, F.T. and NELSON, C. (1972). Cadmium absorption and growth of various plant species as influenced by solution cadmium concentration. J. Environ. Qual. **1**:288–291.

ROOT, R.A., MILLER, R.J. and KOEPPE, D.E. (1975). Uptake of cadmium—Its toxicity and effect on the iron ratio in hydroponically grown corn. J. Environ. Qual. **4**:473–476.

SCHROEDER, H.A. (1965). Cadmium as a factor in hypertension. J. Chron. Dis. **18**:647–656.

SCHROEDER, H.A., NASON, A.P. and BALASSA, J.J. (1967a). Trace metals in rat tissues as influenced by calcium in water. J. Nutr. **93**:331–336.

SCHROEDER, H.A., NASON, A.P., TIPTON, I.H., and BALASSA, J.J. (1967b). Essential trace metals in man: Zinc relation to environmental cadmium. J. Chron. Dis. **20**:179–210.

SHARRETT, A.R., CARTER, A.P., ORHEIM, R.M. and FEINLEIB, M. (1982). Daily intake of lead, cadmium, copper and zinc from drinking water: The Seattle study of trace metal exposure. Environ. Res. **28**:456–475.

SHERLOCK, J.C. (1984). Cadmium in foods and the diet. Experientia **40**:152–156.

STONARD, M.D. and WEBB, M. (1976). Influence of dietary cadmium on the distribution of the essential metals copper, zinc and iron in tissues of the rat. Chem. Biol. Interact. **15**:349–363.

STREET, J.J., LINDSAY, W.L. and SABEY, B.R. (1977). Solubility and plant uptake of cadmium in soils amended wiht cadmium and sewage sludge. J. Environ. Qual. **6**: 72–77.

STRAIN, W.H., FLYNN, A., MANSOUR, E.G., PLECHA, F.R., PORIES, W.J. and HILL, O.A., JR. (1975). Trace element content of household water. In *Trace Substances in Environmental Health,* D.D. Hemphell, ed., pp. 41–46. University of Missouri Press, Columbia, Missouri.

TURNER, M.A. (1973). Effect of cadmium treatment on cadmium and zinc uptake by selected vegetable species. J. Environ. Qual. **2**:118–119.

WASHKO, P.W. and COUSINS, R.J. (1976). Metabolism of ^{109}Cd in rats fed normal and low-calcium diets. J. Toxicol. Environ. Health **1**:1055–1066.

WASHKO, P.W. and COUSINS, R.J. (1977). Role of dietary calcium and calcium binding protein in cadmium toxicity in rats. J. Nutr. **107**:920–928.

WEBB, M. (1979). The Chemistry, Biochemistry and Biology of Cadmium. Elsevier/North-Holland, Biomedical Press, Amsterdam.

WELCH, R.M. and HOUSE, W.A. (1980). Absorption of radiocadmium and radio-selenium by rats fed intrinsically and extrinsically labeled lettuce leaves. Nutr. Rep. Inter. **20**:135–144.

WELCH, R.M., HOUSE, W.A. and VAN CAMPEN, D.R. (1977). Effects of oxalic acid on availability of zinc from spinach leaves and zinc sulfate to rats. J. Nutr. **107**:929–933.

WELCH, R.M., HOUSE, W.A. and VAN CAMPEN, D.R. (1978). Availability of cadmium from lettuce leaves and cadmium sulfate to rats. Nutr. Rep. Inter. **17**:35–42.

WILLIAMS, P.H., SHENK, J.S. and BAKER, D.E. (1978). Cadmium accumulation by meadow voles (*Microtus pennsylvanicus*) from crops grown on sludge-treated soils. J. Environ. Qual. **7**:450–454.

YOST, K.J. (1984). Cadmium, the environment and human health: an overview. Experientia **40**:157–164.

CHAPTER XXV

ABSORPTION OF LEAD FROM DRINKING WATER WITH VARYING MINERAL CONTENT

Robert G. Miller, Daniel Greathouse, Richard J. Bull and James U. Doerger
U.S. Environmental Protection Agency,
Health Effects and Research Laboratory,
Toxicology and Microbiology Division,
26 W. St. Clair Street,
Cincinnati, Ohio

ABSTRACT

Lead (Pb) (200 ppm) was administered via drinking water to rats for nine weeks. In addition, the rats were grouped so that they received 75, 100, 150 and 250% of the minimum daily requirements (MDR) of calcium (Ca), iron (Fe), and magnesium (Mg) as required for normal growth. The exposures were arranged so that no more than one element was varied within the same animal groups, while maintaining 100% of the MDR of all other elements and nutrients.

Blood lead analyses were performed at 0, 1, 2, 3, 7, 8, and 9 weeks after exposure. Food and water consumptions and body weights were measured each week (0–9).

Some gross differences were seen both within and among the groups with respect to milliliters water consumed vs. body weight and grams of food consumed vs. body weight. During the first few weeks of exposure, the mean blood lead in animals fed 75% MDR of Ca, Fe, and Mg appeared less than those receiving 100% MDR of the corresponding elements. There was a decrease in mean blood lead concentration in animals receiving 150 and 250% of the MDR of Fe at the 7–9 week time period; however, this was probably due to a slight decrease in water consumption during this time period. There seemed to be no appreciable differences in mean blood lead concentrations of groups exposed to high concentrations of Ca and Mg. However, analysis of the data after correcting for varying Pb dose points to the conclusion that dietary magnesium has no effect on uptake of lead whereas dietary iron decreases blood lead concentration and calcium only increases blood lead concentration after extended exposure (7–9 weeks).

TABLE I.
Elemental Content of Experimental Rat Diet.

Element	Mg/Kg (ppm)
Calcium	4500
Cooper	5.6
Iron	20
Magnesium	300
Manganese	60
Potassium	2000
Sodium	600
Zinc	13.3
Sulfur	Trace (MDR as per vitamins)
Iodide	.17
Chloride	600
Phosphorous	4400

INTRODUCTION

The possible physiological changes arising from exposure to lead in our environment depend upon the amount of the metal ingested and absorbed and/or retained. Retention of lead in animals varies according to species, ages within species, and nature of the diet. There are some essential dietary components which may have an influence on the retention of lead (Baltrop et al., 1975; Petering, 1980). Calcium was one of the first dietary compounds to be implicated as having a metabolic relationship with lead absorption. An early clinical study was performed by Aub (1953), whereby lead intoxicated human subjects were given high levels of calcium to reduce blood lead levels. However, recent studies by Quarterman et al. (1977) indicate that an increase of dietary calcium to a lead intoxicated rat reduces the actual rate of lead loss from the body rather

TABLE II.
Design of Experimental Animal Groups with
Respect to Supplement Diets with Pb, Ca, Mg and Fe

Low Lead Control (.06 ppm)

Group I

MDR-Fe
MDR-Ca
MDR-Mg

200 ppm Lead in Drinking Water

Group II	Group III	Group IV	Group V	Group VI
MDR-Fe	75% MDR-Fe	MDR-Fe	MDR-Fe	150% MDR-Fe
MDR-Ca	MDR-Ca	75% MDR-Ca	MDR-Ca	MDR-Ca
MDR-Mg	MDR-Mg	MDR-Mg	75% MDR-Mg	MDR-Mg

Group VII	Group VIII	Group IX	Group X	Group XI
MDR-Fe	MDR-Fe	250% MDR-Fe	MDR-Fe	MDR-Fe
150% MDR-Ca	MDR-Ca	MDR-Ca	250% MDR-Ca	MDR-Ca
MDR-Mg	150% MDR-Mg	MDR-Mg	MDR-Mg	250% MDR-Mg

MDR = Minimum Daily Requirement for normal growth

MDR-Calcium = 6000 ppm

MDR-Iron = 25 ppm

MDR-Magnesium = 400 ppm

than increasing lead loss. Other literature suggests that lead affects calcium metabolism. One study by Six et al. (1970) indicates that rats given lead in their drinking water had small decreases in serum calcium levels regardless of their levels of dietary calcium. The study also showed that adding lead to a low calcium diet greatly increased kidney calcium and lead content.

Previous studies by Six et al. (1972) and Barton et al. (1978) have indicated that feeding of an iron deficient diet demonstrated an increased retention of lead in the whole body.

Iron, magnesium and calcium are the major elements of hard water and all have been reported to be readily absorbed in the small intestine and therefore may compete with lead for some common transport system or metabolic interactions as explained by Conrad et al. (1978) and Mahaffey et al. (1980). The present work was undertaken to determine the effects upon lead absorption by increasing the dietary concentration (above normal growth requirements) of those major ions (iron, magnesium and calcium) which constitute water hardness.

TABLE III.
Body Weight, Food and Water Consumption Data
Summary Data Point Week 1-3

Diet	Body Wt. (Gm)	Water (Ml)	Food (Gm)	Ml Water / 100 Gm Body Wt. Per Week	Gm Food / 100 Gm Body Wt. Per Week
75% MDR-Ca	352	175	144	49.7	40.9
100% MDR-Ca	341	167	141	49.6	41.6
150% MDR-Ca	309	149	140	48.9	46.2
250% MDR-Ca	284	148	116	51.8	40.8
75% MDR-Fe	363	178	145	48.6	40.2
100% MDR-Fe	341	167	141	49.6	41.6
150% MDR-Fe	345	184	152	54.9	44.5
250% MDR-Fe	352	148	151	42.0	42.9
75% MDR-Mg	351	149	140	42.5	40.1
100% MDR-Mg	341	167	141	49.6	41.6
150% MDR-Mg	333	153	148	46.8	45.5
250% MDR-Mg	349	158	150	45.2	43.0
No Lead Control	344	189	150	54.9	43.6

METHODS

Diet. Pelleted rat chow was used containing 100% of the minimum daily requirements (MDR) of nutrients and minerals necessary for normal growth and development as recommended by the National Academy of Science (1966) with the exception of calcium, iron and magnesium. These three elements were contained in the chow at a concentration of 75% of MDR. The elemental salt concentration of the rat chow used in this experiment and confirmed by Inductively Coupled Plasma Spectroscopy analysis is found in Table I.

Calcium, iron, and magnesium were added to deionized distilled drinking water at concentrations (assuming a normal water intake) that would provide for a total intake of these elements at 1.0, 1.5, and 2.5 times the MDR for normal growth and development (MDR 25 Mg/Kg for iron, 6000 Mg/Kg for Ca, 400 Mg/Kg for Mg). Lead at 200 ppm was administered via drinking water to all experimental animals except the no lead control group. This Pb dosage has been shown by Six et al. (1970) to be the maximum dose of Pb fed for a ten week period that does not produce significant alterations in hematopoiesis, renal size, histology, and renal function in the rat. The chemical forms of the elements used were $MgCl_2 \cdot 6H_2O$, $CaCl_2 \cdot 2H_2O$, $FeCl_3$ and $PbCl_2$ chloride salts.

Experimental Design. One hundred and ten male albino Sprague–Dawley rats weighing 200–225 grams were divided into eleven groups, ten rats per group, and fed a purified rat diet to contain 75% MDR of the elements Ca, Fe, and Mg supplemented by appropriate amounts in the drinking water to give intakes of the elements indicated in Table II.

TABLE IV.
Body Weight, Food and Water Consumption Data
Summary Data Point Week 7-9

Diet	Body Wt. (Gm)	Water (Ml)	Food (Gm)	Ml Water 100 Gm Body Wt. Per Week	Gm Food 100 Gm Body Wt. Per Week
75% MDR–Ca	487	178	158	36.9	32.4
100% MDR–Ca	480	186	153	39.2	31.8
150% MDR–Ca	453	149	146	32.9	32.2
250% MDR–Ca	420	132	157	31.6	37.5
75% MDR–Fe	502	192	162	38.4	32.3
100% MDR–Fe	480	186	153	39.2	31.8
150% MDR–Fe	508	169	170	33.4	33.4
250% MDR–Fe	493	161	160	32.6	32.4
75% MDR–Mg	503	173	156	34.6	30.9
100% MDR–Mg	480	186	153	39.2	31.8
150% MDR–Mg	471	197	157	41.9	33.3
250% MDR–Mg	485	192	158	40.7	33.0
No Lead Control	480	210	142	43.7	29.6

The animals were housed individually in stainless steel cages for the nine week experimental period. The body weight, food and water consumption for each animal was recorded weekly. Blood samples were collected with heparinized capillary tubes for all animals at the end of 0, 1, 2, 3, 7, 8, and 9 weeks by retro orbital sinus puncture. After collection, each blood sample was immediately transferred into a tube containing Metexchange M reagent of Environmental Science Associates (1982). Lead analyses were performed within 24 hours of collection.

Analytical Methods. Blood lead analyses were performed by the method of anodic stripping voltammetry as outlined by Environmental Science Associates (1978). This method requires only 200 μl of whole blood, making it possible to analyze serial samples from the same animal over a period of exposure time.

RESULTS

One week prior to the start of exposure, the baseline blood lead levels for all animals were determined to be $< 2\mu g\%$. The no lead basal rat diet was analyzed to contain 0.06 ppm lead. These low baseline lead values indicate that any effects obtained could not be attributable to the basal diet or previous lead exposure.

The mean body weights, food and water consumption data for weeks 1–3 and 7–9 of exposure are reported for each group of animals in Tables III and IV.

Since body weight is generally indicative of food and water consumption, the ratios of intake to body weight were calculated. The relative intake of water and food per unit body weight for all exposed groups decreased during the later weeks of the study.

TABLE V.
Effect of Dietary Calcium, Iron and Magnesium
on Blood Lead Absorption

Diet	Blood Lead μg% Week 1-3		Blood Lead μg% Week 7-9	
	Mean	Standard Error	Mean	Standard Error
75% MDA-Ca	53.0	3.3	48.2	1.5
100% MDR-Ca	61.8	3.8	49.8	3.3
150% MDR-Ca	48.5	2.9	45.8	2.3
250% MDR-Ca	51.2	2.7	56.4	5.4
75% MDR-Fe	56.9	4.4	53.9	3.9
100% MDR-Fe	61.8	3.8	49.8	3.3
150% MDR-Fe	54.6	3.1	44.0	2.0
250% MDR-Fe	48.1	4.1	39.4	2.6
75% MDR-Mg	53.3	2.9	48.2	3.0
100% MDR-Mg	61.8	3.8	49.8	3.3
150% MDR-Mg	58.3	3.9	56.6	2.7
250% MDR-Mg	59.2	5.6	52.7	7.9
No Lead Control 100% MDR	4.5		4.8	

The no lead control group appeared to consume slightly more water per unit body weight than those exposed to lead and other experimental elements. This small difference may be attributed to the taste associated with iron and the other elements added to the experimental groups' water.

Table V consists of blood lead data for all experimental groups. Data from weeks 1, 2, and 3 were pooled with the mean blood lead values presented for each diet. Data points at week 7, 8, and 9 were similarly calculated.

Statistically, as would be expected, there was a highly significant difference in the mean blood lead levels of the no lead control group and all other lead exposed experimental groups for both 1-3 and 7-9 weeks time intervals.

In testing the effects of iron, calcium, and magnesium in the diet upon blood lead concentration (assuming an equal number of animals were exposed to each dietary regimen and assuming that lead intake was constant over the different dietary groups), the usual statistical approach would be analysis of variance followed by multiple comparison tests to identify differences in dietary regimens in terms of observed blood lead levels. This approach, however, was not satisfactory since large variations in consumption resulted in significant variations in the intake of dietary constituent intake and lead, both within and among the dietary groups.

Hence, a regression analysis approach was selected with each observation consisting of the blood lead and intake data for one animal during a week. Since food and water intake vary with body weight, weekly intakes were corrected for body weight, i.e., weekly intake for each animal was divided by the body weight of the respective animal. Reflecting the belief that the two observation periods (weeks 1–3 and 7–9) should be summarized separately, mean relative intakes for each period were used in the analysis. The form of the regression model for each period was as follows:

$$Bld\ Pb = b_0 + b_1\,(Ca) + b_2\,(Mg) + b_3\,(Fe) + b_4\,(Pb)$$

where b_0 = intercept
and b_i, $i = 1 - 4$ are coefficients of the constituent and lead intakes

The results of the regression analysis of mean blood lead on the mean relative dietary intake (weekly) is shown in Table VI, indicating a statistical significance for iron at both time periods and for calcium at time period week 7–9.

CONCLUSIONS

When mean blood lead concentration data are observed as dietary groups there were no obvious statistical differences between the groups because of the variability of the data within each group. However, when each animal's data were statistically analyzed as an individual data point, there was some significance in that as the animals were exposed to increased iron in their diets their blood lead levels tended to decrease.

These blood lead data correspond to the lead absorption data findings of Barton et al. (1978), who determined that iron loading above MDR inhibited lead absorption. This could be explained in that iron and lead are absorbed in the duodenum according to Bivin et al. (1979) and may in fact compete for absorption sites in the intestinal mucosa.

TABLE VI.
**Multiple Regression of Mean Blood Lead
on Mean Relative Dietary Intake**

Parameter	Weeks 1–3 Est.	t value	Prob >t	Weeks 7–9 Est.	t value	Prob >t
Intercept	45.466	7.76	0.0001	12.590	2.04	0.045
Ca	−0.002	−1.86	0.067	0.006	3.34	0.001
Mg	0.027	1.30	0.198	0.017	0.77	0.443
Fe	−0.508	−2.10	0.039	−0.685	−2.41	0.019
Pb	0.177	3.54	0.0007	0.407	5.98	0.0001

Overall Model:	F value	Prob >F	F value	Prob >F
	3.02	0.0072	16.20	0.0001

In the case of calcium, blood lead levels in our study increased as the calcium intake increased but only at the 7–9 week period (extended exposure). This differs from the absorption study of Quarterman et al. (1978), as they reported an increase in dietary calcium (200% MDR) at the time of lead exposure would decrease the amount of lead absorbed. Kathryn Six et al. (1979) did demonstrate a 4 fold increase of blood lead with a diet containing much less calcium (15% MDR). Our study did not show any different blood lead levels between those animals receiving 75% and 100% MDR of calcium.

Magnesium seemed to have no effect on blood lead concentrations. This is explained perhaps because of the site of absorption in the small intestine (Bivin et al., 1979). Lead is absorbed primarily in the duodenum while magnesium is absorbed in the ileum; therefore, there is no competition for available mucosae cell sites.

Our study differed from other reported work in that a series of blood samples were taken, over time, from the same animal. Therefore, biological differences due to exposure times were somewhat more realistic although large variations of blood lead values existed for each exposure group.

ACKNOWLEDGEMENT

The research described in this paper has been peer and administratively reviewed by the U.S. Environmental Protection Agency and approved for publication. Mention of trade names or commercial products does not constitute endorsement or recommendation for use.

REFERENCES

AUB, J.C. (1935). The Biochemical Behavior of Lead in the Body. J. Amer. Med. Assoc. **104**:87–90.

BARLTRAP, D. and KHOO, H. (1975). The Influence of Nutritional Factors on Lead Absorption. Postgrad. Med. J. **51**:795–800.

BARTON, JR., CONRAD, M., NUBY, S. and HARRISON, L. (1978). The effects of iron on the Absorption and Retention of Lead. J. Lab. Clin. Med. **92**(4):536–547.

BIVIN, W.S., CRAWFORD, M.P. and BREWER, N.R. (1979). *The Laboratory Rat.* Vol. I, Chapter 4, pp. 79–84. H.J. Baker, J.R. Lindsey and S.H. Weisbroth, eds. Academic Press, Inc., New York.

CONRAD, M. and BARTON, J. (1978). Factors Affecting the Absorption and Excretion of Lead in the Rat. J. Gastroenterology **74**:731–740.

DIRECT ANALYSIS OF LEAD IN BLOOD USING ESA HIGH SENSITIVE ELECTRODE. (1978). Methods Manual of Environmental Science Associates, Inc., Bedford, Massachusetts.

ENVIRONMENTAL SCIENCE ASSOCIATES. A patented antiform hemolyzing reagent. Bedford, MA.

MAHAFFEY, K. and RADER, J. (1980). Metabolic Interactions: Lead, Calcium and Iron. Annal. New York Academy of Sciences. **355**:285–297.

NUTRIENT REQUIREMENTS OF LABORATORY ANIMALS. (1966). National Academy of Sciences—National Research Council, Publication 990, pp. 51–80.

PETERING, H.G. (1980). The Influence of Dietary Zinc and Copper on the Biological Effect of Orally Ingested Lead in the Rat. Annals New York Academy of Science **355**:298–308.

QUARTERMAN, J., MORRISON, J. and HUMPHRIES, W. (1978). The Influence of High Dietary Calcium and Phosphate on Lead Uptake and Release. Environmental Research **17**:60–67.

SIX, K. and GOYER, R. (1972). The Influence of Iron Deficiency on Tissue Content and Toxicity of Ingested Lead in the Rat. J. Lab. Clin. Med. **79**(1):128–236.

SIX, K. and GOYER, R. (1970). Experimental Enhancement of Lead Toxicity by Low Dietary Calcium. J. Lab. Clin. Med. **76**(6):933–942.

CHAPTER XXVI

CHANGES IN MINERAL COMPOSITION OF FOOD FROM COOKING IN HARD AND SOFT WATER

B.J.A. Haring
Ministry of Housing, Physical Planning and Environment
2260 MB Leidschendam
P.O. Box 450
The Netherlands

ABSTRACT

Drinking water softened below a total hardness of 1.5 mmol/l Ca was discouraged because of the negative statistical association found by various investigators between hardness of drinking water and death rate from cardiovascular disease. The causality of the association is still a matter of doubt. A point to consider in this respect is the fact that drinking water used for food cooking can bring about changes in the mineral food composition. In this paper it is demonstrated that the calcium concentration of some vegetables (cauliflower, carrots, endive) decreases upon cooking in soft waters, whereas an increase or lower decrease is found when these foodstuffs are cooked in hard water types. The concentration of magnesium in food is decreased after cooking in both hard and soft water types; this decrease is slightly more pronounced when the vegetables are cooked in the soft water types. The role of trace elements in relation to "the water story" is also investigated.

INTRODUCTION

Many studies have been initiated in the past decade on the relation between inorganic drinking water constituents like Ca, Mg and heavy metals and health. However, the contribution of most of these inorganics in drinking water is usually small compared to the total dietary intake. Therefore if any health related association of inorganics in drinking water is observed in ecological or epidemiological studies, it will be important to consider all possible factors through which drinking water can influence the uptake of these inorganics, including the effect of food cooking. Another important point to consider is the chemical speciation of these inorganics; lead, for instance, is known to be more readily absorbed from water than from food because the chelated form present in food apparently is less available metabolically.

In The Netherlands, Biersteker (1967) found a significant negative association for females between hardness of drinking water and ischemic heart disease (IHD) in 23 communities during the period 1958-1962. A similar result was found for the same communities in the period 1963-1970 (Biersteker and Zielhuis, 1975); the correlation between water hardness and ischemic heart disease for males tended in the same direction but did not reach significance. The outcome of these studies was a reason for the Public Health Counsel to discourage central water softening and recommend further studies on the causal factors underlying these statistical associations.

The objectives of the follow up study were:

1. To investigate, on the basis of recent statistical data, whether an association between hardness of drinking water and death rate from cardiovascular diseases can still be found in The Netherlands.
2. To investigate changes in the mineral composition of food when cooking with waters of different hardness.
3. To investigate the role trace elements in "the water story" with special attention to the metals released from water distribution systems, including the chemical speciation of these metals and the factors affecting their concentration like pH and hardness.

Zielhuis and Haring (1981) reported about the first of these objectives: no significant relations were found over the period 1971-1977 between IHD mortality and hardness of drinking water in 30 communities.

The disappearance of the statistical relation could not be attributed to changes in water hardness. However, investigation of a group of 17 municipalities of which mortality and water quality data are known for three periods, 1958-1962, 1963-1970 and 1971-1977, showed that the inverse statistical relation between I.H.D. mortality and water hardness still existed but with decreasing significance of correlation coefficients. The provisional conclusion of these investigations is that other factors than water hardness overrule to a large extent the potential effect on IHD mortality. Central water softening down to 2-3 meq/1 Ca probably will have no observable effect on mortality.

The second and third objective of the investigations in The Netherlands will be discussed in more detail in this paper.

CHANGES IN MINERAL COMPOSITION OF FOOD FROM COOKING IN HARD AND SOFT WATER

Experimental. Two methods of food preparation were investigated: normal cooking in glass beakers during about 20 minutes until the vegetables and potatoes were well done (Haring and van Delft, 1981) and by cooking in a pressure cooker in accordance with the manufacture's instructions. The ratio of food and water in both experiments was the same (0.6, kg food per litre water). 5

g NaCl was added per litre water. For capacity reasons it was not possible to carry out all the experiments at the same time. In fact, the pressure cooking experiments were carried out in 1983 using water sampled from the same communities and the same kind of foodstuffs.

Water for the cooking experiments was sampled at the tap at five different localities in six selected water supply areas: 1) The Hague, 2) Wageningen, 3) Arnhem, 4) Zutphen, 5) Maastricht and 6) Kerkrade. A mixed sample obtained from 5 houses in each city was analyzed. The general drinking water characteristics in terms of pH hardness, conductivity, etc. are given in Table 1.

The cooking experiments in glass beakers were conducted in duplicate. After draining, the cooked potatoes and vegetables were freeze-dried and ground. Weighted portions (1 g) of the freeze-dry samples of both cooked and uncooked foodstuffs were ashed with sulfuric acid (2 ml 50%) at slowly increasing temperatures up to 500°C, which was maintained for 8 hours.

The resulting ash was treated with concentrated nitric acid at temperatures up to 500°C until a white ash remained which was then dissolved in 1 ml conc. hydrochloric acid and diluted to 50 ml. The water that remained after cooking was adjusted to the original volume with double distilled water to correct for losses by evaporation. These samples were only used for pH measurement. A Perkin Elmer model 373 flame atomic absorption spectrometer was used for determination of Ca, Mg, Fe, Mn, Na, K and Zn. Trace elements i.e. Cd, Pb and Cu were determined by anodic stripping voltammetry using a PAR model 374 polarographic analyser.

Results of cooking experiments in glass beakers. The concentrations of inorganic constituents in the cooked and uncooked foodstuffs are given in Table 2. The data are more conveniently arranged by plotting the concentration changes as shown in Figure 1.

TABLE 1
Drinking water characteristics of six cities selected for investigation of the changes in mineral composition of food as a result of cooking with "hard" and "soft" water

City	HCO_3 mg/1	K_{20}* mS/m	pH	Ca mg/1	Mg mg/1	Pb mg/1
The Hague	201	65	7.70	87	9.4	0.066
Wageningen	99	15.5	7.93	49	2.2	0.012
Zutphen	303	71	7.55	96	10	0.028
Arnhem	82	16.5	7.68	28	2.4	0.003
Maastricht	359	60	7.18	114	19	0.020
Kerkrade	18	16.6	8.72	17	3.6	0.004

* conductivity at 20°C

TABLE 2
Concentration of minerals and metals in food before and after cooking with different types of drinking water.

CADMIUM

City	potatoes		cauliflower		carrots		endive	
	cooked	uncooked	cooked	uncooked	cooked	uncooked	cooked	uncooked
The Hague	0.037	0.052	0.011	0.009	0.027	0.032	0.007	0.008
Wageningen	0.030	0.038	0.023	0.017	0.034	0.043	0.048	0.066
Zutphen	0.037	0.052	0.005	0.007	0.013	0.020	0.009	0.012
Arnhem	0.041	0.052	0.005	0.007	0.013	0.020	0.009	0.012
Maastricht	0.041	0.052	0.005	0.006	0.008	0.011	0.013	0.015
Kerkrade	0.043	0.052	0.006	0.006	0.007	0.011	0.013	0.015

IRON

City	potatoes		cauliflower		carrots		endive	
	cooked	uncooked	cooked	uncooked	cooked	uncooked	cooked	uncooked
The Hague	4.1	5.6	5.5	6.7	1.8	2.0	3.0	4.3
Wageningen	4.4	6.4	5.6	8.1	2.8	4.3	7.3	9.5
Zutphen	3.5	5.6	2.8	4.0	2.8	3.0	2.5	3.2
Arnhem	3.6	5.6	2.3	4.0	2.4	3.0	2.7	3.2
Maastricht	4.8	6.1	3.8	4.2	3.3	4.3	2.5	2.7
Kerkrade	4.9	6.1	3.1	4.2	3.2	4.3	2.6	2.7

COPPER

City	potatoes		cauliflower		carrots		endive	
	cooked	uncooked	cooked	uncooked	cooked	uncooked	cooked	uncooked
The Hague	0.85	0.95	0.60	0.65	0.45	0.40	0.50	0.75
Wageningen	0.70	0.75	0.50	0.70	0.35	0.30	0.45	0.50
Zutphen	0.75	0.95	0.35	0.40	0.25	0.25	0.25	0.30
Arnhem	0.90	0.95	0.30	0.40	0.30	0.25	0.30	0.30
Maastricht	0.90	1.10	0.35	0.40	0.40	0.40	0.20	0.25
Kerkrade	0.90	1.10	0.35	0.40	0.35	0.40	0.25	0.25

All concentrations in mg/kg uncooked food (Data are averages of duplo-analyses.)

The data on Ca and Mg are probably the most important because they support the hypothesis that the deficiency of Ca and Mg in areas supplied with soft drinking water is even more increased because food was found to lose more Ca and Mg when it is cooked in soft water as compared to hard water. A more detailed inspection of the data shows that the concentration of calcium in potatoes, cauliflower and carrots increases when cooked with hard water and decreases (except for potatoes) when soft water was used for cooking. For endive, however, a decrease of calcium is found upon cooking in both hard and

TABLE 2 (continued)

CALCIUM

City	potatoes		cauliflower		carrots		endive	
	cooked	uncooked	cooked	uncooked	cooked	uncooked	cooked	uncooked
The Hague	90	71	167	136	302	294	239	315
Wageningen	71	71	97	114	235	254	282	469
Zutphen	97	71	197	141	232	199	252	340
Arnhem	106	71	116	141	188	199	202	340
Maastricht	107	71	252	155	340	217	308	339
Kerkrade	79	71	150	155	194	217	225	339

MAGNESIUM

City	potatoes		cauliflower		carrots		endive	
	cooked	uncooked	cooked	uncooked	cooked	uncooked	cooked	uncooked
The Hague	158	210	172	207	51	66	50	102
Wageningen	140	192	124	201	39	47	53	124
Zutphen	148	210	69	106	52	71	33	67
Arnhem	162	210	62	106	45	71	32	67
Maastricht	148	213	73	103	80	88	39	66
Kerkrade	155	213	55	103	73	88	34	66

LEAD

City	potatoes		cauliflower		carrots		endive	
	cooked	uncooked	cooked	uncooked	cooked	uncooked	cooked	uncooked
The Hague	0.055	0.027	0.056	0.014	0.137	0.111	0.075	0.040
Wageningen	0.020	0.031	0.009	0.012	0.026	0.030	0.082	0.126
Zutphen	0.023	0.027	0.039	0.020	0.036	0.024	0.046	0.051
Arnhem	0.024	0.027	0.010	0.020	0.023	0.024	0.025	0.051
Maastricht	0.029	0.032	0.033	0.019	0.036	0.030	0.059	0.080
Kerkrade	0.013	0.032	0.016	0.019	0.024	0.030	0.034	0.080

All concentrations in mg/kg uncooked food (Data are averages of duplo analyses.)

soft water types, although the decrease is more pronounced after cooking in soft water.

The change in the calcium concentration of food during cooking appears to be influenced by the pH change during cooking (Table 3). In case of endive, for instance, the decrease of pH by cooking is greater than for the other foodstuffs. The magnitude of this pH decrease is apparently also related to the buffer capacity of the water because all soft water types (with low buffer capacity) show a greater pH decrease upon food cooking than hard water types.

In case the pH does not decrease too much (as is often the case when food is cooked in hard water) precipitation of calcium carbonate onto the boiling foods results in an increase of the calcium concentration.

TABLE 2 (continued)

MANGANESE

City	potatoes		cauliflower		carrots		endive	
	cooked	uncooked	cooked	uncooked	cooked	uncooked	cooked	uncooked
The Hague	0.75	1.00	2.25	2.50	1.00	1.15	0.55	0.85
Wageningen	0.70	0.90	2.10	2.40	1.25	1.40	1.50	2.85
Zutphen	0.70	1.00	1.00	1.35	0.50	0.55	0.30	0.45
Arnhem	0.65	1.00	0.90	1.35	0.50	0.55	0.25	0.45
Maastricht	0.75	1.05	1.35	1.80	0.55	0.60	0.45	0.55
Kerkrade	0.80	1.05	1.20	1.80	0.45	0.60	0.35	0.55

ZINC

City	potatoes		cauliflower		carrots		endive	
	cooked	uncooked	cooked	uncooked	cooked	uncooked	cooked	uncooked
The Hague	2.9	3.6	5.6	7.3	1.4	1.6	0.9	1.6
Wageningen	1.9	2.4	4.5	7.8	1.1	1.6	4.3	6.3
Zutphen	2.7	3.6	1.9	3.2	0.9	1.0	1.1	2.2
Arnhem	2.8	3.6	1.8	3.2	0.8	1.0	1.2	2.2
Maastricht	2.7	3.9	2.2	3.5	1.5	1.8	0.6	1.3
Kerkrade	2.9	3.9	2.2	3.5	1.5	1.8	0.8	1.3

POTASSIUM

City	potatoes		cauliflower		carrots		endive	
	cooked	uncooked	cooked	uncooked	cooked	uncooked	cooked	uncooked
The Hague	2800	4200	2900	3700	800	1100	700	1850
Wageningen	2800	4250	2250	4100	1250	2650	750	2250
Zutphen	2600	4200	1400	2650	1400	2650	900	2900
Arnhem	2850	4200	1350	2650	1300	2650	1050	2900
Maastricht	2500	4100	1550	2900	1950	3100	950	3200
Kerkrade	2500	4100	1500	2900	1800	3100	800	3200

All concentrations in mg/kg uncooked food (Data are averages of duplo analyses

Increased magnesium concentrations in food after cooking were never found; this is not surprising because the solubility of Mg CO_3 is much greater than of $CaCO_3$, and $Mg(OH)_2$ can only precipitate (in the concerned concentration range) at pH above 10.

The interpretation of the lead data is a bit more complicated because lead is known to be easily absorbed into food by the various ligand binding groups that are available within the denatured structure of vegetable proteins (S-H groups by breakdown of S-S bridges). The lead concentrations in food generally were found to be higher after cooking with hard water and lower when soft water was used for cooking. The uptake of lead during cooking in hard water types is probably caused by the higher lead concentrations in the hard water types.

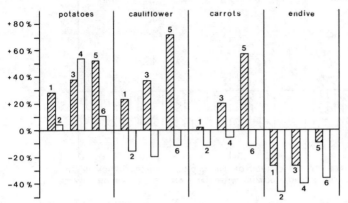

A. PERCENTAGE OF THE CHANGE OF THE CALCIUM CONCENTRATION IN SOME FOODSTUFFS DURING COOKING WITH HARD AND SOFT DRINKING WATER

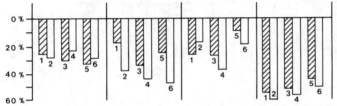

B. PERCENTAGE OF DECREASE OF THE MAGNESIUM CONTENTS IN SOME FOODSTUFFS DURING COOKING WITH HARD AND SOFT DRINKING WATER

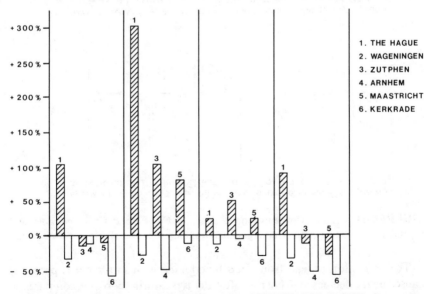

1. THE HAGUE
2. WAGENINGEN
3. ZUTPHEN
4. ARNHEM
5. MAASTRICHT
6. KERKRADE

C. PERCENTAGE OF THE CHANGE OF THE LEAD CONCENTRATION IN SOME FOODSTUFFS DURING COOKING WITH HARD AND SOFT DRINKING WATER

FIGURES 1A, B, C. Concentration changes of Ca, Mg, and Pb in potatoes and vegetables by cooking them in hard (gray bars) and soft (open bars) drinking water types.

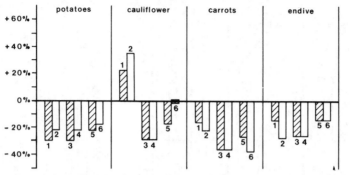

D. PERCENTAGE OF THE CHANGE OF THE <u>CADMIUM</u> CONCENTRATION IN SOME
    FOODSTUFFS DURING COOKING WITH HARD AND SOFT DRINKING WATER

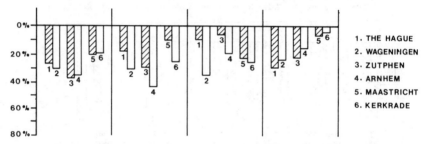

1. THE HAGUE
2. WAGENINGEN
3. ZUTPHEN
4. ARNHEM
5. MAASTRICHT
6. KERKRADE

E. PERCENTAGE OF THE CHANGE OF THE <u>IRON</u> CONCENTRATION IN SOME
    FOODSTUFFS DURING COOKING WITH HARD AND SOFT DRINKING WATER

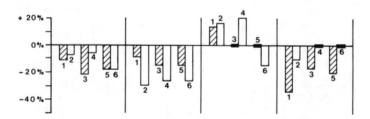

F. PERCENTAGE OF THE CHANGE OF THE <u>COPPER</u> CONCENTRATION IN SOME
    FOODSTUFFS DURING COOKING WITH HARD AND SOFT DRINKING WATER

FIGURES 1D, E, F. Concentration changes of Cd, Fe and Cu in potatoes and
vegetables by cooking them in hard (gray bars) and soft (open bars) drinking water types.

The extraction of lead from food by cooking with soft water is probably
caused by the decreased pH of the soft water types during cooking, compared to
the hard water types which show a smaller pH decrease because of higher buffer
capacities.

The results of the cooking tests, with special reference to the changes in Ca
and Mg concentration when food is cooked in hard and soft water, support the

306

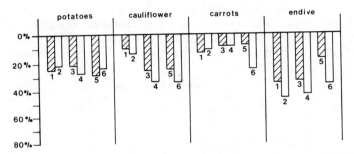

G. PERCENTAGE OF THE CHANGE OF THE <u>MANGANESE</u> CONCENTRATION IN SOME FOODSTUFFS DURING COOKING WITH HARD AND SOFT DRINKING WATER

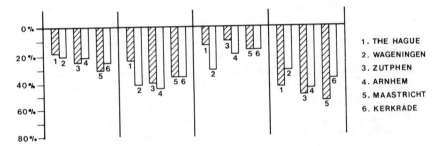

1. THE HAGUE
2. WAGENINGEN
3. ZUTPHEN
4. ARNHEM
5. MAASTRICHT
6. KERKRADE

H. PERCENTAGE OF THE CHANGE OF THE <u>ZINC</u> CONCENTRATION IN SOME FOODSTUFFS DURING COOKING WITH HARD AND SOFT DRINKING WATER

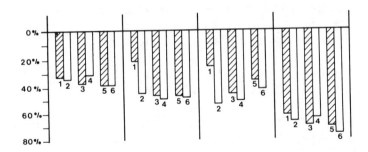

I. PERCENTAGE OF THE CHANGE OF THE <u>POTASSIUM</u> CONCENTRATION IN SOME FOODSTUFFS DURING COOKING WITH HARD AND SOFT DRINKING WATER

FIGURES 1G, H, I. Concentration changes in Mn, Zn and K in potatoes and vegetables by cooking them in hard (grey bars) and soft (open bars) drinking water types.

theory that the statistical inverse relation found between hardness of drinking water and cardiovascular disease mortality is possibly caused by a deficiency of these elements in soft drinking water. Such a deficiency will be further increased by the extraction of Ca and Mg from food by soft waters.

307

TABLE 3
Drinking water pH before and after cooking in glass beakers of potatoes, cauliflower,
carrots and endive in hard and soft water types

city	pH before cooking	pH after cooking			
		potatoes	cauliflower	carrots	endive
The Hague	7,70	7,30	7,44	7,05	6,35
Wageningen	7,93	6,26	7,04	6,35	5,98
Zutphen	7,55	8,00	7,57	7,34	6,45
Arnhem	7,68	6,30	6,96	6,22	6,04
Maastricht	7,18	8,41	7,78	7,62	6,59
Kerkrade	8,72	6,02	7,23	5,92	5,91

The possible effects of other elements is not discussed in detail in this paper
because insufficient information is available at this moment about the effects of
these elements in relation to C.V.D. or because the intake of these elements by
other exposure routes is more important.

Results of cooking experiments carried out in pressure cookers. During food
preparation in a pressure cooker the food is not expected to be enriched with
minerals or metals from water because it only comes into contact with steam.
The decrease of the concentration of calcium and magnesium which was
actually found in the examined foodstuffs in most cases was below about 30%.
The short time of cooking in pressure cookers ($<$ 5 minutes) apparently
prevents greater losses of these nutritionally important elements. In contrast to
the cooking experiments carried out in glass beakers the experiments in pressure
cookers were not carried out in duplicate. For future studies it is recommended
to use neutron activation analysis for the determination of most elements in
foodstuffs, because destruction of samples is unnecessary in that case, decreasing the possibility of contamination of samples during analysis.

TRACE ELEMENTS IN HARD AND
SOFT DRINKING WATER

The role of trace elements in drinking water, especially those released from
distribution systems, has often been discussed in relation to "the water story"
(Calabrese et al., 1980). The actual exposure to these trace elements (Pb, Cd, Cu,
Zn) is determined both by water quality factors (pH, alhalinity, Ca) and by the
stagnation time in the household distribution system prior to consumption. A
special proportional sampling device was developed for the monitoring of the
daily intake of these trace elements (Fig. 2). The proportional sampler is
connected to the kitchen tap during a period of one week and enables people to
sample 5% of the water which is used for consumption purposes. Sampling was
carried out at 1000 households in 20 communities.

A selection of the results is given in Table 4. Data on Cd and Zn are omitted in
this table because the concentrations of these elements are rather low due to the
fact that galvanised iron pipes are seldom applied in The Netherlands.

From the data in Table 3 the mutual relations between plumbosolvency, pH and hardness of drinking water are evaluated. In contrast to the hypotheses found in literature of increased aggressiveness (towards metals like lead and copper) of soft waters as compared to hard water types, the investigations in The Netherlands showed that soft waters generally have a higher pH and a lower plumbosolvency compared to hard water types (Table 5).

An explanation for the observed relation is that Dutch types of drinking water usually are not aggressive vs. $CaCO_3$ which means that the pH of these waters is almost equal to the equilibrium pH at $CaCO_3$ saturation. For soft water types this equilibrium pH is higher than for hard waters. The hypothesis that toxic heavy metals released from distribution pipes in *soft* water areas are the causal factor for the observed negative statistic relation with cardiovascular disease mortality therefore seems (at least in The Netherlands) unlikely.

Lead appeared to be the only trace element in drinking water whose concentration frequently exceeded the maximum allowed concentration of 50 μg/1. The inorganic speciation of lead in The Hague tap water was calculated with the MINEQL computer programme developed by Westall et al. (1976). The $PbCO_3$ complex was found to contribute more than 90% to the total dissolved inorganic lead concentration. Furthermore MINEQL was used to calculate the equilibrium concentration of inorganic lead complexes in equilibrium with hydrocerussite ($Pb_3(OH)_2(CO_3)_2$) which is the solid phase usually found inside lead pipes. This calculation was carried out for different values of pH and total carbonic acid species concentration of the water (Table 6).

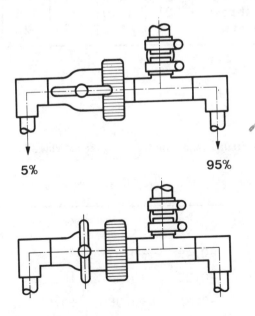

FIGURE 2. Cross section of proportional sampling device.

TABLE 4
Concentration values measured for Ca, Mg, Pb, Cu and pH in 20 water distribution areas

City name	Ca mg/l	Mg mg/l	Pb µg/l	Cu µg/l	pH
Leeuwarden	94	9.1	84	305	7.45
Den Haag	78	8.2	69	52	7.70
Rotterdam	40	7.6	38	40	8.02
Roosendaal	73	4.8	50	259	7.48
Arnhem	25	2.3	10	118	7.68
Tilburg	62	6.1	6	113	7.94
Gouda	87	11.8	26	82	7.65
Haarlem	88	7.1	67	75	7.51
Zwolle	80	9.6	6	141	7.62
Sneek	100	8.8	10	534	7.31
Leiden	140	18.0	48	84	7.53
Utrecht	36	2.5	5	78	7.60
Groningen	59	5.2	37	66	7.73
Maastricht	110	12.2	30	138	7.18
Amsterdam	87	9.2	21	59	8.00
Zutphen	99	10.6	78	220	7.62
Oudenbosch	100	6.7	39	694	7.66
Eindhoven	37	3.2	7	51	8.30
Hoensbroek	107	12.0	12	146	7.48
Brunssum	14	1.2	7	26	8.15

TABLE 5
Correlation matrix for the data given in Table 3 (n = 20).

Parameter	pH	Ca	Mg	Pb
Ca	−0.66			
Mg	−0.49	+0.89		
Pb	−0.32	+0.43	+0.33	
Cu	−0.41	+0.38	+0.06	+0.13

Correlation coefficients (r) > 0,378 or < − 0,378 are significant at 95 percent confidence level.

TABLE 6

Calculated equilibrium concentrations (in mol/1, at 25° C) of total inorganic lead species in relation to pH and C_T for drinking water in equilibrium with hydrocerussite and with a chemical composition similar to that of The Hague tap water.

C_T	pH 6	7	8	9	10	I
$1 \cdot 10^{-3}$	$1,74.10^{-5}$	$1,50.10^{-6}$	$5,87.10^{-7}$	$2,56.10^{-7}$	$1,36.10^{-7}$	$7 \ .10^{-3}$
$2 \cdot 10^{-3}$	$1,24.10^{-5}$	$1,63.10^{-6}$	$7,78.10^{-7}$	$3,43.10^{-7}$	$2,36.10^{-7}$	$9 \ .10^{-3}$
$3 \cdot 10^{-3}$	$1,05.10^{-5}$	$1,77.10^{-6}$	$8,71.10^{-7}$	$4,23.10^{-7}$	$4,66.10^{-7}$	$1,1.10^{-2}$
$4 \cdot 10^{-3}$	$9,51.10^{-6}$	$1,89.10^{-6}$	$9,97.10^{-7}$	$5,06.10^{-7}$	$4,20.10^{-7}$	$1,3.10^{-2}$
$5 \cdot 10^{-3}$	$8,90.10^{-6}$	$2,01.10^{-6}$	$1,10.10^{-6}$	$5,81.10^{-7}$	$5,44.10^{-7}$	$1,5.10^{-2}$
$6 \cdot 10^{-3}$	$8.51.10^{-6}$	$2,12.10^{-6}$	$1,20.10^{-6}$	$6,61.10^{-7}$	$6,83.10^{-7}$	$1,7.10^{-2}$

C_T = total carbonic acid species concentration $[H_2CO_3{*}]+[HCO_3^-]+[CO_3^{2-}]$ (mol/1)

I = ionic strength (mol/1)

High pH and low total carbonic acid species concentrations were found to reduce the plumbosolvency of drinking water. The results were in reasonable agreement with measured equilibrium concentrations (water sampled after 16 hours standstill in lead pipes) of inorganic lead in samples of similar chemical composition (Table 7 and 8).

TABLE 7

Variations in total lead concentrations in early morning samples during repeated sampling at 3 households in The Hague (measured by anodic stripping voltammetry, pH = 2, HNO_3)

Piping material	Number of sampling days	lead conc. in $\mu g/1^{-1}$		
		mean	max	standard deviation
lead	14	232	300	45
lead	14	254	340	46
copper	11	2,8	4,5	1,0

TABLE 8
Results of the speciation study in The Hague tap water sampled
in duplicate from the same tap.

sample	Lead concentrations ($\mu g/l$, in duplicate) as determined by anodic stripping voltammetry (standard addition method)	
acidified (pH=2, HNO_3) ("total lead")	260	260
sample as such (unacidified) ("total lead" minus particulate lead and A.S.V. non labile lead complexes)	100	130
UV irradiated sample (unacidified) ("total lead" minus particulate lead)	140	180

REFERENCES

BIERSTEKER, K. and ZIELHUIS, R.L. (1975). Hard of zacht drinkwater. T. Soc. Geneesk. **53**:3–9.

BIERSTEKER, K. (1967). Drinkwaterzachtheid en sterfte. T. Soc. Geneesk. **45**:658–661.

CALABRESE, E.J., MOORE, G.S., TUTHILL, R.W. and SIEGER, T.L. (1980). Drinking water and cardiovascular disease. Journal of Environmental Pathology and Toxicology 4.

HARING, B.J.A. and VAN DELFT, W. (1981). Charges in the mineral composition of food as a result of cooking in "hard" and "soft" waters. Archives of Environmental Health 36:33–35.

WESTALL, J.C., ZACHARY, J.L. and MOREL, F.M.M. (1976). MINEQL: a computer program for the calculation of chemical equilibrium composition of aqueous systems. MIT Department of Civil Engineering, Technical Note No. 18.

ZIELHUIS, R.L. and HARING, B.J.A. (1981). Water hardness and mortality in The Netherlands. The Science of the Total Environment 18:35–45.

CHAPTER XXVII

SUMMARY AND CONCLUSIONS OF RESEARCH CONDUCTED AND A STATEMENT OF RESEARCH NEEDS

Edward J. Calabrese
Division of Public Health
University of Massachusetts
Amherst, MA 01003

The ideas that I've formulated over the last 2½ days with regard to where the research should go in relation to inorganics in drinking water and cardiovascular disease are as follows. In terms of sodium, it seems that, if you take a look at what has been published and presented, almost exclusively the findings have been presented on school-aged children, involving third grade up to senior high school. An obvious gap is that we haven't looked at adults within the population. When we initiated our Massachusetts Blood Pressure Studies, high school students were not selected because we thought they were at increased risk, but because they presented fewer confounding variables in the sense of a lower percentage of the population with obesity and fewer years of smoking and also because they were truly a captive population that one could evaluate very quickly with a very limited budget. But it didn't necessarily indicate that this group would be one that would be affected within their relatively limited number of years by elevated levels of sodium.

A comment by Dr. McCauley indicated that the physiologic regulation of sodium as well as phosphorous and some other ions are tightly controlled by the body. It is possible that as one ages our regulatory capability may begin to deteriorate slightly and our capacity to handle low level excesses of sodium or other types of substances may begin to lose some of their resiliency or gain. If we are to find some particular epidemiologic effect of sodium, it may well be found in an older population. By using this type of paradigm it is not unexpected that the epidemiologic studies with children were equivocal. Thus, concluding that there isn't any effect within the human population at these low levels may be premature given the fact that we may not have taken a look at the most sensitive populations. Consequently, I would advocate that subsequent research be conducted with an adult population.

A second point is that most of the sodium epidemiologic studies have been of

313

a cross-sectional nature. Clearly, the intervention type of studies (i.e. quasi-experimental studies) are much stronger from a methodologic perspective. A study that I would recommend would be to have someone attempt to replicate in different communities the bottled water study that Dr. Robert Tuthill and I directed. In this particular case, you can actually attempt to measure in a controlled fashion whether a decrease in the water sodium levels will be reflected in blood pressure. We clearly had what appeared to be an effect with girls and not with boys. It appears to me that this is a better approach than attempting to add sodium to the diet as we did in our subsequent studies (Massachusetts Blood Pressure study—Part 4), and it is much stronger than the cross-sectional methodology. It also appears from the clinical literature that one can diminish blood pressure much more quickly than one appears to be able to increase it, given only modest levels of exposure. So I think that if an intervention study was to be conducted that would be a reasonable approach.

Another area that I think is important to consider is the general concept of missed opportunities in research. I think all of us have had numerous missed opportunities. Unfortunately, many of them are not salvageable once you realize that they existed. For example, when I saw the EPA studies with regard to barium levels in teeth, I was interested in whether there was any possibility that the investigators could have taken other non-invasive measures (e.g. hair measurements) by which they try to correlate the amount of barium in the teeth with body burden. If you wanted to try to monitor exposure over a prolonged period, you're not going to be able to ask an adult to have teeth removed or even children who have now had their secondary teeth. Developing a readily available and non-invasive indicator of body burden would have been a good idea to have added to that study.

There are some situations where missed opportunities still can be salvaged. For example, Dr. Ben Douglas' studies suggest that a decrease in calcium ingestion may be a predisposing factor for sodium-induced high blood pressure. These findings made me think back to missed opportunities within our own Massachusetts studies. But we have, within our high sodium community, very detailed dietary records. It seems that we could go back into our data and determine if there were variations in blood pressure associated with differences in calcium intakes. This may provide us with some type of independent attempt to validate the work that Dr. Ben Douglas has shown in his animal models.

There have been several papers recently published which suggest that chloride and not sodium may be the culprit with respect to blood pressure. Traditionally, the research community has always dismissed chlorine as insignificant in favor of sodium. Now we're being forced to rethink that hypothesis in light of at least some animal studies.

How does one get at this problem epidemiologically? There are some possible opportunities. In fact this is going to force me to review our data because in the town of Reading, Massachusetts, our high sodium community, one source of water that has elevated sodium contamination was contaminated by sodium chloride—road salt—but the other wells in the town had sodium hydroxide (NaOH) for pH control process. This raised the sodium levels from 30 to 120

314

ppm. The chlorine levels in the NaOH treated water have to be considerably less than those from the wells contaminated with road salt. There may be a possibility of differentiating one population from another epidemiologically. Consequently, there may be a way to try to get a handle on the purported chlorine phenomenon.

I think that the agency should be strongly encouraged to bring the research granting office into better coordination with the enforcement branch because there are naturally occurring experiments which take place seemingly every year, with communities adopting a new well, new well sources, or new treatment strategy. In such situations, natural experiments of a new technology/treatment could be carried out. Unfortunately, there are numerous opportunities lost that could provide much useful data for the regulatory branch. I think that taking advantage of the natural experiment is much more socially acceptable than EPA trying to carry our intervention studies.

Another idea that has not been considered in a specific paper was suggested by Lee McCabe. He noted that blacks have a higher incidence of hypertension and they are a population that hasn't been considered within the context of the sodium and drinking water hypothesis. It is possible that they may be a subgroup within the population which has, for a variety of potential reasons, some predispositions. If we are concerned with establishing our standards based upon protecting sizeable high risk segments of the population, this may be an area that could be looked at.

Another sizeable subgroup of the population that may have some unique predisposing factors with respect to accumulation of some of the heavy metals such as lead, cadmium and possibly other substances is menstruating women. We heard Dr. Michael Moore mention that it is fairly common to find women having higher body burdens of some of the heavy metals. In support of this idea was an interesting study that was published out of McGill University a few years ago. In this study men and women of varying iron stores were fed 25 micrograms of radioactively labeled cadmium, and then assessed for what their cadmium absorption rates were. The absorption rate in the individuals who had normal iron stores was approximately 1–2%, but in people with marginal iron stores the absorption of cadmium was 8–9%—a four-fold increase. A difference of this magnitude may be potentially significant.

Another high risk group which EPA hasn't looked at in a systematic fashion and that deals in terms of heavy metals is diabetics. Diabetics comprise 5% of the population, a very sizeable subgroup. They also suffer from a high degree of renal nephropathies. Their glomerular filtration becomes less efficient over time with age. In addition, lead is excreted principally via glomerular filtration. Whether diabetics, in fact, have a higher retention of lead is not known, but it is known that in fluoridated communities diabetics have a higher level of fluoride in their plasma than nondiabetics, suggesting a problem with excretion. Whether and to what extent this particular subgroup of the population may be adversely affected is a legitimate public health question of sizeable proportions, and one which hasn't been addressed to date.

Another idea that hasn't been discussed is the relationship of blood pressure to cancer. There are several epidemiological studies which have associated elevated diastolic blood pressure with the occurrence of a variety of cancers. In addition, research has related elevated blood pressure to increases in pollutant-induced DNA repair synthesis as well as in pollutant-induced chromatid breaks. Whether one can associate environmentally induced hypertension with not only increasing one's risk to coronary heart disease, but also increasing one's risk to environmentally induced cancer may be of some considerable interest. There seem to be a theoretical basis and some underlying data for some link between the two. It is a link that wasn't investigated in this conference, but I think that it may be worthy of further study.

Another area that I think is worthy of following up on was the work presented by Dr. Wilkins dealing with his predictions of the significance of a 3–5 mm Hg increase in blood pressure and what that means in public health terms. His predictive outcomes were in terms of the numbers of people that can be affected. It seems that efforts should be made to validate that model in population studies. This model may also have the capability of being extended into the area of cancer risks as well, especially tied into the relationship with blood pressure.

Finally, if you consider the American population, especially those who are below the poverty level, 9 out of 10 Black and Caucasian children below the poverty level get less than their RDA for iron. Approximately 15% of children below the poverty level get less than the RDA for vitamins A and C. Approximately 40% of the Black children under the poverty levels get less than their RDA for calcium while it's not quite as large a percentage for the poor white. These data were derived from fairly recent surveys and they mirror the findings of studies 15 years ago. And as Jay Wilkins talked about the tracking phenomenon with respect to blood pressure, there appears to be a tracking phenomenon of inadequate diets. American adults also display comparably inadequate diets in terms of the RDA. Whether these dietary factors involving marginal deficiencies may have a potentially significant influence on the occurrence of pollutant-induced toxicity needs further assessment.

CHAPTER XXVIII

REGULATION OF DRINKING WATER IN CANADA

P. Toft
Department of National Health and Welfare
Ottawa, Canada

I would like to thank the organizers for inviting me to this most stimulating conference. I have had an interesting and rewarding two and half days and I would like to congratulate the organizers for bringing together some of the leading scientists in this field.

I have been asked to speak about the regulatory implications of the work presented here in the Canadian context. The legal framework for regulating drinking water in Canada differs from that in the United States. There is no Canadian legislation which corresponds to the United States Safe Drinking Water Act. In Canada the provinces have the primary authority to legislate in the area of public water supply. On the other had the federal Department of National Health and Welfare has been given the responsibility to investigate and conduct programs related to public health. The net result is that drinking water is a shared federal-provincial jurisdiction. The provinces play the lead role in providing an adequate and safe supply of drinking water, while the federal government provides leadership in conducting research and in developing standards and guidelines for water quality to protect human health.

Canadian standards or guidelines exist to limit the concentration of many of the substances which are found in drinking water. They are based upon scientific criteria developed for the purpose, within the context of prevailing social and economic factors tempered by practical considerations such as the availability of technological means to produce water of the desired quality. The 1978 national guidelines are used by federal, provincial, and territorial authorities; they are not legally enforceable with respect to public water supplies unless promulgated by the appropriate provincial or territorial agency. At present two provinces have regulations based on the Federal-Provincial Guidelines.

The current guidelines were published in 1978; they were developed by a Federal-Provincial Working Group set up in 1974. Some 61 parameters were reviewed and guideline values were derived for 51 of them (6 physical, 2 microbiological, 1 radiological, and 42 chemical). Two types of limits were defined in the 1978 Guidelines. Firstly, a "Maximum Acceptable Concentration" (M.A.C.) was defined as the upper limit for each parameter. Water containing a substance at concentrations higher than the M.A.C. may cause disease or may be aesthetically unpleasant to consumers. Conversely, water which contains substances at concentrations below the M.A.C. values is considered acceptable for life-long consumption. Secondly, a more stringent or "objective" level was defined as the ultimate quality goal for both health and aesthetic purposes. It was felt that this would provide a yardstick by which to judge water quality and would serve to discourage pollution.

For those substances whose ingestion may cause adverse health effects the "objective" limit was generally set at the detection limit obtainable by a good laboratory using conventional analytical techniques. For aesthetic parameters the "objective" concentrations was often rather vaguely described as being "less than the M.A.C."

An exception was made for fluoride, for which the beneficial effects on dental health warranted recommending an objective concentration of 1.0 mg/L. This is achieved in many cases, of course, by adding fluoride ions at the water works to obtain the desired concentration.

Hardness is considered to be both an aesthetic and a health parameter. Too much hardness leads to consumer complaints and results in incrustation of pipes. There is some epidemiological evidence that there is an inverse correlation between water hardness and cardiovascular disease, and we have heard yesterday from several speakers about further advances in this field. If this relationship is confirmed it raises the interesting question as to whether it would be desirable to have a *minimum* value for hardness in public drinking supplies, always assuming that we know which characteristics of hardness are responsible for the beneficial effects on the cardiovascular system. Or alternatively, as Dr. Pocock mentioned yesterday, at least whether we should have a minimum value below which hard water should not be softened. In fact the Canadian Guidelines do not specify any recommended value for hardness, recognizing that public acceptance of hardness, from an aesthetic viewpoint, varies according to local conditions. The Guidelines, however, do recommend that where consumers use water softening devices, a separate unsoftened supply be retained for drinking and cooking purposes.

Water softeners replace the calcium and magnesium ions present in hard water with sodium ions, and levels as high as 500 mg/L of sodium may be attained. Even with such high sodium concentrations in water, whether from softening or as naturally present, however, food still appears to be the most significant source of sodium, accounting for about 4000 mg per day for the average adult assuming no addition or removal of sodium during food preparation. Nevertheless, we have heard this morning that considerable quantities of salt may be absorbed into food during cooking. This will be particularly significant for persons on salt restricted diets. As in the United States, the current Canadian Guidelines recommend that local health authorities be notified when the sodium concentration of the drinking water supply exceeds 20 mg/L, as a guide to physicians who are treating patients suffering from hypertension or congestive heart failure. There is no recommended maximum value for sodium and no plans to develop one, although the new W.H.O. Drinking Water Guidelines include a standard for sodium of 200 mg/L, based on taste considerations.

I was particularly interested in the papers presented this morning on the absorption of sodium, lead and cadmium from drinking water during the cooking of food, and the impact of mineral content on the absorption rate. The current Canadian M.A.C. for cadmium is 0.005 mg/L which was reduced in 1978 from the previous value of 0.01 mg/L. Recent surveys have demonstrated that Canadian ingestion of cadmium via food is in the range of 52-80 μg per day, very close to the FAO/WHO provincial guideline of 57-72 μg per day. Drinking water containing 0.005 mg/L would contribute about 15% of the tolerable intake. In fact, water quality data demonstrate that public water supplies contribute only about 1% of ingested cadmium.

The work on barium presented yesterday afternoon was interesting but I think more data are needed before the current maximum value of 1 mg/L is reassessed.

Of more potential significance is the possible link between chlorine in drinking water and the absorption of cholesterol We shall be closely watching the outcome of further research in this field.

As I mentioned earlier, drinking water is not the only source of exposure to many of the substances found in our drinking water supplies; due accout must be paid to exposures that result from food, air, occupation, and lifestyle factors (such as smoking). For most Canadians the major source of exposure to trace metals is from food; for lead and cadmium, for example, the contribution from water is only about 1% or less. In the case of some substances such as trihalomethanes, however, water is the major source.

To assess the contribution that drinking water makes to exposure to chemicals, a knowledge of the tap water consumption habits of the population is required. Although an average adult requires about 2.5 litres of water per day, only part of this is derived from tap water; the remainder is obtained from foodstuffs and other beverages. There is surprisingly little information on tap water consumption. In the development of the 1978 Guidelines a figure of 2 litres per day was used as an average figure. In order to obtain more precise and complete data on tap water consumption in Canada, we carried out a national survey using interview and questionnaire techniques. A total of 970 persons from 295 households took part. All regions of Canada except Newfoundland and the Territories were included in the survey. The same households were surveyed twice, once in the summer and again in the winter. The information collected included age, sex, type of plumbing and age of house. Participants were asked to record for one week day and one weekend day all tap water drunk and in what form, i.e., whether consumed in the raw form or in beverages such as tea, coffee, home-made beer or wine, or in soups or other water-based food.

The results showed a wide variation in daily consumption of tap water, ranging from virtually zero to more than 4 litres. The average daily consumption differed only slightly between summer and winter, being 1.31 and 1.37

litres/day, respectively. Consumption by men was slightly higher than by women. Eighty-four percent of the population drank less than 2 litres/day.

The distribution appears to follow a log-normal pattern. About 32% reported their consumption to be in the range 1.0 to 1.5 litres/day. There is a steady increase in consumption from 0.61 litres/day for ages less than 3 to 1.57 litres/day for ages over 55. Consumption appears to be slightly higher for males than for females. However, this is reversed when body weight is accounted for. For most age groups females drank more tap water per kilogram of body weight than males. It is also important to note that tap water consumption per kilogram of body weight is highest for children.

The survey also showed that 17% of persons never flush the tap when drawing water for drinking and that about one-third of all persons use water directly from the hot water line for preparing hot drinks. This would expose them to the greater possibility of finding higher concentrations of chemicals dissolved from the piping system.

We will be using this consumption information to assist us in the revision of the Canadian Drinking Water Guidelines now in progress. Last year the Department of National Health and Welfare recognized that there was a need to revise the 1978 Guidelines in light of new knowledge, and the Federal-Poivincial Working Group was reconvened in June 1983. Much of the effort of this revision will be directed towards developing new guidelines for a range of organic substances not currently included. However, we will not ignore the more traditional inorganics in the revision and, in this regard, this Conference is therefore particularly timely. I shall be very pleased to bring the papers presented here to the attention of my colleagues. And once again I would like to express my thanks to the organizers for inviting me.

REFERENCES

HEALTH AND WELFARE CANADA. (1978). Guidelines for Canadian Drinking Water Quality 1978. Supporting Documentation. Supply and Services Canada, Ottawa.

HEALTH AND WELFARE CANADA. (1981). Tapwater Consumption in Canada. Supply and Services Canada, Ottawa.

CHAPTER XXIX

REGULATORY IMPLICATIONS OF THE CONFERENCE—U.S. PERSPECTIVE

Joseph A. Cotruvo
U.S. Environmental Protection Agency
Office of Drinking Water

There has been substantial progress made in this area in the five years since the last meeting. There was new information and some consensus building also occurred. I would like to discuss a few of those topics as I heard them, and also the direction of our work at the Environmental Protection Agency in the next few years as we apply some of these and other data to revising National Drinking Water Regulations.

As with the Canadians, the USEPA is in the process of revising our National Regulations—it is mandated in the Safe Drinking Water Act. The interim regulations were published initially in 1975 and there were later iterations between 1976 and 1980 that added substances such as radionuclides and trihalomethanes. The original interim regulations were based on data that were not much more current than 1962 because they were derived directly from the Public Health Service Standards of 1962. The intent of the Congress was for EPA to codify those guidelines very quickly into enforceable regulations and then undertake a detailed scientific review and provide more scientifically based standards; those will be the revised regulations.

Development of the revised regulations is a formidable task as was learned by the National Academy of Sciences. They were commissioned to do a detailed review of existing scientific data, occurrence information, and toxicology, and to actually provide recommended levels (no effect-levels) for significant drinking water contaminants. EPA was to derive its regulatory program from those National Academy recommendations. The Academy concluded that it wasn't their role but rather that of the regulators to make those kinds of determinations. The scientific background was not complete then and it still isn't, but EPA still must make judgments based on what is known and then defer some for later as new data are developed.

EPA's regulatory program is divided into four phases. The first deals with volatile organics; the second deals with other organics, mostly pesticides, inorganics and biological contaminants; the third will deal with radionuclides; and the fourth will cover the disinfection-related toxicology and chemistry.

This meeting's discussion relates primarily to Phase II and to a lesser degree

Phase IV. The paper presented by Revis on chlorination and its toxicology obviously is very significant to our forthcoming Phase IV work, although that will not occur until 1986.

Our Phase II effort is well underway. Proposal of the comprehensive Phase II Recommended Maximum Contaminant Levels (RMCLs) is due by early 1985 and most of the technical work is now complete. RMCLs are defined in our law as "the level at which no known or anticipated adverse effects on health would occur with a margin of safety." From those recommended levels, which are the goals, EPA must establish actual enforceable regulations and those are to take into consideration feasibility and technology and cost. Sodium and hardness were subjects of this symposium that are of immediate interest as well as barium, lead and cadmium. In addition we will be examining asbestos, antimony and tin, and all of the other inorganics that are in the current regulations, such as arsenic and nitrates.

Drinking Water Contributions to Ions in Food

One of the very important sessions was the discussion of drinking water as an indirect contributor to human exposure to inorganic ions through the processing of food in water. Processing water has not been considered as a contributor to the total dose that drinking water produces. However, as drinking water standards are written today they assume 2 liters consumption which is probably relatively high for most persons in the population. Perhaps there is an adequate margin of safety automatically built into the current 2 liter assumption that provides some cushion to cover some of that extra exposure that comes from food processed in the water.

Sodium in Drinking Water and Hypertension

From the discussions of the last few days there seemed to be a good consensus among this group and among many scientists that sodium intake does relate to an increase in blood pressure in at least some significant portion of the population. The question for our concern is what does drinking water sodium contribute to the total sodium intake and then further, what should EPA do about drinking water sodium, if anything?

Drinking water is generally a minor source of exposure to sodium (usually much less than 10%) but nevertheless it is a systematic incremental contribution and a very large population is exposed. There are possibilities of significant levels of effects projected from even relatively low risk events occurring in large populations. So obviously this possible risk is something that cannot be ignored. But given the fact that drinking water is such a small contributor, and that the costs of altering drinking water to reduce sodium are substantial, perhaps there are non-regulatory routes that may be the more appropriate way to deal with that subject.

Thus an MCL is not planned at this time. Perhaps prevention through public information would be the best approach. EPA could provide guidance that could address minimizing the presence of sodium in drinking water through source selection and protection and avoidance of water treatment procedures that unnecessarily add sodium.

The existing EPA guideline is 20 miligrams per liter of sodium with monitoring the notification requirement and that probably that will continue into the future.

Water Hardness and Cardiovascular Disease

There seemed to be a fairly good consensus that there is some kind of inverse relation between a population's cardiovascular disease risk and elevated hardness of water. Apparently the magnitude of that effect is small compared to many other risk factors that contribute to CVD rate in populations. The British heart study report has helped to us focus even better on beginning to approximate some upper limit of the risk that may be involved relative to typical levels of hardness in water.

It appeared that the consensus of the group was that it is more probable that the effect that is being observed, if any, is one of protection from some component, perhaps calcium in the hard water, as opposed to significant detriment from components of soft water or lack of substances in soft water.

The conclusion that I would draw tentatively because of the structure of the Safe Drinking Water Act is that there may not be a direct regulatory role for EPA in this area. There are indirect ways in which one can deal with these kinds of issues such as through regulations that deal with corrosion by-products or by issuing guidance for public water systems and consumers. Perhaps the best route to take is similar to the Canadian and EEC concept of a guidance along the lines of avoiding unnecessary softening of drinking waters, encouraging the non-softening of cold water in homes, and perhaps putting some recommended lower limit on the extent of softening when it is practiced. The 1.5 millimole recommendation of the EEC was probably related to the cut-off that was observed in the British heart study around 60 milligrams per liter of calcium where there appears to be a leveling of the CVD risk curve. It does seem to be a reasonable idea and again something that perhaps EPA can better deal with through guidance as opposed to regulatory action.

In water hardness, as well as in the case of sodium, I agree with the speakers including Dr. Pocock and Dr. Masironi of WHO that additional epidemiological studies are not likely to be productive. However, perhaps there will be some targets of opportunity that may be found where changes of water quality are being contemplated in public water supplies and where there is an inexpensive opportunity to collect before and after data. That may be a very efficient way of gathering more information to help us to refine these suggestions in the future. The paper by Dr. Revis may provide some new and important insights on this subject.

Regulatory Status of Various Substances

EPA has a current standard of 50 parts per billion for lead in drinking water. Lead in drinking water is principally a problem of corrosion of lead products in drinking water distribution systems. These sources include pipe, service connections, solders and fixtures. EPA is conducting a reevaluation of that standard and whatever the decision it will be highly controversial, I am sure. We are seriously considering lowering the standard. The NAS recommended a reduction from 50 to 25 parts per billion. We are trying to determine the minimum indication of adverse effects from lead. It is indicated by blood-lead levels? How does that relate to adverse effects per se? Is it a neurological effect or learning disorder? Our goal is to reduce unnecessary human exposure to lead from drinking water.

Cadmium. The cadmium standard is 10 parts per billion. We do not believe there are very many people within the U.S. who are exposed to nearly as much as 10 parts per billion from drinking water. The proposed revised standard is probably going to fall somewhere in the same range, perhaps slightly lower but probably not significantly. The data to date seem to be pretty much revalidating the existing standard.

Barium. Barium was another subject discussed at the first conference. I am pleased that so much work has occurred since then on barium. There were four papers presented at this conference. The epidemiology study reported by Dr. Brenniman, completed before the last conference, did not detect significant differences in blood pressure or CVD risk rates between two communities with high and low barium levels in drinking water. Dr. Miller demonstrated that people who consume water that has high barium do accumulate more barium (e.g., in teeth), which was a question at one time. The toxicology issues appear to have been explored but they are not much clearer than they were at the last meeting. We can probably conclude that under the conditions of Dr. Perry's study in rats barium was shown to be hypertensinogenic. The question is how is that related to human exposure risk, and that is going to be a matter of further study in the near future. The other toxicology data appeared to be generally negative, at least at levels reasonably close to human exposures in drinking water.

The current standard is one milligram per liter. It appears that the state-of-the-art is somewhat more confused than a few years ago, given some of the conflicting data. We will have to study the data more carefully and see what the next steps can be. I do encourage continuation of work in the area, particularly in the direction of the controlled exposure clinical investigations.

Chlorine and Hypertension. Dr. Revis' presentation impressed all of us with its indications of perhaps significant alterations of cholesterol occurring in the test animals at levels of exposure to chlorine that were close to levels that occur in drinking water supplies in many countries of the world. Probably 150 million people in the U.S. alone drink water that is chlorinated either with free or combined chlorine. The other risk factors that Dr. Revis showed to be significant were high-fat diet and low calcium, and there are probably many people who fit one or both of these characteristics.

This is the area of imminent need for extensive scientific study. I strongly enourage accelerated work in all related areas, including speciation of the causal agent in the animal studies and a rapid parallel set of studies to determine whether similarly used water treatment chemicals like chlorine dioxide, chloramines and ozone can lead to similar kinds of effects. We need to know the toxic mechanism for the effects that occur in the animals. If they can be replicated, obviously there is epidemiology work given the variety of study opportunities that one can choose from. I think studies of a clinical nature are essential with controlled exposures to individuals who are being carefully monitored for the effects that may be occurring. All aspects of disinfection that will be examined in the Phase IV regulatory actions will begin in late '85 and will continue into '86 and '87.

Future Research

There is certainly a role for all of the different kinds of investigations that can be done to examine drinking water health risks, including both toxicology and epidemiology, and of course clinical work which is a form of epidemiology. Each has its optimum place is the process of health risk evaluation. There are situations where one or more should be the preferred direction to take. I think it is important, however, to try to approach these studies in a more organized and planned way in the future than they have been in the past. Therefore, it is necessary for us, EPA and prospective researchers to work closely together in the planning stages of these projects to decide the kind of work that should be done and the sequence in which it should be done, along with careful assessments of experimental designs.

It is also essential that proposed studies include a very careful quantitative analysis of the objective and carefully design and analyses to be able to project the statistical power of the study that is being proposed. In that way one would not arrive two years later at the point of concluding that even under the best of circumstances the study that was carried out did not have the remotest possibility of demonstrating the effect that it was searching for.

Another research area involved radon in drinking water and inhalation exposure and there are some beginnings of work along those lines but I hope some of you will be moved to examine populations that are being exposed to high levels of radon from this source. Similar work should be done on the inhalation exposure to volatile organic chemicals from drinking water.

In closing, I think the conference did take us a considerable distance from where we were five years ago. Although it has not unequivocally answered many of the questions, it has helped us arrive at several important working hypotheses on a number of them and it will help EPA's Drinking Water Office make several important decisions in our regulatory programs. Of course there is more work to be done in the future along several different technical lines that were discussed here.

Let me express my appreciation to the Chairman, Dr. Ed Calabrese, and the sponsors—EPA/HERL—for another excellent and productive conference that will assist EPA's Drinking Water Office carry out its regulatory responsibilities. This and similar events are some of the ways that good communication is fostered between EPA and the scientific community, leading to better and more efficient use of the limited research funds that we have available.

EDITORS' BIOGRAPHIES

Edward J. Calabrese

Edward J. Calabrese, Ph.D. is a board-certified toxicologist who is Professor of Toxicology at the University of Massachusetts School of Public Health, Amherst. He has researched extensively in the area of host factors affecting susceptibility to pollutants. He is the author of more than 180 papers in refereed journals and eight books, including *Principles of Animal Extrapolation, Pollutants and High Risk Groups, Methodological Approaches to Deriving Environmental and Occupational Health Standards, Nutrition and Environmental Health, Volumes 1 and 2, Ecogenetics,* and *Toxic Susceptibilities: Male/Female Differences,* all published by Wiley-Interscience. He has been a member of the U.S. National Academy of Sciences (NAS), the NATO Countries Safe Drinking Water Committees and the NAS Committee on Air Cabin Safety and has consulted extensively with governmental and private agencies.

Robert W. Tuthill

Robert W. Tuthill, Ph.D. received his doctoral training in epidemiology at the University of North Carolina. He is currently a professor and chair of the Biostatistics/Epidemiology Department of the School of Public Health at the University of Massachusetts. He is widely published, with his recent work in environmental epidemiology including: sodium in drinking water and blood pressure; chlorine dioxide in drinking water and newborn health; trihalomethanes and cancer; woodburning stoves and respiratory disease; formaldehyde in the home and respiratory illness; and heavy metal concentrations in inner city children. Other recent work includes a comprehensive review of the literature on the health effects of video display terminals, and an evaluation of the effectiveness of the Massachusetts Childhood Lead Screening Programs in achieving deleading of the dwellings of children with high lead levels.

In conjunction with his research, Dr. Tuthill teaches courses in principles of Epidemiology, Epidemiologic Investigation, Environmental Epidemiology and Psycho-Social Epidemiology. In addition, he has served on national review committees and state commissions and referees manuscripts for several professional journals. He is a member of the American College of Epidemiology, the Society for Epidemiologic Research and the American Public Health Association, and also belongs to the Delta Omega and Sigma Xi national honor societies.

Lyman W. Condie

Lyman W. Condie, Ph.D. has been a research toxicologist and Branch Chief of the Target Organ Toxicology Branch, Toxicology and Microbiology Division, Health Effects Research Laboratory at the U.S. Environmental Protection Agency in Cincinnati, Ohio. Dr. Condie has served on numerous government committees and has been an invited speaker at several EPA workshops. Previously, he was a Regional toxicologist for the EPA's Toxic Substances Offices in Chicago. Before joining the EPA in 1978, he was a research associate at the Environmental Health Sciences Center, Oregon State University. His current research interests include environmental toxicology, hazard assessment of complex mixtures, and mechanisms of interaction between drinking water contaminants.

Dr. Condie received his B.S. in Pharmacy from the University of Utah and his Ph.D. in Pharmacology from the University of Iowa. Author of numerous technical publications and several review articles, he is a member of several professional societies. He has been an invited participant in symposia and conferences in Europe and the United States.

ABOUT THE SERIES EDITOR

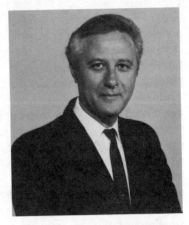

Myron A. Mehlman

Dr. Myron A. Mehlman is the Director of Toxicology and Manager of the Environmental and Health Sciences Laboratory at Mobil Oil Corporation. Born in 1934, Dr. Mehlman was educated at the City College of New York (B.S., 1957), the Massachusetts Institute of Technology (Ph.D., 1964), the University of Wisconsin (Post-Doctoral Fellow, Institute for Enzyme Research, 1967), and Harvard Business School (Program for Health Systems Management, 1974). His academic appointments include Associate Professor of Biochemistry at Rutgers University and tenured Professor of Biochemistry at the University of Nebraska Medical School. He was appointed Adjunct Professor of Medicine at the Mt. Sinai School of Medicine (1980-1986).

Dr. Mehlman was Chief of Biochemical Toxicology (1972-1973) at FDA, Special Assistant for Toxicology, Environmental Affairs, and Nutrition (1973-1975) at Office of Assistant Secretary for Health, HEW, and Special Assistant for Program Planning and Evaluation, and Interagency Liaison Officer, Office of Director at National Institutes of Health (1975-1977).

In addition to serving as Chairman of the First and Second National Meetings of the American College of Toxicology, he has chaired symposia at Rutgers University, the University of Nebraska, FASEB, NIH, FDA, EPA, and the Collegium Ramazzini. His professional memberships include the American Society of Biological Chemists, the American Physiological Society, the American Institute of Nutrition, American Society for Experimental Therapeutics and Pharmacology, the American Chemical Society, the Society of Toxicology, the American College of Toxicology, the American Industrial Hygienist Society, and the Collegium Ramazzini.

Dr. Mehlman is also the founding editor of the Journal of Toxicology and Environmental Health and the Journal of Environmental Pathology and Toxicology, and has been series editor for Advances in Modern Nutrition, Advances in Modern Toxicology, Symposium on Metabolic Regulations, and Advances in Modern Environmental Toxicology. From 1977-1979 Dr. Mehlman was the first and founding president of the American College of Toxicology.

Since 1962, Dr. Mehlman has published 180 articles in the fields of biochemistry, toxicology, nutrition and human health. He has edited and co-edited approximately 40 books.

SUBJECT INDEX

VOLUME VIII

OCCUPATIONAL AND INDUSTRIAL HYGIENE: CONCEPTS AND METHODS

Edited by Nurtan A. Esmen and Myron A. Mehlman

Princeton Scientific Publishing Co., Inc.

VOLUME VI

Applied Toxicology of Petroleum Hydrocarbons

Edited by H.N. MACFARLAND, Gulf Oil Corporation
C.E. HOLDSWORTH, American Petroleum Institute
J.A. MACGREGOR, Standard Oil of California
and M.L. KANE, American Petroleum Institute

Princeton Scientific Publishing Co., Inc.

VOLUME IV
Carcinogenicity and Toxicology of Benzene

Edited by M.A. MEHLMAN, Mobil Oil Corporation

Princeton Scientific Publishing Co., Inc.

VOLUME III

Assessment of Reproductive and Teratogenic Hazards

Edited by M.S. CHRISTIAN, Argus Research Laboratories, Inc.
W.M. GALBRAITH, U.S. Environmental Protection Agency
P. VOYTEK, U.S. Environmental Protection Agency
and M.A. MEHLMAN, Mobil Oil Corporation

Princeton Scientific Publishing Co., Inc.

ADVANCES IN MODERN ENVIRONMENTAL TOXICOLOGY

VOLUME II
Occupational Health Hazards
of Solvents

Edited by A. ENGLUND, Bygghalsan, Construction Industry's Organization
for Working Environment, Safety and Health, Stockholm
KNUT RINGEN, Worker's Institute for Safety and Health, Washington, D.C.
M.A. MEHLMAN, Mobil Oil Corporation

Princeton Scientific Publishing Co., Inc.

VOLUME I

Mammalian Cell Transformation by Chemical Carcinogens

Edited by N. MISHRA, U.S. Food and Drug Administration
V. DUNKEL, U.S. Food and Drug Administration
M.A. MEHLMAN, Mobil Oil Corporation

Princeton Scientific Publishing Co., Inc.